STATISTICS FOR HEALTH POLICY AND ADMINISTRATION USING MICROSOFT EXCEL

STATISTICS FOR HEALTH POLICY AND ADMINISTRATION USING MICROSOFT EXCEL

James E. Veney

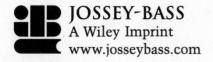

JOSSEY-BASS
A Wiley Imprint
www.josseybass.com

Published by Jossey-Bass
A Wiley Imprint
989 Market Street, San Francisco, CA 94103-1741   www.josseybass.com

Jossey-Bass books and products are available through most bookstores. To contact Jossey-Bass directly
call our Customer Care Department within the U.S. at 800-956-7739, outside the U.S. at 317-572-3986
or fax 317-572-4002.

Jossey-Bass also publishes its books in a variety of electronic formats. Some content that appears in print
may not be available in electronic books.

ISBN 0-7879-6458-1

FIRST EDITION
PB Printing   10 9 8 7 6 5 4 3 2 1

THE JOSSEY-BASS HEALTH CARE SERIES

CONTENTS

PREFACE

I first studied statistics as a graduate student back in the dark ages before computers. Most of the problems we worked with were carried out either with pencil and paper or with electric mechanical calculators that took up the entire top of the desk and literally minutes to multiply. We couldn't take square roots directly with these calculators so we used a cybernetic process—also appropriately called trial and error, where we entered some number we thought should be close to the square root of whatever number we wanted the square root of and multiplied it by itself. If the result was greater than the initial number, we reduced the original entered number. If the result was less than the initial number, we increased the original entered number. Then we multiplied again. After a few or many tries, we could arrive at the square root of any number to any number of decimal places we desired. But it often took several minutes to get the answer.

The study and use of statistics have come a long way since then. Particularly, computers have reduced both the effort and the time involved in the statistical analysis of data. But this ease of use has been accompanied by some difficulties. As computers became more and more proficient at carrying out statistical operations of increasing complexity, the actual operations—and what they actually meant and did—became more and more distant from the user. It became possible to do a wide variety of statistical operations with a few lines or words of commands to the computer. But the average student, even the average serious user of statistics, found the increasingly complex operations increasingly difficult to access and understand.

But sometime in the late 1980s, Microsoft Excel became available, and with it came the ability to carry out a wide range of statistical operations—and to understand the operations that were being carried out—in a spreadsheet format. My first introduction to Excel was a revelation. I discovered that Excel was not only a powerful statistical tool but also, more important, a powerful *learning* tool. When I began to teach the introductory course in statistics for the master's degree students in our health policy and administration department, Excel seemed to me to be the obvious medium for the course. But there were no books devoted to statistics using Excel that also provided health-related examples. And so this book was born.

This book was designed as an introductory statistics text for students at the advanced undergraduate level or for a first course in statistics at the master's degree level. It was designed to stand alone as the book for the only course a student may have in statistics, but the material is presented in terms that should provide a good foundation for other more advanced courses as well. Furthermore, since the book relies on Excel for all the calculations of the statistical applications, it was also designed to provide a statistical reference for people working in the health field who may have access to Excel but not to other dedicated statistical software.

The book is organized into two major sections. The first major section, Chapters One through Six, provides an introduction to the use of statistics in health policy—and health administration—related fields, to Excel as a statistical tool, to data preparation and the data display capabilities of Excel, and to probability, the foundation of statistical analysis. For students and other users of the book truly familiar with Excel, much of the material in Chapters Two, Three, and Four, particularly, could be covered very quickly. The second section of the book is devoted to the subject of hypothesis testing, the basic function of statistical analysis. Chapter Seven provides a general introduction to the concept of hypothesis testing. Each subsequent chapter, Chapter Eight through Fourteen, provides a description of the major hypothesis testing tool for a specific type of data. Chapter Eight, on the chi-square statistic, discusses the use of this statistic for assessing data for which both the independent and dependent variables are categorical. Chapter Nine, on *t* tests, discusses the use of the *t* test for assessing data where the independent variable is a two-level categorical variable, whereas the dependent variable is a numerical variable. Chapter Ten is devoted to analysis of variance, which provides an analytical tool for a multilevel categorical independent variable and a numerical dependent variable. Chapters Eleven through Thirteen are devoted to several aspects of regression analysis, which deals with numerical variables both as the independent and the dependent variables. The final chapter, Chapter Fourteen, deals with numerical independent variables and dependent variables that are categorical and take on only two levels, and it introduces the use of Logit.

Each section of the book is structured around examples demonstrated extensively with the use of Excel displays. Most sections include step-by-step discussions of how statistical problems are solved using Excel. Each section of the book is followed by exercises that address the material covered in the section. Most of these exercises include the replication of examples given in the section, so that the student has an immediate reference with which to compare his or her work as a way of determining whether he or she is able to correctly carry out the procedure involved. Additional exercises are provided on the same subjects for further practice and to reinforce the learning gained from the section. Data for all the exercises are included on the Web at http://www.josseybass.com/go/veney, and it may be accessed by the file reference given in the examples themselves.

There will be a supplemental package available to instructors that will include all answers to the exercises at the end of each section of the book. In addition, the supplemental package will contain exam questions with answers and selected Excel spreadsheets that can be used for class presentations, along with suggestions as to how these materials might be presented in a classroom setting. However, the book can be effectively used for teaching without the additional supplemental material.

Users of the book who would like to provide feedback, suggestions, corrections, examples of applications, or whatever else can e-mail me at veney@unc.edu. The Web site where additional resources and information can be found is at http://www.josseybass.com/go/veney. Please feel free to contact me and provide any comments you feel are appropriate. I plan to teach this course many times in the future, so any suggestions are welcome.

There are many people who contributed to this book as it now appears. In particular, I want to mention several faculty colleagues at the University of North Carolina who contributed to this book in various ways. Jim Porto deserves particular thanks as the person who got me involved in teaching introductory statistics for master's degree students in the first place, and he provided the opportunity for me to learn that it perfectly matched my interests and skills. Jim also spent many hours with me discussing the meaning and best presentation of a number of the concepts in this book, including, in particular, type I and type II error, and he was kind enough to read and comment on sections that were difficult in the writing. Jim is also an Excel wizard. Numerous other faculty colleagues provided ideas, insights, and inspiration, of whom Kerry Kilpatrick, Bill Zelman, and Edward Norton specifically deserve mention.

I must also thank students who helped me in various ways with this project. In particular, I thank the many students who have taken my class and, in so doing, have forced me to improve and clarify my ideas and their presentation. And I must thank all the students in my classes in Fall 2002, who were forced to deal with the drafts of the manuscript as their text. Their comments have been invaluable in improving the presentation and catching many typos and thinkos. I must also thank students who contributed more directly to the writing of the book. Samruddhi Thaker carefully read and corrected early drafts of several of the chapters and provided better wordings in many places. She also contributed numerous ideas for problems and data to use for problems. Several students, working as my teaching assistants, have also contributed to the final product. There have been many teaching assistants, but I should particularly mention Wang Hua. Finally, I want to thank the several students who contributed directly to the examples used in the book by providing either specific ideas or data. These students include Lee Boles, LeRoy Oakley, and Bill Shepley. There are others I should thank by name, but I am chagrined to say I cannot remember their names.

Last and far from least, I want to thank my wife, who put up with me during the many days that I ignored other things to concentrate on this one task.

Chapel Hill, N.C.   James Veney
December 2002

To my students

STATISTICS FOR HEALTH POLICY AND ADMINISTRATION USING MICROSOFT EXCEL

CHAPTER ONE

INTRODUCTION

S tatistics is a subject that for many people is pure tedium—a little bit like eating hay. For others, it is more likely to be anathema. The last thing they want to do in their life is have to take a course in statistics. Of course, there are those strange souls who find statistics interesting, even stimulating. But they are usually in the minority in any group.

This book is posited on the recognition that in the health field, as indeed among people in any discipline, there are at least these three different views of statistics, and that any statistics class is likely to be made up more of the former two groups than the latter. It is the goal of this book to provide an introduction to statistics in health policy and administration that will be relevant and useful, and perhaps finally interesting, to people in the first two groups, while still being challenging and informative to the people in the latter.

Section 1.1 How This Book Differs from Other Statistics Texts

The primary difference between this statistics text and most others is that this text uses Microsoft Excel as the tool for carrying out statistical operations and understanding statistical concepts as these relate to health policy and health administration issues. This is not to say that there are no other texts in statistics that use Excel. Levin, Stephan, Krehbiel, and Berenson (1999) have produced a very useable text entitled *Statistics for Managers Using Microsoft Excel*. But that book focuses almost exclusively on non-health-related topics. In many years of teaching statistics, especially to mid-career professionals, it is clear that the closer the applications of statistics are to the real-life interests and experiences, the more effective students will be in understanding and using statistics. Consequently, this book focuses its examples entirely on subjects that should be immediately recognizable to people in the health sciences.

Microsoft Excel, which most people will know as a spreadsheet program for creating budgets, comparing budgeted and expended amounts, and generally fulfilling accounting needs, is also a very powerful statistical tool. Chapter Two is devoted specifically to the ways in which Excel can be used as a statistical tool. Books that do not use Excel for teaching statistics (and, as has been said, this is most other books) generally leave the question of how to carry out the actual statistical operations in the hands of the student or the instructor. It is often assumed that relatively simple calculations, such as means, standard deviations, and t tests, will be carried out by hand or with a hand calculator. For more complicated calculations, the assumption is usually that a dedicated statistical package such as SAS, SPSS, STATA, or SYSTAT will be used. There are at least two problems with this approach that the current book hopes to overcome. First, hand calculations, or even the use of a hand calculator, can make the simple statistical operations overly tedious and prone to errors in arithmetic. Second, because dedicated statistical packages are designed for use rather than for teaching, they often obscure the actual process of calculating the statistical results, which comes between the student and an understanding of both how the statistic is calculated and what the statistic means.

In general, this is not true with Microsoft Excel. It is true that a certain amount of time in using this book must be devoted to the understanding of how to use Excel as a statistical tool. But once that has been done, Excel makes the process of carrying out the statistical procedures under consideration relatively clear and transparent. It is hoped that the student will end up with a better understanding of what the statistic means, through an understanding of how it is calculated, and not simply with the ability to get a result by entering a few commands into a statistical package. This is not to say that Excel cannot be used to shortcut many of the steps needed to get particular statistical results. As discussed in Chapter Two, a number of statistical tests and procedures are available as add-ins to Excel. However, using Excel as a relatively infallible, powerful, but transparent calculator can lead to a much clearer understanding of what the statistic means than that which can be obtained by other methods.

Section 1.2 Examples of Statistical Applications in Health Policy and Health Administration

In many iterations of teaching statistics to health policy and health administration students, the same question arises. Every semester sees students who say something like, "All these statistics are fine, but how do they apply to anything I am concerned with?" The question is not only a reasonable one, but it also points directly to one of the most important and difficult challenges for a statistics teacher, a statistics class, or a statistics text. How can it be demonstrated that these statistics have any real relevance to anything that the average person working in the health field ever needs to know or do? Happily, it has seemed that by the time a student has finished one of the courses that is the inspiration for this book, he or she usually sees how the knowledge of statistics can be useful. But it would be nice to be able to provide this kind of insight at the very beginning of a book, or course, as a way of getting rid of at least one stumbling block in the process of learning statistics.

To work toward a better understanding of why and when the knowledge of statistics may be useful to someone working in health policy or health administration, six examples have been selected of situations in which statistical applications can play a role. All six of these examples were inspired by real problems faced by students in classes in statistics, and they represent real statistical challenges that students have faced and hoped to solve. In virtually every case, the person who presented this problem recognized it as one that could probably be dealt with using some statistical tool. But also in every case, the solution to the problem was not obvious in the absence of some understanding of statistics. Although these case examples are not likely to resonate with every reader, perhaps they will give many readers a little better insight into why knowledge of statistics might be useful.

Documentation of Medicare Reimbursement Claims

The Pentad Home Health Agency provides home health services in five counties of an eastern state. The agency must be certain that its Medicare reimbursement claims are appropriately and correctly documented in order to ensure that Medicare will reimburse these claims in a timely manner. Appropriate documentation requires that all physician orders, including medications, home visits for physical therapy, home visits of skilled nursing, and any other orders for service be correctly documented on a form 485. Inappropriate documentation can lead to rejection or delay in processing of the claim for reimbursement by the Medicare administration.

The Pentad Agency serves about eight hundred clients in the five-county region. In order to assure themselves that all records are appropriately documented, the administration runs a chart audit of one in ten charts each quarter. The audit seeks to determine (1) whether all orders indicated in the chart have been carried out and (2) if they have been correctly documented in the form 485. Orders that have not been carried out, or orders incorrectly documented, lead to follow-up training and intervention appropriate to ensure that the orders and documentation are carried out correctly in the future.

Historically, the chart audit has been done by selecting each tenth chart, beginning at the beginning or at the end of the chart list. Typically, the chart audit determines that the majority of charts are correctly documented, usually 85 to 95 percent. But there are occasionally areas, such as skilled nursing care, where correct documentation may fall below that level. When this happens, the administration initiates an appropriate intervention.

One of the questions of the audit has been the selection of the sample. Because the list of clients changes relatively slowly, the selection of every tenth chart often results in the same charts being selected for audit from one quarter to the next; therefore, a different strategy for chart selection is desirable. It has been suggested that a strictly random sample of the charts might be a better way to select them for quarterly review, as this selection would have a lesser likelihood of resulting in a review of the same charts from quarter to quarter. But how does one go about drawing a strictly random sample from any population? Or, for that matter, what does strictly random actually mean and why is it important beyond the likelihood that the same files may not be picked from quarter to quarter? These are questions that are addressed by statistics, specifically the statistics associated with sample selection and data collection. They are the subjects of Chapter Three.

Another question related to the audit is the question of when to initiate an intervention. Suppose a sample of one in ten records is drawn (for eight hundred clients, that would be eighty records) and it is discovered that twenty of the records have been incorrectly documented. Twenty of eighty records incorrectly documented would mean that only 75 percent of the records were correctly documented. This would suggest that an intervention should be initiated to correct the documentation problem. But it was a sample of the eight hundred records that was examined, not the entire eight hundred. Suppose that the twenty incorrectly documented records were, by the luck of the draw, so to speak, the only incorrectly documented records in the entire eight hundred records. That would mean that only 2.5 percent of the cases were incorrectly documented.

If the intervention to correct the problem were expensive—a five-day workshop on correct documentation, for example,—the agency would not want to initiate that intervention when 97.5 percent of all cases are correctly documented.

But how would the agency know from a sample what proportion of the total eight hundred cases might be incorrectly documented, and how would they know the likelihood that fewer than, say, 85 percent of all cases was correctly documented if 75 percent of a sample was correctly documented? This, again, is a subject of statistics and is discussed particularly in Chapter Five, which deals with probability.

Emergency Trauma Color Code

The emergency department (ED) of a university hospital was the site of difficulties arising from poor response time to serious trauma. Guidelines indicate that a trauma surgeon must attend for a certain level of trauma severity within twenty minutes and that other trauma, still severe, but less so, should be attended by a trauma nurse within a comparable time. Less serious trauma did not require such immediate response. In general, it had been found that the response time for the ED in the university hospital was more or less the same for all levels of severity of trauma—too long for severe cases and often quicker than necessary, given competing priorities for less severe cases.

The ED director knew that when a trauma case was en route to the hospital, a call was put in from the ambulance to the ED to indicate that the emergency was on the way. Part of the problem as perceived by the director of the ED was that the call-in did not differentiate the trauma according to severity. The ED director decided to institute a system whereby the ambulance attendants would assign a code red to the most severe trauma cases, a code yellow to less severe trauma cases, and no color code to the least severe trauma cases. The color code of the trauma would be made known to the ED as the patient was being transported to the facility. The object of this coding was to ensure that the most severe traumas were attended within the twenty-minute guidelines. This in turn was expected to reduce the overall time from admission to the ED to discharge of the patient to the appropriate hospital department (all trauma cases at the red or yellow level of severity are transferred from the ED to a hospital department).

A major concern of the director of the ED was whether the new system actually reduced the overall time between admission to the ED, treatment of the patient in the ED, and discharge to the appropriate hospital department. The director of the ED has considerable information about each ED admission going back a period of several months before the implementation of the new color coding system and six months of experience with the system after it was implemented. This information includes the precise time that each trauma patient was admitted to the ED and the time that the patient was discharged to the appropriate hospital department.

It also includes the severity of the trauma at admission to the ED on a scale of 0 to 75, gender, age, and, of course, whether the admission occurred before or after the color coding system was implemented. The ED director also has information about the color code assigned after the system was initiated that can generally be equated to the severity score assigned at admission to the ED. Trauma scoring 20 or more on the scale would be assigned code red, below 20, code yellow, and those not on the scale would not be assigned a color.

The question the ED director wishes to address is how she can use her data to determine whether the color-coding system has reduced the time spent by trauma victims in the ED before discharge to the appropriate hospital department. At the simplest level, this is a question that can be addressed by using a statistic called the *t* test for comparing two different groups. The *t* test is discussed in Chapter Nine. At a more complex level, the ED director can address the question of whether any difference in waiting time in the ED can be seen as related somehow to changes in severity levels of patients before or after the color coding scheme was introduced. She can also examine whether other changes in the nature of the people who arrived as trauma victims before and after the introduction of the color-coding scheme might be the cause of possible differences in waiting time, if these are found. These questions can be addressed by using regression analysis, which is presented in Chapters Eleven through Thirteen.

It might be useful at this point to mention two caveats to the use of statistics that apply directly to this example. The first of these caveats is that no statistical analysis may be needed at all if the difference in waiting time after the initiation of the color-coding scheme is clearly shorter than the waiting time before. Suppose, for example, that the average waiting time before the color-coding scheme was three hours from admission to the ED to transfer to hospital department. Suppose also that after the initiation of the scheme the average waiting time was forty-five minutes. In this scenario, no statistical significance tests would be required to show that the color-coding scheme was associated with a clear decline in waiting time. Furthermore, it is likely that the color-coding scheme would not only become a permanent part of the ED armamentarium of the university hospital but would be adopted widely by other hospitals as well.

However, suppose that after the initiation of the color-coding scheme the average waiting time in the ED was reduced from three hours to two hours and fifty minutes. A statistical test (probably the *t* test, discussed in Chapter Nine) would show whether 170 minutes waiting was actually less, statistically, than 180 minutes. Although such a small difference may seem to have little practical significance, it may be a statistically significant difference. Then the administrator would have to decide whether to retain an intervention that had a statistical, but not a practical, effect.

The second caveat to the use of statistics is the importance of understanding that a statistical test cannot establish causality. It might be possible, statistically, to show that the color-coding scheme was associated with a statistical reduction in waiting time. But in the absence of a more rigorous study design, it is not possible to say that the color-coding scheme actually caused the reduction in waiting time. In a setting such as this, where measurements are taken before and after some intervention (in this case, the color-coding scheme), a large number of things other than the color-coding scheme might have accounted for a reduced waiting time. The very recognition of the problem and consequent concern by ED physicians and nurses may have had more effect on waiting time than the color-coding scheme itself. But this is not a question that statistics, per se, can resolve. Such questions may be resolved in whole or in part by the nature of a study design. A double-blind, random clinical trial, for example, is a very powerful design for resolving the question of causality. But, in general, statistical analysis alone cannot determine whether an observed result has occurred because of a particular intervention. All that statistical analysis can do is establish whether two events (in this case, the color-coding scheme and the reduction in waiting time) are or are not independent of each other. This notion of independence will come up many more times, and, in many ways, it is the focus of much of this book.

Length of Stay, Readmission Rates, and Cost Per Case in a Hospital Alliance

Because of the skyrocketing costs of providing hospital services, every hospital administrator is interested in any mechanism that can be found to account for the rise in costs and that can be used to control this rise as it occurs. The Sea Coast Alliance, an alliance of eight hospitals, is as interested in mechanisms to control costs as any other hospital or group of hospitals, and the administrators of the alliance hope to be able to use the case experience of the Alliance to provide guidance about how to accomplish costs controls. Because the Alliance has the experience of eight hospitals, it has a substantial volume of case data that the administrators believe can be used to move ahead in understanding areas in which costs can be controlled.

There are, in particular, three measures of hospital performance related to costs that the staff of the Alliance are concerned about: length of stay (LOS), readmission rates, and cost per case. One of the initial questions is whether there are real differences between the eight hospitals in these three cost-related measures of hospital performance. The question of what is a real difference is, of course, critical. If the average LOS in one of the hospitals of the Alliance is five days for all hospital stays over the past year, while the average LOS for another one of the hospitals is six days, is this a real difference? Given certain assumptions about what the average LOS for a year in these two hospitals represents, this is a question that can be answered with statistics.

If the interest is in comparing two hospitals to one another, the statistic that could be used would be a t test. As indicated earlier, the t test is discussed in Chapter Nine. In general, though, the real interest would be in deciding if there was any difference between all eight hospitals, taken simultaneously. This question can be examined in a couple different ways. One would be to use analysis of variance (ANOVA), which is discussed in Chapter Ten. Another would be to use multiple regression, which is discussed in Chapters Eleven through Thirteen. If it is determined that the hospitals are different on LOS, using any of these statistical techniques, efforts could be directed toward determining whether lessons could be learned from the better performers about how to control costs that might be applied to the poorer performers. The same approach could be applied to understanding readmission rates and cost per case.

One particular focus of the Alliance administrators is diagnostic-related groupings (DRG) that have especially high costs. In addition to looking at the performance across the eight hospitals on high-cost DRGs, the Alliance would like to be able to examine the question of whether individual physicians seemed to stand out in LOS, readmission rates, or cost per case. The identification of individual physicians who have unusually high LOS, readmission rates, or cost per case can allow the Alliance to engage in selective educational efforts toward reduced costs. But an important question in looking at individual physician differences is whether what may appear to be unusually high values for LOS, readmission rates, or cost per case actually are unusual. Again, this question can be answered with statistics. In particular, predicted values for LOS, readmission rates, and cost per case can be determined by using regression analysis. If individual physician averages are relatively far from the predicted values (which is determined by the probability of being relatively far), then these physicians could be statistically determined to be unusually high—or unusually low, as the case may be.

Regression can also be used to assess whether differences that may exist across hospitals or across individual physicians could be attributed to differences in the mix of cases or patients that the hospitals accept or the physicians see. Such differences may be attributable statistically to such characteristics of patients as sex, age, and payer, which may differ across the eight hospitals or the numerous physicians. There might also be differences across cases such as severity or multiple diagnoses. If these were differentially distributed among hospitals or physicians, they could account for differences that are seen. All of these questions can be addressed (although not necessarily answered in full) by using multiple regression analysis, which is discussed in Chapters Eleven through Thirteen.

A Hospital Billing Change

At the Carteret Falls regional hospital, the emergency department has instituted a major change in how physicians are contracted to provide services and consequently how services are billed in the ER. Prior to January 1 of a recent year, emergency department physicians were employed by the regional hospital and the hospital billed for their services. Beginning January 1, the physicians became private contractors working within the emergency department, essentially working on their own time and billing for that time directly.

While the physicians bill on their own behalf for emergency room services, the bills are still submitted to Medicare by the hospital. Bills are submitted to Medicare under five different levels that correspond to the level of reimbursement Medicare provides. The higher the coding level, the more that is actually reimbursed for the service. Despite the fact that physicians are now billing for their own services, the Medicare administration still views the hospital, which is actually submitting the bills, as having final responsibility for the accuracy of billing codes.

The chief financial officer of the hospital is concerned that he will begin to see the billing level creep, as physicians begin billing for their own services. As the distinction between levels is frequently a matter of judgement, the CFO is concerned that physicians may begin, even without conscious decision making, to upgrade the level of the coding because it is directly tied to their reimbursement. The question the CFO faces is how to decide if the physicians are upgrading their codes, consciously or not, after the initiation of the new system. If they are, the hospital needs to take steps, either to ensure that the coding remains constant before and after the change in billing, or to have very good justification for Medicare as to why it should be different.

The first problem is to determine if the billing levels have changed from before the change in billing to after the change. But it is not simply enough to say that there is a change, if one is seen to have occurred. It is critical to be able to say that this change is or is not a change that would have been expected, given the pattern of billing in the past. In other words, is any change seen large enough to be deemed a real change and not just a chance occurrence? If a change has occurred, and if it is large enough to be viewed as a real change, then the second problem arises. The second problem is to determine whether there is anything in the nature of the ER cases before and after the billing change that might account for the difference and thus be the explanation of the difference that will satisfy the Medicare administration.

Both of these problems can be examined by using statistics. In regard to the first problem, a difference between the distribution of billings across the five categories before and after the change in billing source can be assessed by using the chi-square statistic that is discussed in Chapter Eight. Or, because the amount of a bill is constant within the five categories, it is also possible to compare the two groups, before and after using the t test that is discussed in Chapter Nine. The second problem, of whether any difference can be attributed to changed characteristics of the cases seen in the ER, can be assessed by using regression—when the cost of the bills before and after is the measure of change. Regression is discussed in Chapters Eleven through Thirteen.

A Study of the Effectiveness of Breast Cancer Education

A resident at a local hospital has been asked by the senior physician to develop a pilot study on the effectiveness of two alternative breast cancer education mechanisms, both aimed at women coming to a women's health center. The first alternative is a brochure on breast cancer given to the women when they arrive at the clinic. The second is time specifically allocated during a clinic visit where the physician spends five to ten minutes with a women, giving direct information and answering questions on the same topics covered in the brochure.

The student-resident recognizes that a study can be designed in which one group of women would receive the brochure and a second group would participate in a session with a physician. She also believes that a questionnaire can be developed to measure the knowledge women have about breast cancer before the distribution of the brochure or session with the physician and after either event, to assess any difference in knowledge. She also has concern about the possibility of the need for a control group of women to determine whether either method of information dissemination is better than no intervention at all. And perhaps she is interested in whether the brochure and discussion with the physician together would be better than either alternative separately.

Although she has been asked to design a pilot study only, the student-resident wishes to be as careful and thoughtful as possible in developing her study. There are a number of different alternatives she might consider. One alternative would be a simple t test of the difference between a group of women who received the brochure and a group of women who participated in the sessions with a physician. The measurement for this comparison could be the knowledge assessment administered either after the distribution of the brochure or after the physician encounter. Such a t test is discussed in Chapter Nine.

But the student-resident may very well not be satisfied with the simple t test. One problem is that she wants to include a control group of women who received no intervention at all. She may also wish to include another group of women— those who received the brochure *and* participated in a session with the physician.

Again, the measurement of the effect of any intervention (or of none) could be done using her previously developed knowledge assessment, administered after the fact. This assessment could be carried out using a one-way analysis of variance (ANOVA), which is discussed in Chapter Ten.

Again, however, the student-resident may not be entirely satisfied with either the t test or the one-way analysis of variance. She might wish to be sure that in her comparison she is not simply measuring a difference between women that existed prior to the receipt of the brochures or the physician sessions. To ensure this, she might wish to measure women's knowledge both before and after the interventions, at both times using her knowledge assessment questionnaire. This assessment could be carried out using a two-way analysis of variance, which is also discussed in Chapter Ten.

Whether the student-resident decides to go with a t test, a one-way ANOVA, or a two-way ANOVA, one of the more important aspects of the study will be to randomly allocate women to the experimental or control group. When measuring knowledge only after the intervention, the student-resident will be able to ensure that prior knowledge is not responsible for any differences she might find only if she is certain that there is only a small chance that the groups of women receiving different interventions were not different to begin with. The only effective way to ensure this is through random assignment to the groups. Random selection and random assignment are discussed in Chapter Three.

Calculating a Standard Hourly Rate for Health Personnel

In an article published in *Healthcare Financial Management,* Richard McDermott (2001) discusses the problem and importance of establishing standard hourly labor rates for employee reimbursement. He points out that many compensation systems have been worked out over a number of years by different human resource directors, each with his or her own compensation philosophy. As a result, these systems may fail to reflect market conditions and may be inconsistent in their treatment of differing categories of labor. McDermott suggests a regression approach to calculating labor rates that have both internal consistency and external validity.

The approach McDermott (2001) suggests for establishing labor rates is based on an example in which he provides data for ten different positions. Each position is assigned a score from 0 to 5 based on the degree of complexity in the job in five separate categories, such as level of decision making, amount of planning required, educational requirements, and so on. He does not indicate specifically which five characteristics are employed in the example. The assigned scores on each category would have been developed through an examination of the requirements of the job by a compensation consultant after interviews with the incumbent of each position. Each of the ten positions also includes an actual hourly wage.

Regression analysis, discussed in Chapters Twelve and Thirteen, was used by McDermott (2001) to assess the relationship between each of the five characteristics of the job and the actual hourly compensation. The regression analysis indicates both the relationship between any one of the five characteristics (when all characteristics are considered simultaneously) and hourly compensation, and it provides a set of coefficients by which to translate assigned values on any set of characteristics into a *predicted* hourly compensation. This, then, becomes a relatively objective means to determine hourly compensation for a person in any position.

There are purely statistical problems in using this regression approach, at least as discussed by McDermott (2001), to propose hourly compensation. Particularly, ten observations (the jobs assessed) are rarely considered by statisticians to be an adequate number to assess the relationship between five predictor variables (the characteristics) and a sixth predicted variable (the hourly compensation). While there are no absolute rules for the number of observations needed relative to the number of variables assessed, it is often accepted that there should be at least three times as many observations as variables, and some statisticians suggest a ratio of as many as ten observations to each variable.

A second problem with this approach to assigning hourly compensation is inherent in the fact that many jobs are essentially the same, with similar job titles and expectations. If such jobs are included in an analysis of the type discussed here, one of the basic premises of regression analysis—that there is no correlation between observations—will be violated. This can be overcome, in part, by the use of dummy variables, which is also discussed in Chapter Thirteen.

Exercises for Section 1.2

1. Look in familiar magazines or journals that might deal with subjects relevant to your current work situation or your planned area of work. Can you find discussions that involve statistics? If so, briefly describe these and how the statistics are applied.

2. Consider experience you have had or a situation that you are familiar with in your work or planned area of work. Can you imagine any way that this experience or situation could be benefit from the application of statistics? Briefly describe this experience or situation.

3. On the basis of you current knowledge of statistics (even though it might be quite limited), suggest possible ways in which statistics might be applied to your experience or situation.

Section 1.3 What Is the Big Picture?

Having discussed several specific examples of why a health worker might be interested in knowing statistics, and having suggested some ways in which this book will aid in that knowledge, it is now desirable to step back and ask, What are we actually trying to do? Put in another way, what is the big picture? The big picture is basically this: in any situation in which statistics may be applicable and useful, the beginning is the question for which an answer is sought. Are our Medicare claims properly completed? Does a color coding scheme for emergencies reduce emergency room time? Do the hospitals in a region differ in costs? Will an education strategy work?

In attempting to answer any of these questions, it is generally true that not all the data that might bear on the answer will ever be available. In some cases, though it might be possible to access all the relevant data, it might just be too costly to do so. This would be true, for example, with regard to Medicare claims in a home health agency. Because it would be very costly to examine every claim, the answer must rely on a subset of the claims. In other cases, it might never be possible to access all records or all people who might be necessary to provide a definitive answer. In regard to the question of whether an education intervention will increase the knowledge women have of breast cancer, it would be physically impossible to assess all women who might ever be potential subjects of such an education effort.

The consequence of this inability to access all the data that may be relevant to a decision means that it will be necessary, generally, to rely on only a subset of the data—a sample—to make whatever decision is called for. Statistics is about the rules and procedures for using a subset of the data to make the decisions desired. In learning statistics, one learns these rules and procedures, when and to what types of data to apply, and the confidence that one can have in using the results of the sample data to make inferences about the total population. This is the basic function of statistics.

In considering the function of statistics as the process of using a sample to make inferences about a larger population, it is important to point out that in many cases this is the only way, and often the best way, to reach decisions. In the case of the acceptability of Medicare claims, for example, it is highly likely that if the staff of a home health agency were required to review every one of the files, they would become tired, bored, and generally unhappy with the process. They might make mistakes or errors in judgement that they would perhaps not make if working with only a sample of records. When they had finished their audit of the entire population of claims, they could very well have less useful information than they would have had under the limitations of a sample. And, in any case, the cost would be prohibitive.

Even if the entire population appeared to be available for assessment and the assessment could be made for the entire population easily and at relatively low cost, statistics would still be useful. For example, the chief financial officer of a hospital that has changed billing procedures so that a concern about billing creep might arise probably has machine-readable records for every hospital charge before and after the change in billing. Suppose he examines these bills and discovers that before the change, the average charge was $250, but afterward it was $500. He would probably be pretty confident that there had been billing creep. But what if the average charge before the billing change was $250 but afterward was $265? Is this a difference that might be expected on the variation in the data? Should he or should he not see this difference as a chance occurrence or as the mark of a real change? Furthermore, and very much to the points made previously, even though the financial officer has all the billing records at a given point in time, he will never have the billing records for cases yet to be seen. One function of statistics is to take what is available now, assuming that this information is similar to all that will become available, and make inferences about all the data.

The big picture, then—the purpose of statistics—is to take information about limited portions of a population and use that information to make judgements about the entire population. Through the course of this book, that purpose of statistics will continue to be stressed and examined.

Section 1.4 Some Initial Definitions

Before proceeding much further in this discussion, it is essential to make certain that everyone is clear about a number of terms that will crop up again and again in this text.

Populations and Samples

Populations are those groups of entities about which there is an interest. Populations may be made up of people—for example, all citizens of the United States or all patients who have or ever will show up at a specific emergency room clinic. Populations may be made up of organizations—for example, all hospitals in the United States, or all long-term care facilities in New York state. Populations may be made up of political entities—for example, all the countries in the world or all the counties in California. Populations might be made up of all the persons who might ever receive a particular type of treatment—for example, all people who have had an MRI are a population, but also all people who ever will have an MRI could be considered another population, or together, these two groups could be considered a population.

In general, we are interested in characteristics of populations as opposed to characteristics of samples. We might wish to know the average cholesterol level of all persons aged fifty-five or older (a population). We might wish to know the daily bed occupancy rate for hospitals in the United States (a population). Or we might wish to know the effect of a specific drug on cholesterol levels of some group of people (a population). If we knew these specific pieces of information, we would know a *parameter*. Parameters are information about populations. In general, except for some data collected by complete census of the population (even most complete censuses are not complete), we do not know parameters. The best we can usually do is estimate parameters based on a subset of observations taken from populations.

Samples are subsets of populations. If a population of interest consists of all patients who have or ever will show up at a specific emergency room clinic, a sample from that population could be all the patients who are there on a specific afternoon. If a population of interest consists of all long-term care facilities in New York state, a sample from that population might be all these facilities in Buffalo, Syracuse, and Albany. If a population of interest is all persons who have or ever will use a cholesterol-reducing drug, a sample from that population might be all persons who received prescriptions for such a drug from a specific physician. An individual member of a sample might be referred to as an *element* of the sample, or, more commonly, as an *observation*.

Information from samples can be used to make estimates of information about populations (parameters). When a specific value from a sample is used to make an estimate of the same value for a population, the sample value is known as a *statistic*. Statistics are to samples what parameters are to populations. If the parameter of interest is, for example, waiting time in emergency rooms, an estimate of that parameter could be the average waiting time for a small, carefully selected group of emergency rooms. The estimate would be a statistic. In general, we can know values of statistics but not parameters, even though we would wish to know the values of parameters.

Random and Nonrandom Samples

Samples are subsets of populations. These subsets may be selected in a random manner or in a nonrandom manner. All patients in an emergency room on a specific afternoon would probably not constitute a random sample of all people who have used or will use an emergency room. All the hospitals in Buffalo, Syracuse, and Albany might be a random sample of all hospitals in New York state, but they probably would not be. All persons who received prescriptions for a cholesterol-reducing drug from a specific physician would, in general, not be a random sample of all persons who take such drugs. All of these examples would probably be considered nonrandom samples. Nonrandom samples may be drawn in many ways. In general, however, we are not interested in nonrandom samples. The study of statistics is based on and assumes the presence of random samples. This requires some discussion of what constitutes a random sample.

A *random sample* is a sample drawn in a way in which every member of the population has a known probability of being selected. At a minimum, this means that all members of the population must be identifiable. Frequently, there is a gap between the population of interest and the population from which the sample is actually drawn. For example, suppose a health department wished to draw a random sample of all families in its area of responsibility to determine what proportion believed that the health department was a possible source of any type of health services—prevention, treatment, advice—for members of the family. The *target population* is all families in the area of responsibility. If we assume that this is a county health department, a random sample would assign a known probability of selection to each family in the county. In general, this would mean that each family in the county would have an equal probability of selection. If there were, for example, thirty thousand families in the county, each one would have a probability of 1/30,000 of being selected as a member of the sample.

But, in general, it would be very difficult to be certain that every family in the county had exactly a 1/30,000 probability of being selected for the sample. The difficulty arises from the problem of devising an economically feasible mechanism of identifying and contacting every possible family in the county. For example, one relatively inexpensive way of collecting the information desired would be to contact a sample of families by telephone and ask them questions from a short questionnaire by phone. But some families do not have phones, making their probability of selection into the sample not 1/30,000 but simply zero. Other families may have more than one phone, and if care is not taken to ensure that the family is not contacted twice, some families might have twice the chance (or more) of being selected into the sample. Still other families—especially in the present age of telemarketing—would refuse to participate, which would make their probability of being included zero, as well.

Other mechanisms of identifying all families in a county or other area have equal difficulties. Voter rolls contain only registered voters. Tax rolls contain only persons who pay taxes. Both of these rolls also contain single persons. A decision would have to be made about whether a single person was a family. In summary, then, it is very often nearly impossible, or at least very expensive, to draw a truly random sample from a target population. What often happens instead is that the sample drawn is actually from a population very close to the target population but not the target population exactly. Instead of all the families in the county being the population from which the sample is drawn, the population may be all families with telephones. The population from which the sample is actually drawn is known as the *sampled population*. Inferences from the sample to the population are always to the sampled population, although it is certainly hoped that these inferences hold for the target population as well.

Given that the population sampled may not be exactly the target population desired, there still needs to be a mechanism for assuring that each member of the population to be sampled has a known probability—generally equal—of being selected. There are lots of ways of assuring randomness in specific settings. Shuffling cards is a way of assuring that each person has an equal chance of getting the good cards and the bad cards during the deal—essentially a random distribution of the cards. Rolling dice is a way of ensuring a random distribution of the faces of a die. Flipping a coin is a way of ensuring the random appearance of a head or a tail.

But sampling from a population of all families served by a health department is more complicated. One workable mechanism might be to put every family's name on equal-sized slips of paper, put all the slips of paper in a box, shake them up, and without looking at the slips of paper, draw out the number of slips desired. But this approach, although it would produce a random sample of families, would be both cumbersome and time-consuming. Happily, Excel provides several mechanisms that can be used to draw random samples. The question of random sampling will be treated at several points in the text, but a workable approach to drawing a random sample using Excel is discussed specifically in Chapter Three.

Types of Random Samples

There are basically four different types of random samples. These are systematic samples, simple random samples, stratified samples, and cluster samples.

Systematic samples are samples drawn by first dividing the population into subsets equal to the number of observations ultimately desired in the sample and then drawing a specific observation from each subset. If the total population of interest consisted of thirty thousand families and the sample to be drawn was to consist of a hundred families, the first step in drawing a systematic sample would be to divide the total population into a hundred subsets. If the thirty thousand families were on a list, say, in alphabetical order, the common way to divide the families into a hundred subsets would be to take the first three hundred families as the first subset, the second three hundred as the second subset, and so on to the end of the list.

The next step in drawing a systematic sample would be to select randomly one family from the first subset of three hundred. Then, the corresponding family from each of the other ninety-nine subsets would be selected to fill out the sample. For example, if the family in position 137 in the alphabetical list were selected at random, then family number 437 (the 137th family in the second subset of three hundred) would be taken as the next member of the sample and family number 737 would be selected as the third member, all the way to family number 39,837. This would produce a sample of a hundred families, all of whom are spaced three hundred families apart in the alphabetical list.

A systematic sample actually represents a single observation in statistical terms, because once the selection is made from the first subset, all other observations are fixed. If a sample of one hundred is to be selected systematically from a population of thirty thousand, three hundred different samples can be selected, corresponding to each of the three hundred families that can be selected as the first element of the sample. Because systematic samples are samples made up from a single random selection, the results expected from statistics do not actually apply to systematic samples. Nevertheless, systematic samples are often treated as if statistics do apply appropriately to them, and this is generally considered acceptable for drawing inferences about populations.

Simple random samples are samples drawn in such a way that every possible sample of a given size has an equal likelihood of being selected for the sample. If the total population of interest consisted of thirty thousand families and the sample to be drawn was to consist of a hundred families, every possible sample of a hundred families would have an equal likelihood of being drawn in a simple random sample. Before the widespread availability of computers, simple random samples were typically drawn by associating each element of the population with a number from a *random number table*. If the number in the random number table was in a certain range, the element was included in the sample; if not, the element was not included in the sample. The advent of computers, and especially such programs as Microsoft Excel, has eliminated the need for random number tables. Excel can generate lists of random numbers that can be used to select simple random samples. This is discussed in detail in Chapter Three.

Whereas there are only three hundred different systematic samples of size 100 that could be drawn from a population of thirty thousand families, there are far more simple random samples of size 100. The number of different simple random samples of a hundred families that can be taken from a population of thirty thousand families is so large, it would take about three lines of text to write it out completely. It is approximately the number 46,815 followed by 285 zeros. And each one of this very large number of samples has an equal likelihood of being selected as the one simple random sample taken.

Stratified samples are samples drawn by dividing the total population into two or more groups, or *strata,* and then drawing a specified proportion of each strata for the sample. The specified portion might be proportional to the strata size, or it might be equal to the number drawn from other strata, whether the strata sizes are equal or not. Within each strata, the sample may be drawn by simple random sampling or by systematic sampling, but it is typically drawn by simple random sampling.

Consider how a stratified sample might apply to our sample of a hundred families from a population of thirty-thousand families. Suppose we know that within our population of thirty thousand families, three thousand have Hispanic surnames. If we want to draw a stratified sample that would guarantee that we had proportional representation of families with Hispanic surnames in our sample, we could first divide the total population into two strata—those with Hispanic surnames and those with other surnames. Then we could take a sample of ten families from among those with Hispanic surnames and a sample of ninety families from among those who do not have Hispanic surnames.

In general, stratified samples are drawn either because the researcher wishes to ensure that the groups represented by the strata are appropriately represented in the final sample or because there is reason to believe that the subject of interest to the study is closely related to the characteristics upon which the strata are based. In the latter case, for example, if a health worker wished to estimate average height among teenagers seventeen to nineteen years of age, it would probably be useful to stratify on sex, because at this age, males are likely to be taller than females. At preadolescence, it might be useful to stratify on sex because females are likely to be taller than males.

Cluster samples are samples drawn by first dividing the sample into several groups, or *clusters.* The sampling then proceeds in two or more stages. This discussion is only of a two-stage cluster sample. In the first stage, a set of the clusters is drawn using either systematic or simple random sampling, although simple random is most commonly employed. In the second stage, either all members of the cluster or a sample of members of the cluster are selected to be included in the final sample.

In the case of our sample of a hundred families from among thirty thousand, it might be that the families to be selected could be divided into zip code areas first, with a sample of zip code areas randomly selected in the first stage. In the second stage, families could be selected randomly from the zip codes selected in the first stage to fill out the sample of one hundred. Typically, cluster samples are used when the collection of data from a simple random sample would involve a great deal of travel time. The use of clusters limits the travel required for data collection only to those clusters selected. A major drawback of cluster sampling is that it is likely to increase the variability of those statistics about which estimates are to be made.

Cluster samples and stratified samples differ from one another in that in cluster samples only a few of the groups or clusters actually have members represented in the final sample, whereas in stratified samples, all groups, or strata, have members represented in the final sample. *While it is important to know that these different types of samples exist, the material presented in this book universally assumes that the data were drawn in what would be considered either a simple random method or a stratified method with the number of observations drawn from each strata proportional to strata size.*

Variables, Independent and Dependent

Throughout this book there are frequent references to the term *variable*. A variable is a characteristic of an observation or element of the sample that is assessed or measured. A value for a variable across all members of a sample (such as the average height of preadolescent teens) is typically referred to as a statistic. The comparable value for the population is a parameter. Most statistical activities are either an attempt to determine a value for a variable from a sample (and thus to be able to estimate the population value) or to determine whether there is a relationship between two or more variables.

In order to show a relationship between two or more variables, the variables must vary. That is to say that they must take on more than one value. Any characteristic of a population that does not vary is a *constant*. There can be no relationship between a constant and a variable. This is equivalent to saying that there can be no way of accounting for the value of any variable by referring to a constant. For example, if we wished to describe variations in adult onset diabetes rates among persons with Hispanic surnames, it would be useless to employ Hispanic surname as an explanation, because it is constant for all these people. It cannot explain differences. But if we wished to describe differences in adult onset diabetes among all the people living in New Mexico, Hispanic surname or non-Hispanic surname might be a useful variable to employ.

Variables are typically classified as either of two types: categorical or numerical. Numerical variables are further classified as either discrete or continuous. These distinctions are important for the type of statistic that may effectively be employed with them.

Categorical variables are variables, the levels of which are distinguished simply by names. Hispanic and non-Hispanic surname is a two-level categorical variable that roughly distinguishes whether a person is of Hispanic ancestry. Sex is a two-level categorical variable that in general divides all persons into male or female. Categorical variables can take on more levels as well. Type of insurance coverage, for example, is a multilevel categorical variable that may take on the values— Medicare, Medicaid, voluntary not-for-profit, for-profit, self-pay, and other. Other categorical variables may take on many levels.

Although a variable may be represented by a set of numbers, such a representation does not automatically mean that it is not a categorical variable. The ICD9 code is a categorical variable, even though the codes are represented as numbers. The numbers simply classify diagnoses into numerical codes that have no actual numerical meaning. Another type of categorical variable that is assigned a number is the *dummy variable*. The dummy variable is a two-level categorical variable (such as sex) that is assigned a numerical value, usually the values 1 and 0. The value 1 might be assigned to female and 0 assigned to male, or vice versa. Although this type of variable remains a categorical variable, it can be treated as a numerical variable in some statistical applications that require numerical variables. However, a categorical variable with more than two levels, such as the ICD9 code, can be treated as a numerical variable in analysis only by dividing the multilevel categorical variable into a number of two-level categorical variables that can be treated as dummy variables.

Numerical variables are, as the name implies, variables whose values are designated by numbers. But unlike ICD9 codes, the numbers have some meaning relative to one another. At the very minimum, a numerical variable whose value is, for example, 23 is presumed to be larger than a numerical variable whose value is 17. Numerical variables may be measured on three scales: the ordinal scale, the interval scale, and the ratio scale.

The *ordinal scale* is a scale in which the values assigned to the levels of a variable simply indicate that the levels are in order of magnitude. A common ordinal scale is the *Likert* scale, which requests a response to one of usually five alternatives: *strongly agree, agree, undecided, disagree,* or *strongly disagree.* These responses are then assigned values of 1 to 5, or 5 to 1 and treated as values of a numerical variable. Treating Likert scale responses as numerical variables assumes that the conceptual difference between strongly agree and agree is exactly the same, for example, as the conceptual difference between undecided and disagree. If that cannot be assumed, then ordered variables, such as Likert scale variables, even if assigned numerical values, should not be treated as numerical variables in analysis but must be treated as categorical variables.

The *interval scale* is a scale in which the values assigned to the levels of a variable indicate the order of magnitude in equal intervals. The commonly employed measures of temperature, Fahrenheit, and centigrade are interval scales. For centigrade, for example, the value of 0 refers not to the complete absence of heat, but simply to the temperature at which water freezes. One hundred on the centigrade scale refers to the temperature at which water boils at sea level. The distance between these two has been divided into one hundred equal intervals. Because this is an interval scale measurement, it is possible to say that the difference between 10 degrees centigrade and 15 degrees centigrade is the same as the distance between 20 degrees centigrade and 25 degrees centigrade. But it is not possible to say that 20 degrees centigrade is twice as warm as 10 degrees centigrade.

The *ratio scale* is a scale in which the values assigned to the levels of a variable indicate both the order of magnitude and equal intervals, but, in addition, assumes a real zero. The real zero represents the complete absence of the trait that is being measured. Temperature measured on the Kelvin scale has a real zero, which represents the complete absence of heat. At a more prosaic level, the number of patients in an emergency room is measured on a ratio scale. There can be zero patients in the emergency room, representing the complete absence of patients, or there can be any number of patients. Each new patient adds an equal increment to the number of patients in the emergency room. In general, any variable that is treated as numeric for statistical analysis is assumed to be measured on at least an interval scale and most commonly on a ratio scale.

Discrete numerical variables are variables that can take on only whole number values. Discrete numerical variables are typically the result of the counting of things, persons, events, activities, and organizations. The number of persons in an emergency room is a discrete numerical variable. There must always be a whole number of persons in the room—for example 23. There can never be 23.7 persons in an emergency room. The number of children born to a single woman, the number of organizations that are accredited by a national accrediting body, the number of physicians on a hospital staff, the number of health departments in a state—these are all discrete numerical variables.

Continuous numerical variables are variables that can take on any value whatsoever. They can be whole numbers, such as forty-seven, or they can be numbers to any number of decimal places, such as one-third (which is .33333 . . . and so on forever). The amount of time that a person spends in an emergency room is a continuous variable that can be stated to any level of precision (in terms of minutes, seconds, parts of seconds) that we have the ability and interest to measure. Body temperature, pulse rate, height, weight, and age are all continuous numerical variables. Measures that are created as the ratio of one variable to another, such as cost per hospital admission or cost per day, or proportion of children fully immunized, are also continuous numerical variables.

Probabilities of occurrence of discrete or continuous numerical values cannot be found in the same ways. In general, it is possible to find the exact probability of the occurrence of a discrete outcome based either on an a priori distribution or on empirical information. Probabilities of outcomes for continuous numerical variables, however, can only be approximated. Despite this, the distribution of continuous numerical variables has been extensively researched and in the form of the normal distribution: particularly, it forms the basis of most statistical analyses for numerical variables, whether the variables are measured as discrete or continuous.

Exercises for Section 1.4

1. For each of the following sets of entities, decide whether you think the set is more likely to be a population or a sample, and explain why.
   a. All hospitals in the United States
   b. All patients in the emergency room of a given hospital on a given day
   c. One hospital from each of the fifty largest cities in the United States
   d. Sixteen health departments selected from among those in a state
   e. The patients who visit a single physician
   f. Operating room procedures for February 11 in a single hospital

2. What mechanisms might you use to obtain a list of all members of the following target populations, and how successful might you be?
   a. Emergency room visitors for the past six months at a single hospital emergency room
   b. Hospitals in the United States
   c. Health department clientele for a single health department
   d. All food service facilities in a health department catchment area
   e. All people in a single hospital catchment area
   f. People who will dial 911 in the next six months in a given municipality

3. Determine whether each of the following is a systematic sample, a simple random sample, a stratified sample, a cluster sample, or a nonrandom sample, and say why.
   a. A sample drawn by randomly selecting fifty pages from a telephone book and taking the fifth name on each page
   b. A sample drawn by dividing all persons visiting an emergency room in the last six months into male and female and randomly selecting a hundred from each group

   c. A sample drawn by selecting the person who arrives at a doctor's office at
      a time closest to a randomly selected time of day (say, 9:10 A.M.) and each
      person coming closest to that time on forty subsequent days
   d. Any five cards drawn from a well-shuffled deck
   e. A sample drawn by randomly selecting six health departments from among
      those in a state and then randomly selecting six staff members from each
      of the six health departments
   f. A sample taken by selecting twenty hospitals in such a way as to ensure that
      they are representative of the types of hospitals in the United States

 4. For each of the following random variables, determine whether the variable
    is categorical or numerical. If the variable is numerical, determine whether
    the phenomenon of interest is discrete or continuous.
    a. The number of clients at a health department MCH clinic
    b. The primary reason for an MCH clinic visit
    c. The length of time in minutes spent by a client waiting to be seen at the clinic
    d. Whether children at the clinic have the recommended immunizations
    e. The weight of children seen at the clinic
    f. The income of families of clients seen at the clinic

 5. Determine whether each of the following scales is nominal, ordinal, interval,
    or ratio, and say why.
    a. The classification of patients into male and female
    b. The designation of male patients as 0 and female patients as 1
    c. The number of live births to a woman coded 0, 1, 2, 3, or more.
    d. The measured pulse rate
    e. The number of staff members in a health department

Section 1.5 Five Statistical Tests

This book is divided into two sections. The first section, which comprises the
first six chapters, is essentially preparatory material designed to equip the user of
the book for the second section. The first section includes this introduction, a chapter on the use of Excel for statistical analysis, a chapter on data acquisition and
preparation for statistical analysis, a chapter on descriptive presentation of data
and Excel's graphing capability, a chapter on probability, and a chapter on the examination of data distributions.

   The second section of the book, which comprises Chapters Seven through
Fourteen, is concerned with hypothesis testing. Hypothesis testing is essentially the
act of determining whether data from a sample can be seen to support or not

support a belief in independence between two or more variables in a population; one is commonly considered a dependent variable and the other or others are thought of as independent variables.

Five separate statistical tests that address this question of independence are discussed in this book. They are the chi-square test, the t test, analysis of variance (ANOVA), regression analysis, and Logit. In practical terms, each of these tests can be thought of as testing whether sample values for two or more variables could have been drawn from a population in which the variables are independent of one another. Without considering specifically what independence means in regard to any one of these tests, it is possible to distinguish between these five tests on the basis of the type of data for which they are able to assess independence.

The chi-square test can be used to assess the independence of two variables, both of which are categorical. Either of the two variables may take on two or more levels or categories, but the data itself is measured simply as named categories. For example, the chi-square can be used to determine whether coming to an emergency clinic for a true emergency or for a visit that is not an emergency (a two-level categorical variable) is independent of whether one comes during the day or during the night (another two-level categorical variable). Or a chi-square test could be used to determine whether the desire of women for an additional child (a two-level, yes-no variable) is independent of the number of children she already has in the three categories—for example; one, two or three, and four or more. The chi-square can be used on variables that take on larger numbers of values as well, but in practical terms, it is unusual to see a chi-square that involves variables having more than three or four levels. The chi-square test is discussed in Chapter Eight.

The t test can be used to assess the independence of two variables, one being a numerical variable measured either in discrete or continuous units and the other being a categorical variable taking on only two values. For example, the t test can be used to determine whether the score people receive on a test of knowledge about breast cancer measured on a 20-point scale (a numerical variable) is independent of whether those people were specifically and consciously exposed to knowledge about breast cancer or were not (a two-value categorical variable). Or a t test could be used to determine whether the cost of a hospital stay (a numerical variable) was independent of whether the patient was a member of an HMO or not (a two-level categorical variable). The t test is discussed in Chapter Nine.

Analysis of variance is an extension of the t test. Analysis of variance (ANOVA) can be used to assess the independence of two or more variables, one being a numerical variable measured either in discrete or continuous units and the others being categorical variables that may take on any number of values rather than only two. Analysis of variance, for example, could be used to assess not only whether a knowledge score about breast cancer was independent of exposure to knowledge about breast cancer but also whether the score might be independent of several different types of exposure—that is, the reading of a brochure, a one-on-one discussion with a physician, both, or neither. Analysis of variance could also be used to determine whether the length of a hospital stay (a numerical variable) was independent of the hospital in which the stay took place over five separate hospitals (a categorical variable taking on five values). Analysis of variance is discussed in Chapter Ten.

Regression is a logical last stage in this progression, in that regression is a technique that can test the independence of two or more numerical variables measured either in discrete or continuous units. Regression may also include one or more categorical variables, any one of which can take on only two values (in which case, it is often referred to as analysis of covariance). Regression, then, could test the independence, for example, of the cost of a hospital stay (a numerical variable) and the length of a hospital stay (a second numerical variable) across an essentially unlimited number of hospitals. Or it could assess the independence of the dollar value of all hospital billings (a numerical variable) and the number of patients admitted (a second numerical variable) for a sample of for-profit and not-for-profit hospitals (a categorical variable taking on two values). Regression analysis is discussed in several chapters, including Chapters Eleven, Twelve, and Thirteen.

Logit is an extension of regression that can examine the independence of two or more variables where the dependent variable is a dichotomous categorical variable and the independent variable or variable set may be categorical (taking on only two values) or numerical—either discrete or continuous. Logit could be used, for example, to assess the independence of the outcome of an emergency surgical procedure (measured as successful or unsuccessful) and such variables as the degree of presurgery trauma, the length of time between the emergency and the surgical procedure, the age of the patient, and so on. Logit is discussed in Chapter Fourteen.

Exercises for Section 1.5

1. Consider which type of analysis could be used to assess independence for each of the following sets of data and state why this would be so (the dependent variable is given first).
   a. Hospital length of stay per admission and insurance type, including Medicare, Medicaid, private not-for-profit, private for-profit, and self-pay

  b. Cost per hospital stay and sex, age, and whether medical or surgical

  c. Whether a woman desires an additional child and the number of children now living categorized as none, one or two, and three or more

  d. Blood pressure readings for a group of people before and after the initiation of a six-week exercise and diet regimen

  e. Hospital length of stay per admission for the first digit of the ICD-9 code

  f. Birth weight for newborns measured as low or normal and gestational age, mother's age, and whether she is a smoker or nonsmoker

2. Suggest a dependent variable and at least one independent variable for a question that could be analyzed using each of the following:

  a. Chi-square analysis

  b. A t test

  c. Analysis of variance

  d. Regression

  e. Logit

Section 1.6 Outline of the Book

This book includes fourteen chapters. The following paragraphs give a brief overview of each chapter, including this one.

Chapter One: Introduction

This chapter introduces the book and presents several examples of problems that may be faced by health workers that can be solved, or at least considered, using statistical analysis. These problems are real problems faced by health administrators, managers, policymakers, and planners, having been developed from questions raised or comments made by students in the class who are actually mid-career health workers. Examples of the types of problems raised by the students and briefly outlined in this chapter include sampling problems, data preparation problems, and displaying data. Examples using hypothesis testing include comparing two groups or more than two groups to one another with both categorical and numerical outcome variables, predicting trend lines, and describing the relationships between several numerical variables.

Chapter Two: Excel as a Statistical Tool

This chapter introduces Excel as a statistical tool. It begins with a very basic introduction to the use of Excel. It then focuses on various Excel statistical features, including the various built-in Excel statistical and mathematical functions that are useful to statistical analysis, introductory material on using the Excel graph function, sorting data, and the pivot table. The chapter also briefly introduces the Excel statistical analysis add-ins that provide a powerful source of data analysis potential. It concludes with a discussion of Excel functions, such as =MMULT() and =MINVERSE() that produce results in more than one worksheet cell. The chapter includes examples and exercises relevant to health services.

Chapter Three: Data Acquisition: Sampling and Data Preparation

This chapter deals with various aspects of getting ready to use statistical analysis. The primary focus is on several issues relative to acquisition and preparation. The chapter discusses methods of sample selection and the ways in which random numbers can be generated and a random sample can be selected using Excel. It briefly discusses data collection, especially as this relates to the ways in which data are analyzed. It deals with the types of data that may be collected and how these data can be modified when necessary to meet the needs of the statistical analysis that might be most appropriately applied. The chapter also deals with some of the strategies for treating missing data and transforming data from numerical to categorical data or from categorical data to data that can be used with statistics (such as regression) that require numerical variables. All of this discussion draws upon the capabilities of Excel in random number generation and in the ability to implement decisions in data handling and modification. The chapter includes examples and exercises relevant to health services.

Chapter Four: Data Display: Descriptive Presentation, Excel Graphing Capability

This chapter considers the extensive graphing capabilities of Excel for displaying and presenting data, including bar charts, column charts, line graphs, and xy scatter plots. It also considers the special graph capabilities of Excel, such as the creation of Paretto charts and dual axis charts. The chapter also focuses on the ways in which Excel can be employed to prepare data for plotting, such as the construction of frequency distributions, using the frequency function in Excel and using the pivot table function. The chapter includes examples and exercises relevant to health services.

Chapter Five: Basic Concepts of Probability

This chapter considers probability concepts important to understanding categorical data probabilities, including marginal probabilities, joint probabilities, and conditional probabilities. It discusses discrete probability functions useful in statistical analysis, particularly the binomial and poisson distributions, and shows how exact probabilities for these distributions can be obtained from Excel and how they apply to realistic health related problems. The chapter also introduces the normal distribution as the most important continuous distribution considered in statistical analysis. Included are examples and exercises relevant to health services.

Chapter Six: Measures of Central Tendency and Dispersion: Data Distributions

This chapter introduces the mean, variance, and standard deviation as measures of central tendency and dispersion and demonstrates their calculation. It also distinguishes between the population mean and the sample mean and shows how the means of many samples tend toward normality, no matter what the distribution of the original data. It introduces the standard error of the mean and demonstrates how the standard error is a measure of the standard deviation of a large group of sample means. The chapter includes examples and exercises relevant to health services.

Chapter Seven: Confidence Limits and Hypothesis Testing

This chapter focuses on the setting of confidence limits and what they mean for hypothesis testing. It discusses the nature of hypotheses and how they are tested. It includes a discussion of Type I and Type II errors and what these mean in hypothesis testing and draws upon the graphing capabilities of Excel to demonstrate the notions of Type I and Type II errors in relation to sampling distributions. The chapter also introduces the concept that all statistical tests are essentially the test of independence between two or more variables. The chapter includes examples and exercises relevant to health services.

Chapter Eight: Statistical Tests for Categorical Data

This chapter discusses the chi-square distribution and the chi-square test as a test for independence between two or more categorical variables. It examines two-by-two contingency tables, two-by-n contingency tables, and n-by-n contingency tables and demonstrates how chi-square may be calculated and interpreted in each setting. It also discusses issues related to small cell frequencies in any contingency table and discusses the Yates correction for calculating probabilities of distributions in two-by-two tables with small cell frequencies. The chapter also demonstrates the use of the various Excel functions relevant to the chi-square, in particular showing that the =CHITEST() function produces the probability for the chi-square rather than the chi-square value itself. The chapter will include examples and exercises relevant to health services.

Chapter Nine: *t* Tests for Related and Unrelated Data

This chapter discusses the *t* test as a test of independence between a numerical dependent variable and a categorical independent variable that takes on only two values. These values may be, for example, experimental and control, intervention, and nonintervention groups, or they may be characteristics such as sex or membership in some category of service payment (which assumes two levels). The values of the categorical variable may also be measurement before or after some particular intervention, whether specifically planned or naturally occurring. The chapter discusses both equal and unequal variance assumptions when conducting *t* tests and the *F* test to assess this. It demonstrates the use of these various tests as made available by the Excel data analysis add-ins. And it demonstrates the Excel add-in for related (before and after) data. The chapter includes examples and exercises relevant to health services.

Chapter Ten: Analysis of Variance

This chapter discusses analysis of variance as a test of independence between a numerical dependent variable and one or more categorical independent variables that may take on multiple values. The chapter examines one-way and two-way analysis of variance with and without repeated measures. It discusses the *F* test as the statistical test for assessing the results of the analysis of variance and the distribution of *F*. It includes a discussion and demonstration of the use of the analysis of variance add-ins for Excel and shows how each of the results from the add-ins are derived. Included in the chapter are examples and exercises relevant to health services.

Chapter Eleven: Simple Linear Regression

This chapter introduces simple linear regression as a mechanism for examining the null hypothesis of independence between a numerical dependent variable and a numerical independent variable. It discusses the nature of the linear assumption and demonstrates the use of the Excel graphing capability to examine this assumption visually. It presents the calculation of the coefficients of the regression equation as given by the standard simple linear regression formulas and follows with a demonstration of the use of the Excel regression add-in to carry out linear regression. The chapter provides a discussion of the source and calculation of all the statistics provided by the add-in. This includes the R^2, the standard error of the regression line, the sums of squares due to regression and the sums of squares error, the F test for the overall regression, the t test for the coefficients, and the probabilities of these test results. It also includes a discussion of the underlying assumptions of regression, including linearity, equal variance, and independence of observations. And it includes examples of data sets that do not fit the linear regression model. The chapter includes examples and exercises relevant to health services.

Chapter Twelve: Multiple Regression: Concepts and Calculation

This chapter introduces the use of multiple regression as a mechanism for examining the null hypothesis of independence between a numerical dependent variable and multiple numerical independent variables. It demonstrates the logical progression from the minimization of the squared difference between the actual and predicted values of the dependent variable to the simultaneous equations needed to solve for the regression coefficients, although it does not assume knowledge of calculus. It demonstrates the solution of the multiple regression problem, solving the simultaneous equations with both successive elimination and the use of Excel's matrix functions that allow the direct solution of the $(X'X)^{-1}X'y = b$ formula. It shows the use of the multiple regression add-in in multiple regression and demonstrates through calculations the source of all the results in the Excel add-in printout. The chapter includes examples and exercises relevant to health services.

Chapter Thirteen: Extensions of Multiple Regression

This chapter takes up a number of different topics in multiple regression. Curve fitting includes a discussion of the use of data transformations and alternative formulations of the regression equation (such as second-degree curves) to fit nonlinear data. It includes a discussion of dummy variables in regression and the effect of both a dummy and dummy—continuous variable interaction. It shows the use of the graphing capabilities of Excel to visually examine the effect of dummy variables and interaction terms.

Chapter Fourteen: Analysis with a Dichotomous Categorical Dependent Variable

This chapter examines the null hypothesis of no relationship between a categorical dependent variable that takes on two values and one or more independent variables that may be either numerical or categorical. The chapter considers the linear probability model (ordinary least squares applied to a 0, 1 dependent variable), weighted least squares, and Logit. The chapter shows how Excel, and the Excel add-in Solver, can be used to solve the maximum likelihood equations needed to find the Logit solution, and it discusses the meaning of the output of this analysis in comparison with both the linear probability model and weighted least squares. The chapter includes examples and exercises relevant to health services.

References

Levine, D. M., Stephan, D., Krebbiel, T. C., and Berenson, M. L. Statistics for Managers Using Microsoft Excel. (2nd ed.) Upper Saddle River, N.J.: Prentice Hall, 1999.

McDermott, R. E. Using Multiple Regression to Establish Labor Rates. *Healthcare Financial Management,* Sept. 2001, pp. 49–60.

CHAPTER TWO

EXCEL AS A STATISTICAL TOOL

Most people, if they have used Excel at all, have used it as a spreadsheet for financial management, for budget keeping, or for maintaining lists. They have probably not used it as a statistical medium. But Excel has powerful statistical capabilities. This book uses these statistical capabilities for examples and for problem sets. But to ensure that the user will have some facility with Excel from the outset, this chapter provides a basic introduction to most of what Excel will do as a statistical tool. Readers who are already comfortable with the use of Excel might skip Section 2.1 and Section 2.2. However, anyone not currently carrying out statistical applications with Excel is likely to benefit from the material in the later sections of the chapter.

Section 2.1 The Very Basics

Excel is a spreadsheet application. This means that it is made up of columns that are designated by letters (A through IV) and of rows that are designated by numbers (1 through 65,536). There are 256 columns and 65,536 rows in Excel 2000. Figure 2.1 shows an initial Excel spreadsheet window. The intersection of each row and column (for example, column C and row 12, designated C12 in Excel) is a cell in which, generally, one piece of information can be stored, viewed, and manipulated. This means that there are potentially over sixteen million data cells

FIGURE 2.1. INITIAL EXCEL SPREADSHEET.

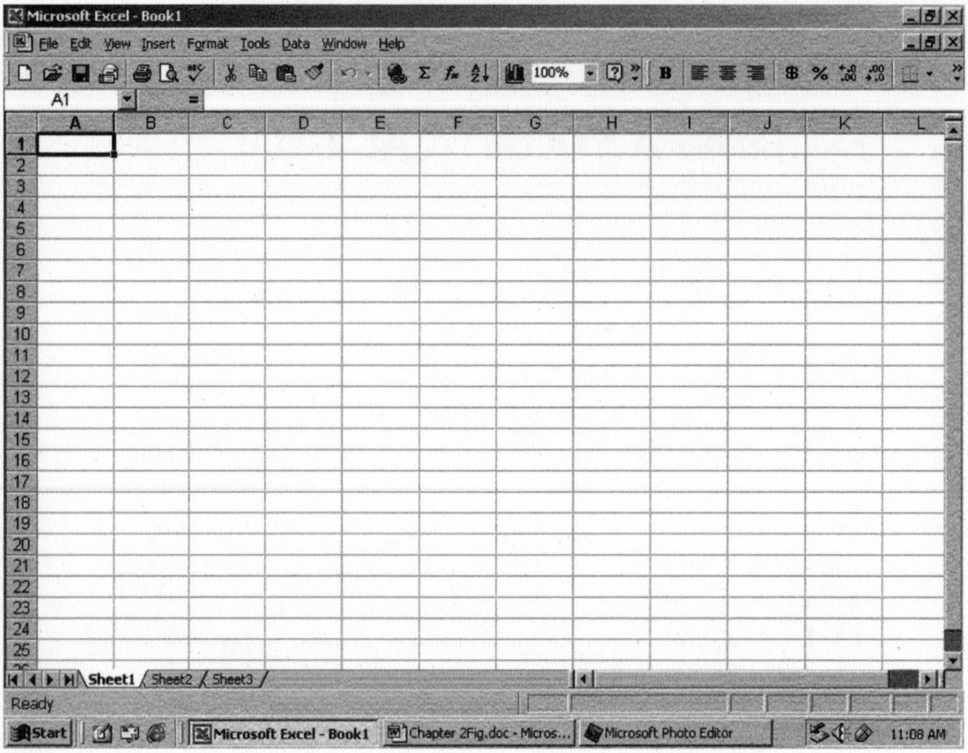

available on a single spreadsheet. In practical terms, though, it is probably not likely that any statistical application will use all the space on a single spreadsheet. In fact, it is not clear that Excel would function in any reasonable amount of time if it had to manipulate data in a completely full spreadsheet. However, in the vast majority of statistical applications using Excel, it is unlikely that more than a small fraction of the spreadsheet, probably less than 5 percent, will actually be used.

Spreadsheets can be put together in what Excel calls workbooks. Any actual application might consist of a workbook of several spreadsheets, one containing an explanation of the application, a second containing the data, and a third or additional sheets containing the statistical analyses conducted using the data. If a large amount of data—say, two or three thousand observations—are subjected to analysis using several spreadsheets, the data file may become quite large. It is possible to develop a data file that may actually exceed the size of a standard high-density floppy disk, making portability from one computer to another something of a problem. Nevertheless, for most statistical applications, this will not be the case.

As shown in Figure 2.1, the Excel spreadsheet includes a menu bar across the top (with the words File, Edit, Insert, Format, and so on) and the two additional menu bars with various icons representing possible actions and operations. The two additional menu bars shown are referred to as the "standard" and the "formatting" menu bars. The standard menu bar contains three icons that are particularly useful to statistical applications. These are the icon Σ, the icon fx, and the chart icon. The Σ icon automatically provides the sum of a set of contiguous numbers. The fx icon calls up an extensive menu of special Excel functions, including statistical and mathematical functions. The chart icon allows the user to create a wide variety of charts from one or a number of data entities.

Excel allows the user to carry out all mathematical operations within cells. In doing this, Excel can refer to other cells for values needed for the arithmetical operations, or actual numbers can be included in cells. Figure 2.2 shows all the important arithmetical operations that will be considered in this book. Row 2 shows the addition of the numbers 5 and 2. As shown in columns D and E, this can be done in two different ways. The addition can be carried out by referencing the cells B2 and C2, in which the values of 5 and 2 are found (cell D2) or it can be carried out by simply putting the numbers 5 and 2 into the addition equation (cell E2). It should also be noted that Excel arithmetical operations must always begin with the equal sign (=) in order for Excel to recognize that an arithmetical operation is to be carried out. Addition and subtraction use the plus sign (+) and minus sign (−), respectively. Multiplication uses the star (∗), which appears above the number eight on most keyboards. Division uses the right leaning slash (/), which is the last key on the right in the bottom row on most keyboards. Raising a number to a power uses the caret (^), which is found above the six on most keyboards (the caret, incidentally, is almost universally called *hat* by statisticians).

FIGURE 2.2. EXCEL ARITHMETICAL CONVENTIONS.

	A	B	C	D	E	F
1						
2	Addition	5	2	=B2+C2	=5+2	7
3	Subtraction	5	2	=B3-C3	=5-2	3
4	Multiplication	5	2	=B4*C4	=5*2	10
5	Division	5	2	=B5/C5	=5/2	2.5
6	Raise to power	5	2	=B6^C6	=5^2	25

Exercises for Section 2.1

1. Carry out the following arithmetical operations in an Excel spreadsheet:
   a. $= 6 + 6$
   b. $= 22 - 16$
   c. $= 11 \times 5$
   d. $= 14/7$
   e. $= 4\wedge3$

2. Enter the following numbers into the indicated cells and carry out the operations given by referencing the cells:
   a. A1, 11; B1, 13: add
   b. A2, 16; B2, 5: subtract B2 from A2
   c. A3, 21; B3, 15: multiply
   d. A4, 36; B4, 4: divide
   e. A5, 16; B5, 2: raise A5 to the power in B5

Section 2.2 Working in and Moving Around in an Excel Spreadsheet

One difficulty faced by most novice users of Excel is not knowing how to move around in a spreadsheet and select specific cell references for operations. A second difficulty most new Excel users face is not knowing how to let Excel do the work. This includes allowing Excel to correct mistakes, allowing Excel to enter formulas in multiple cells, and knowing the easy ways to move data around in an Excel spreadsheet. There is absolutely no substitute for actual hands-on experience in learning what the capabilities of Excel are, but some initial hints should be helpful.

Consider the spreadsheet shown in Figure 2.3. That figure might show a small data set of fifteen records for people who had used the services—for example, of an ambulatory clinic. The variables shown are a separate ID or identifier, age of the patient, number of visits to the clinic, total cost of all clinic visits, and average cost per visit. The figure also shows three different types of moves that can be easily made within a data set using Excel. Assuming a starting point at cell A2, holding down Ctrl and Shift, and pressing the right arrow highlights the entire row 2 to the first blank column. This also works with Ctrl/Shift/down arrow, left arrow, or up arrow. Again, assuming a starting point in cell A2, holding down Ctrl alone, and pressing the down arrow moves the cursor from cell A2 to the last cell in column A that contains data, cell A16. This also works with Ctrl/right arrow, left arrow, and up arrow. The final move shown in Figure 2.3 is the move

FIGURE 2.3. MOVING AROUND A DATA SET.

	A	B	C	D	E	F
1	ID	Age	Visits	Total Cost	Cost/Visit	
2	1	30	1	$ 59.77	$ 59.77	
3	2	69	3	$ 323.02	$ 107.67	
4	3	73	1	$ 92.82	$ 92.82	
5	4	22	5	$ 589.40	$ 117.88	
6	5	15	4	$ 530.60	$ 132.65	
7	6	29	2	$ 170.31	$ 85.16	
8	7	50	3	$ 386.58	$ 128.86	
9	8	47	1	$ 117.03	$ 117.03	
10	9	17	8	$1,078.59	$ 134.82	
11	10	63	2	$ 143.70	$ 71.85	
12	11	48	2	$ 77.92	$ 38.96	
13	12	70	6	$ 175.55	$ 29.26	
14	13	8	1	$ 135.68	$ 135.68	
15	14	38	8	$ 213.42	$ 26.68	
16	15	41	5	$ 637.49	$ 127.50	
17						
18						

that highlights both the current cell and the one next to it. Holding down Shift and pressing the down arrow will highlight both the initial cell (A2) and A3. This, too, works with Shift/left arrow, Shift/right arrow, and Shift/up arrow. These operations can also be combined in virtually any order, so, for example, from a starting point of cell A2, Ctrl/Shift/right arrow followed by Shift/down arrow/down arrow would highlight cells A2 to E4. Or, as a further example, from a starting point in cell A2, Ctrl/Shift/right arrow followed by Ctrl/Shift/down arrow would highlight cells A2 to E16.

Any contiguous group of cells can be highlighted in Excel by left-clicking in any corner cell of the area to be highlighted and dragging the cursor to all the cells that are to be highlighted. Two short cuts can be used when highlighting cells to make this task much easier. The first of these is Cntl/Shft/Arrow. Cntl/Shft/Arrow (right arrow, left arrow, down arrow, up arrow) will highlight every cell from the selected cell to the last contiguous cell containing data. For example, Figure 2.4 shows the result of the use of Cntl/Shift/right arrow when the cursor starts in cell A5. At this point, it is possible to highlight cells A5 to E16 with the use of Cntl/Shift/down arrow. The value of this capability is, perhaps, not evident when the data set consists of only sixteen rows and five columns. But when the data comprises, for example, 357 rows and forty-two columns, it is much easier to use Cntl/Shift/arrow to highlight all of a row or of a column than to drag the highlight with the cursor.

FIGURE 2.4. RESULT OF CNTL/SHIFT/RIGHT ARROW.

	A	B	C	D	E	F
1	ID	Age	Visits	Total Cost	Cost/Visit	
2	1	30	1	$ 59.77	$ 59.77	
3	2	69	3	$ 323.02	$ 107.67	
4	3	73	1	$ 92.82	$ 92.82	
5	4	22	5	$ 589.40	$ 117.88	
6	5	15	4	$ 530.60	$ 132.65	
7	6	29	2	$ 170.31	$ 85.16	
8	7	50	3	$ 386.58	$ 128.86	
9	8	47	1	$ 117.03	$ 117.03	
10	9	17	8	$1,078.59	$ 134.82	
11	10	63	2	$ 143.70	$ 71.85	
12	11	48	2	$ 77.92	$ 38.96	
13	12	70	6	$ 175.55	$ 29.26	
14	13	8	1	$ 135.68	$ 135.68	
15	14	38	8	$ 213.42	$ 26.68	
16	15	41	5	$ 637.49	$ 127.50	
17						

The second shortcut that is useful in highlighting is the ability to highlight an entire row (256 cells) or an entire column (65,536 cells). Clicking either on the letter that represents the column or the number that represents the row can highlight an entire row or an entire column. For example, Figure 2.5 shows the first eighteen rows for column B. Clicking the B at the head of the column has highlighted the entire column, from cell 1 to cell 65,536. It is also useful to know that the entire worksheet can be highlighted at one time by clicking in the empty cell at the top of the row-number column (or to the left of the column-letter column).

Another important capability of Excel is its ability to copy one cell to a range of other cells. For example, Figure 2.6 shows the data in Figure 2.3, but before the E column was completely filled in. While the actual spreadsheet from which both Figure 2.3 and Figure 2.6 were taken has numbers in columns A through D (entered by hand), cell E2 represents a simple formula (shown in the formula line above the spread sheet of Figure 2.6) that simply divides cell D2 (Total Cost) by cell C2 (Visits). The result is the average cost per visit. Rather than typing the same formula in each cell from E3 to E15, or even copying and pasting the formula in each cell, it is possible either to drag or to double-click the formula in E2 to all the cells E3 to E15. To do either, it is necessary to put the cursor on the lower right-hand corner of the cell E2, as shown in Figure 2.6. When this is done, the cursor will turn into a small black cross. With the cursor as a small black cross, physically dragging with the mouse will copy the formula to each successive cell

FIGURE 2.5. HIGHLIGHTING AN ENTIRE COLUMN.

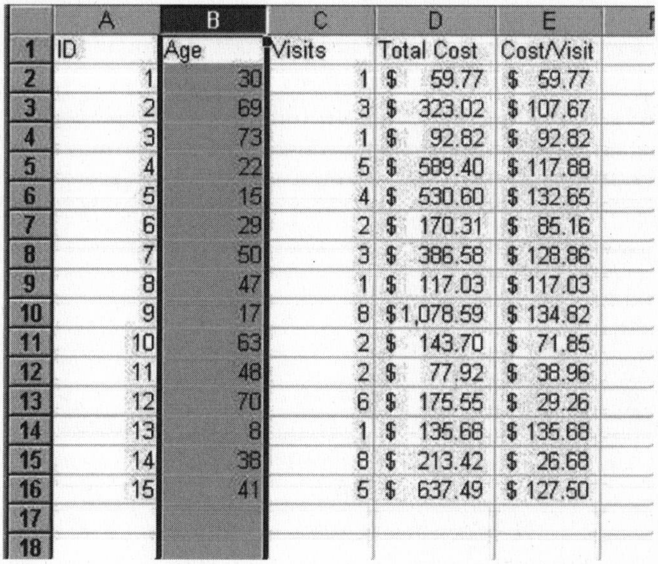

	A	B	C	D	E	
1	ID	Age	Visits	Total Cost	Cost/Visit	
2	1	30	1	$ 59.77	$ 59.77	
3	2	69	3	$ 323.02	$ 107.67	
4	3	73	1	$ 92.82	$ 92.82	
5	4	22	5	$ 589.40	$ 117.88	
6	5	15	4	$ 530.60	$ 132.65	
7	6	29	2	$ 170.31	$ 85.16	
8	7	50	3	$ 386.58	$ 128.86	
9	8	47	1	$ 117.03	$ 117.03	
10	9	17	8	$1,078.59	$ 134.82	
11	10	63	2	$ 143.70	$ 71.85	
12	11	48	2	$ 77.92	$ 38.96	
13	12	70	6	$ 175.55	$ 29.26	
14	13	8	1	$ 135.68	$ 135.68	
15	14	38	8	$ 213.42	$ 26.68	
16	15	41	5	$ 637.49	$ 127.50	
17						
18						

FIGURE 2.6. COPYING A FORMULA TO SEVERAL CELLS.

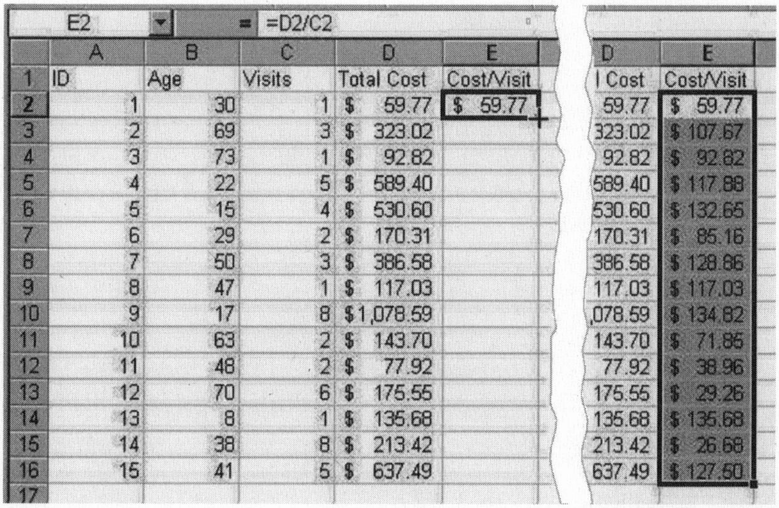

E2			=	=D2/C2				D	E
	A	B	C	D	E			l Cost	Cost/Visit
1	ID	Age	Visits	Total Cost	Cost/Visit				
2	1	30	1	$ 59.77	$ 59.77			59.77	$ 59.77
3	2	69	3	$ 323.02				323.02	$ 107.67
4	3	73	1	$ 92.82				92.82	$ 92.82
5	4	22	5	$ 589.40				589.40	$ 117.88
6	5	15	4	$ 530.60				530.60	$ 132.65
7	6	29	2	$ 170.31				170.31	$ 85.16
8	7	50	3	$ 386.58				386.58	$ 128.86
9	8	47	1	$ 117.03				117.03	$ 117.03
10	9	17	8	$1,078.59				,078.59	$ 134.82
11	10	63	2	$ 143.70				143.70	$ 71.85
12	11	48	2	$ 77.92				77.92	$ 38.96
13	12	70	6	$ 175.55				175.55	$ 29.26
14	13	8	1	$ 135.68				135.68	$ 135.68
15	14	38	8	$ 213.42				213.42	$ 26.68
16	15	41	5	$ 637.49				637.49	$ 127.50
17									

down the E column. Or, still with the cursor as a small black cross, double-left-clicking the mouse will fill the entire E column to the last occupied cell in the D column.

The double-left-click on the lower left corner can be used to copy a formula down a column as far as the last filled cell in a column on either the right or the left of the column to be filled. But if there is a blank cell on the left of a column, even with a filled column on the right, it is necessary to drag the formula to the end of the data set, because the double-click will go only to the first empty cell on the left. Also, if you wish to copy a formula or other data across columns, or up columns, this can only be done with the drag on the lower left corner of the master cell.

Moving data around in Excel is made easy with the drag and drop. A highlighted area (as shown as cells A1:A15 in Figure 2.7) can be moved anywhere in the spreadsheet simply by placing the cursor on the highlight outline and pulling it to the spot where it is to be placed. This process is illustrated in Figure 2.7 as the highlighted area, cells A1:A15 is moved with the drag and drop to cells G1:G15. When the drag and drop is completed, the data will no longer be in cells A1:A15. If a drag and drop is executed, any formulas that either referenced or were referenced by the data when the data was in column B will now reference the data correctly in column G.

FIGURE 2.7. DRAG AND DROP TO MOVE A DATA RANGE.

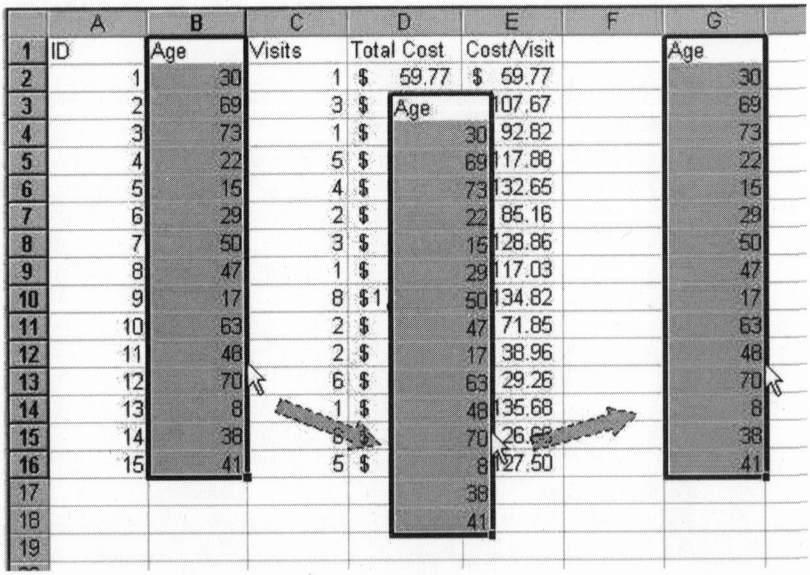

FIGURE 2.8. EXCEL UNDO BUTTON.

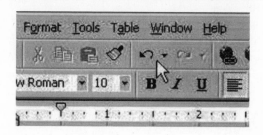

A very useful tool in Excel is the undo button. Suppose there is a large Excel spreadsheet in which a great amount of data has been entered and, perhaps, a number of complex operations have been carried out. Just as you are about to save the entire spreadsheet, you somehow inadvertently erase the whole thing. Is it the appropriate time to slit your wrists? No. You can recover the spreadsheet exactly by going to the Standard toolbar, where you will find an arrow that circles counterclockwise. This arrow is shown in Figure 2.8. Clicking on this arrow allows you to back up through a series of up to sixteen operations. So if you inadvertently cleared an entire data sheet, you could just click on the counterclockwise arrow and the spreadsheet would be reconstituted.

Exercises for Section 2.2

1. Enter the identifiers for each column and the data for columns A through D, as shown in Figure 2.3 (or use the data in the file Chpt 2–1.xls) and do the following:
   a. Start in cell A2 and depress Ctrl/Shift/down arrow.
   b. Start in D3 and depress Ctrl/Shift/left arrow.
   c. Start in C1 and depress Ctrl/down arrow.
   d. Start in A1 and depress Shift/right arrow.
   e. Start in A1 and depress Shift/right arrow, followed by Ctrl/Shift/down arrow.
   f. Left-click the A column head; the 2 row head.

2. Using the data from Exercise 1 of Section 2.2, do the following:
   a. Type the label Cost/Visit in cell E1. Type the formula =D2/C2 in cell E2 and hit return.
   b. Put the cursor in the lower right-hand corner of the cell E2 (the cursor will become a black cross) and double-left-click the mouse.

   c. Confirm that the resulting data are the same as given in column E of Figure 2.3.

   d. Highlight column E by left clicking the E above the column, and with the cursor on the edge of the highlighted area, drag it to column G.

   e. Confirm that the formulas in the cells still refer to columns D and C.

   f. Left-click the undo arrow in the Standard toolbar.

Section 2.3 Excel Functions

Left-clicking the *fx* icon calls up the Paste Function window. The Paste Function window is shown in Figure 2.9. On the left side of this window there are ten different function categories, and on the right are the different functions available in each function category. When a function is selected, the bottom of the window shows the name of the selected function and a brief description of what it does. To use a particular function, select it and left-click the OK button. Excel will then lead you through a short sequence of steps that designate the cells in which the numbers are found for the calculation for the selected function. As an example, the =AVERAGE() function will produce the average value for a series of numbers contained in several Excel cells.

To look at the working of the =AVERAGE() function, suppose the Excel spreadsheet contains a column of five numbers in cells B4 through B8 and you

FIGURE 2.9. PASTE FUNCTION WINDOW.

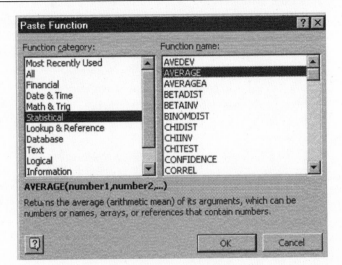

FIGURE 2.10. AVERAGE CALCULATION WINDOW.

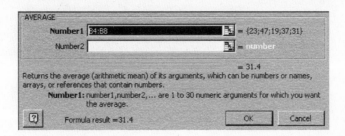

wish to calculate the average of those five numbers in cell B9. When you click the OK button, as shown in Figure 2.9, the =AVERAGE() function window, shown as Figure 2.10, will come up. Several things about the =AVERAGE() function window are worth discussing. First, the highlighted area designated Number 1 shows the five cells—B4 to B8—that are being averaged. These cells are shown by using the standard Excel convention for designating a set of contiguous cells, which is to display them as B4:B8. Directly to the right of the cells being averaged is an equal sign and the actual numbers that are in the cells. If there had been, for example, twenty cells being averaged, the window would have displayed only the first few. The area marked Number 2 can be ignored in this calculation, and, in general, it can be ignored in function windows. Below the areas designated Number 1 and Number 2 is some additional information. The number 31.4 is the actual value of the average that will be put into cell B9 when the calculation is completed. If no number appears there, it means that Excel does not have the information needed from you, the user, to calculate a result. Below the result is a brief statement of what the function actually does. Clicking the OK button will put the result of the formula into the selected cell (in this case B9).

Figure 2.11 shows a portion of the spreadsheet in which the average function has been employed. The representation is a record of total clinic visits for a single outpatient clinic for a five-day period. The purpose is to determine the average number of persons coming to the clinic over these five days. In cell B9 is shown the actual function being calculated by Excel. When OK is clicked in Figure 2.10, the function statement will be replaced by the value 31.4. In addition to the average function being shown in cell B9, it is also shown in the line just above the spreadsheet area. This area is known as the formula line or formula bar. In general, if you wish to know if a value in a particular cell is a number or a formula, clicking on the cell of interest will reveal which one it is in the formula line, and if it is a formula, it will give the formula for the cell in terms of cell references, as shown in Figure 2.11.

FIGURE 2.11. CALCULATION OF AVERAGE.

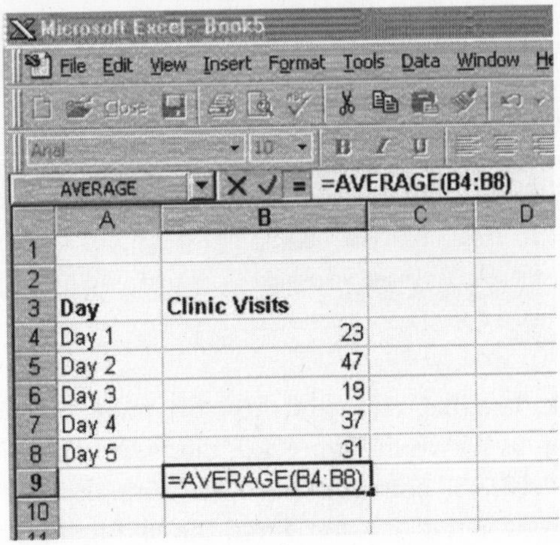

It should be noted that the numbers that are actually being averaged in cell B9 in Figure 2.11 are shown as cell references within the parentheses following the name of the function. This indication of cell references is called an *argument* of the function. The =AVERAGE() function takes only one argument, the reference to the cells in which the data to be averaged are found. Other Excel functions may take more than one argument, and some functions—for example, =RAND(), which returns a random number between 0 and 1, and =PI(), which returns the value of pi to fourteen decimal positions—take none. If a function takes more than one argument, commas are used to separate the arguments when they are given within the parentheses.

There are eighty separate statistical functions built into Excel, most of which you will never use. Excel also has several mathematical and trigonometric functions that are useful in doing statistical analyses. It may be useful to look at the various Excel statistical and math and trig functions (click on *fx* and scroll through the functions on the right side of the Paste Function window) as a means of getting an initial notion of what the functions do. It is likely right now that most of them will be obscure, but as you work through this book you will become increasingly familiar with many of the functions.

Functions can be invoked in Excel without using the *fx* icon. If you know the correct spelling of the function name, you can type the function directly into the cell in which it is to be applied. For example, to enter the =AVERAGE function directly into an Excel spreadsheet, it is necessary to begin with an equal sign (=). This informs Excel that you are going to enter a formula, and it is why functions are referred to throughout this text by the inclusion of the = sign. *(The same convention holds if you want to carry out any mathematical operation, such as adding the numbers in two cells together; the addition command must begin with an equal sign for Excel to recognize the input as a mathematical formula.)* The equal sign is followed immediately (no spaces) by typing AVERAGE (it does not have to be in caps), which is followed by a left parenthesis. At this point, you can directly type the cell references in which the numbers to be averaged are found, or you can highlight the cells with the cursor. A right parenthesis completes the formula, and pressing return calculates the result of the formula, which appears in the selected cell. If the function name is misspelled, Excel will let you know by showing #NAME? in the cell where the function was to be calculated.

In general, any of the Excel functions will operate on any contiguous set of cells. For a number of Excel functions, such as the average function already discussed, the sum function (activated by the Σ icon on the standard menu bar), and a number of others, the numbers do not have to be in contiguous cells. However, if noncontiguous cells are to be the subject of the operation, it is necessary to use the Excel convention of depressing the Ctrl key before highlighting any second or subsequent set of noncontiguous cells that are part of the operation. For example, if the spreadsheet were as shown in Figure 2.12, the two columns B and D, representing the clinic visits for the five days of two different weeks, could be summed with the =SUM() command, as shown in the equation line. Entering the actual cell references directly into the cell from the keyboard, rather than highlighting the areas with the help of the Ctrl key, will also produce this result. If the cell references were entered from the keyboard, a comma would be used to separate the two different sets of cell references.

FIGURE 2.12. SUMMING TWO NONCONTIGUOUS AREAS.

AVERAGE	X ✓ =	=SUM(D4:D8,B4:B8)	
	A	B	C	D
1				
2		Week 1		Week 2
3	Day	Clinic Visits	Day	Clinic Visits
4	Day 1	23	Day 1	23
5	Day 2	47	Day 2	32
6	Day 3	19	Day 3	39
7	Day 4	37	Day 4	16
8	Day 5	31	Day 5	25
9				:D8,B4:B8)
10				

Exercises for Section 2.3

1. A well-baby clinic recorded the weight for the infants receiving services during one workday. The weight of the infants is given below in lbs. Enter the data into an Excel spreadsheet (or take it from the file Chpt 2–2.xls, worksheet Infants) and do the following:

10.7	18.2	17.8	16.0	17.8	15.9	21.5
17.1	20.6	18.8	15.4	20.8	19.8	18.3
17.2	15.8	10.8	19.6	17.9	17.8	14.5

   a. Use the Excel =COUNT() function to confirm that there are twenty-one infants.
   b. Use the Excel Σ function to obtain the total weight of all infants coming to the clinic on the given day.
   c. Use the Excel =AVERAGE() function to determine the average weight of infants coming to the clinic.
   d. Use the Excel =MAX() function to determine the weight of the heaviest child coming to the clinic on the given day.
   e. Use the Excel =MIN() function to determine the weight of the lightest child coming to the clinic on the given day.

2. Over the course of several days, the number of inpatients in Mercy Hospital was recorded in the accounting office. The inpatient totals for those days are given below. Enter the data into an Excel spreadsheet (or use Chpt 2–2.xls, Worksheet Days) and do the following:

89	92	93	93	92	100	97
100	102	95	91	103		

   a. Use the Excel =COUNT() function to confirm that there are records for twelve days.
   b. Use the Excel Σ function to obtain the cumulative total of inpatient days represented by the data.
   c. Use the Excel =AVERAGE() function to determine the average inpatient census for the twelve days.
   d. Use the Excel =MAX() function to determine the highest inpatient census for the twelve days.
   e. Use the Excel =MIN() function to determine the lowest inpatient census for the twelve days.

3. A dentist kept track of the time he spent with each patient in a single morning of visits. The total time in minutes that he spent with each is given below. Enter the data into an Excel spreadsheet (or use the file Chpt 2–2.xls, worksheet Time and do the following:

9	18	9	13	11	5	7
13	15	10	10	18	13	16
9	14	5				

   a. Use the Excel =COUNT() function to confirm that there are records for seventeen patients.
   b. Use the Excel Σ function to obtain the cumulative total of minutes he spent with patients during this morning.
   c. Use the Excel =AVERAGE() function to determine the average time in minutes he spent with each patient.
   d. Use the Excel =MAX() function to determine the most time he spent with a patient.
   e. Use the Excel =MIN() function to determine the least time he spent with a patient.

Section 2.4 The =IF() Function

The =IF() function is a particularly useful Excel function that provides a way to make decisions within an Excel spreadsheet. The =IF() function tests a condition and produces one result if the condition is true and a different result if the condition is false. For example, suppose that we have the data as shown in Figure 2.13, where we have twelve patients identified by the numbers 1 through 12 in column A and the minutes they spend waiting in the emergency room identified in column B. In column C, we want to assign a 1 or a 0, depending on whether each patient spent more or less than the average time patients spend in the waiting room. Excel allows us to do this with the =IF() function. Column C in Figure 2.13 already has the values of 1 or 0 assigned, using the =IF() function.

The way the function is written is shown, for cell C2, in the formula line in the figure. As can be seen there, the =IF() function is written with three arguments. The first of the arguments is the decision. In this case, Excel is asked to decide whether the value in B2 is greater than (>) the value in $B$15 (the average for all twelve values in column B). The $ convention is used for cell B15 because we want to compare each of the twelve values in column B to the same value, the average for all twelve, which is found only in B15 (see Section 2.9). The

FIGURE 2.13. =IF( ) FUNCTION.

	C2	▼	=	=IF(B2>$B$15,1,0)	
	A	B	C	D	E
1	Patient	Minutes (x)			
2	1	2	0		
3	2	8	0		
4	3	11	1		
5	4	12	1		
6	5	6	0		
7	6	10	1		
8	7	7	0		
9	8	8	0		
10	9	14	1		
11	10	8	0		
12	11	7	0		
13	12	14	1		
14					
15	Mean(x)	8.92			

second argument, always separated from the first by a comma, is a 1, and the third argument, again separated by a comma, is a 0. The =IF( ) function operates by evaluating the relationship in the first argument. If that relationship is true, it assigns the value of the second argument to the cell in which the function is invoked. If it is false, the =IF( ) function assigns the value of the third argument to the cell in which the function is invoked. The way the function works can be stated as follows: if the value in cell B2 is greater than the value in cell B15, put a 1 in cell C2; otherwise, put a 0 in cell C2. This same function is copied to all cells C2 through C13 and automatically produces the desired decision.

In the example in Figure 2.13, the =IF( ) function is used to make only a single decision. Nested =IF( ) functions can be used to make more complex decisions. For example, instead of assigning a 1 or a 0, depending on whether the waiting time was above or below the average, suppose we wished to determine whether the waiting time was short, long, or medium. For the sake of the example, let us say that a short waiting time is anything under five minutes and a long waiting time is anything more than ten minutes. That would leave any waiting time from five to ten minutes as medium.

Figure 2.14 shows one =IF( ) function nested within another so that the computer can simultaneously make both decisions. What the decision statement (shown in the formula line for cell C2) does, is the following: if B2 is greater than 10 (shown now as the actual value of 10, and not as a cell reference), the =IF( ) function assigns the word "Long" to the cell C2. If B2 is not greater than 10, a

FIGURE 2.14. NESTED =IF( ) FUNCTIONS.

	C2	▼	**=** =IF(B2>10,"Long",IF(B2<5,"Short","Medium"))			
	A	B	C	D	E	F	G
1	Patient	Minutes (x)					
2	1	2	Short				
3	2	8	Medium				
4	3	11	Long				
5	4	12	Long				
6	5	6	Medium				
7	6	10	Medium				
8	7	7	Medium				
9	8	8	Medium				
10	9	14	Long				
11	10	8	Medium				
12	11	7	Medium				
13	12	14	Long				
14							

second =IF( ) function is assessed by Excel. This second =IF( ) function asks if B2 is less than 5, and if so, it assigns the word "Short" to the cell C2 (which is what it actually assigned). If B2 is not less than 5, the =IF statement assigns the word "Medium" to cell C2. Excel will operate on up to sixteen nested =IF( ) statements, but it is hard to imagine why anyone would want so many. It is also useful to mention that the exact way in which the nested =IF( ) function is developed in Figure 2.14 is not the only possible way such a function could be developed to assign the appropriate term to each waiting time. An alternative nested =IF( ) function as; =IF(B2>5, IF(B2>10, "Long," "Medium"), "Short") will produce exactly the same result as produced by the statement actually used in the figure.

Figure 2.14 also shows one additional important point: it is possible to produce a number as the result of a decision or it is possible to produce an alphabetic character (or, for that matter, any printable character). But if the result to be produced is not a number, it must be contained in quotation marks in order for the function to work. The function =IF(B2>10, Long, IF(B2<5, Short, Medium)) would result in an Excel error message, which in this case would be to put the message #NAME! in the cell in which the function was invoked.

Exercises for Section 2.4

1. Use the data from Exercise 1 of Section 2.3 and do the following:
   a. Create an =IF( ) statement that determines whether the infant is greater or less in weight than the overall average and assign a 1 to those greater and a 0 to those less.

b. Create an =IF() statement that determines whether the infant is less than fifteen lbs., greater than twenty lbs., or between the two extremes and assign a "low" to the lightest group, a "high" to the heaviest group, and a "medium" to the middle group.

c. Create an =IF() statement that determines whether the infant is the lowest weight or the highest weight in the group and assign a 1 to the lowest and highest and a 0 to all others.

d. Create an =IF() statement that divides the infants into four-lb. age groups (beginning at 10 lbs.) and assign a 1 to the lowest group, a 2 to the second, and so on.

2. Use the data from Exercise 2 of Section 2.3 and do the following:

a. Create an =IF() statement that determines whether the day has more or fewer inpatients than the overall average and assign a 1 to days with more and a 0 to days with fewer.

b. Create an =IF() statement that determines whether the day has fewer than ninety inpatients or more than a hundred inpatients, or is between the two extremes, and assign a "low" to the days with fewest patients, a "high" to the days with most patients, and a "medium" to the middle group of days.

c. Create an =IF() statement that determines whether the day had the fewest inpatients or the most and assign a 1 to the lowest and highest and a 0 to all others.

d. Create an =IF() statement that divides the days into four patient groups (beginning at 88 patients.) and assign a 1 to the lowest group, a 2 to the second, and so on.

3. Use the data from Exercise 3 of Section 2.3 and do the following:

a. Create an =IF() statement that determines whether the dentist spent more or less time with a patient than the overall average and assign a 1 to patients with whom the dentist spent more time and a 0 to patients with whom the dentist spent less.

b. Create an =IF() statement that determines whether the dentist spent less than nine minutes or more than fifteen minutes with a patient, or was between the two extremes and assign a "low" to the patients with whom the dentist spent the least time, a "high" to patients with whom the dentist spent the most time, and a "medium" to the middle group of patients.

c. Create an =IF() statement that determines whether a patient had the fewest minutes of the dentist's time or the most and assign a 1 to the patients with the fewest and most minutes and 0 to all others.

    d. Create an =IF() statement that divides the patient into three-minute groups (beginning at five minutes) and assign a 1 to the lowest group, a 2 to the second, and so on.

Section 2.5 Excel Graphs

The Excel graph function is exceedingly valuable for an understanding of how data actually look. This can be useful to gain a better understanding of the data, or for helping to assure that the data conform to the assumptions of particular statistical operations. The graph function is invoked with the Chart Wizard icon on the standard menu bar (it looks like a little column chart), or it can be invoked by using Insert/Chart. Either option produces the same result.

    Figure 2.15 shows the first window of the Chart Wizard, whether invoked through the Chart Wizard Icon or through Insert/Chart. Several things might be noted in regard to this first window. For example, there are eleven types of

FIGURE 2.15. CHART WIZARD, SCREEN 1.

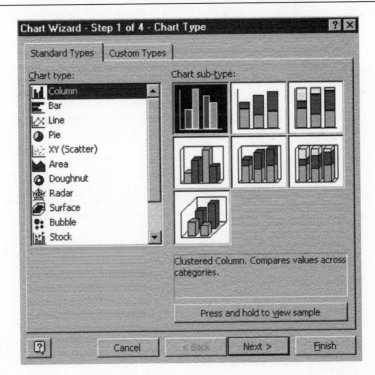

standard charts (shown on the left side of the window). Each of these eleven standard types can be represented by several different chart subtypes within the standard types, these being shown on the right side of the window. Highlighting the chart type of interest on the left shows the subtype of charts that can be produced within that chart type option. The window also contains two tabs. The initial window comes up on the Standard charts, but it is also possible to select from among twenty custom types by left-clicking the Custom tab. When the appropriate chart type has been selected, you can continue by choosing the Next> button or finish the chart directly by choosing the Finish button. It is also possible to terminate the entire operation with the Cancel button.

If the Next button is selected, the second sheet of the Chart Wizard is as shown in Figure 2.16. Figure 2.16 also shows several things. The most important part of the second screen is the place to identify the data to be shown in the chart. The data making up this chart are the same data that were used to find the average

FIGURE 2.16. CHART WIZARD, SCREEN 2.

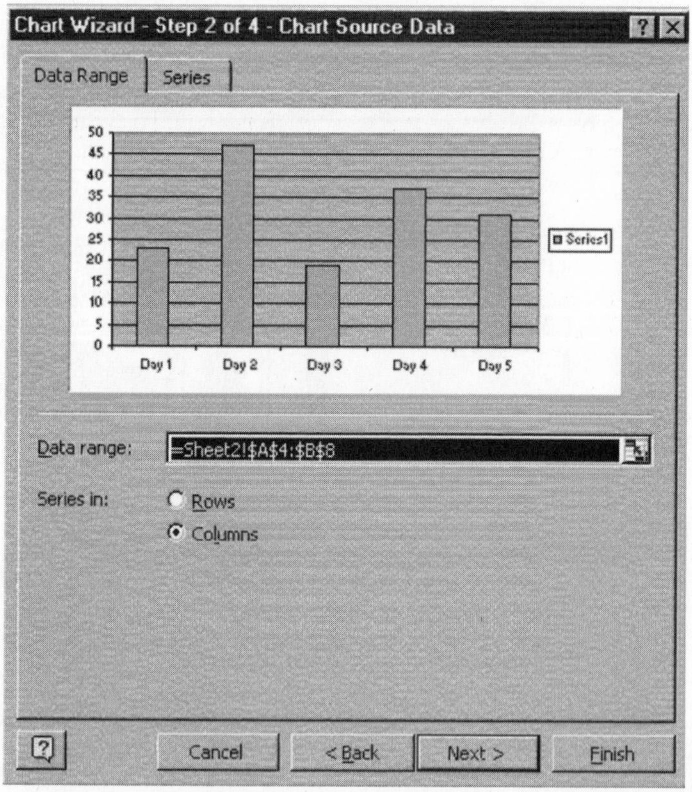

in Figure 2.11. It is interesting to note the way in which it is identified in the second window of the Chart Wizard. The identification of the data is given as =Sheet2!\$B\$4:\$B\$8. There are a couple points to make with regard to this designation when used by Excel to identify specific cells. First, the Sheet2! identifies the data in the table as coming from sheet number 2 of the Excel Workbook. This is useful because not only is it possible to use data from a sheet different from the one that may be active at the time the Chart Wizard is invoked, but it is also possible to use data from more than a single worksheet. The second point of importance relates to the dollar signs that appear before both the alphabetic column references and the numerical row references. The dollar sign convention, with regard to cell references, is discussed in detail in Section 2.9.

A second point to note with regard to the second window in the Chart Wizard is that it shows a preview of what the finished chart will look like once the data have been specified. If the chart does not look like you expect it to or does not show what you expect it to show, it is possible to choose the button labeled <Back to return to the previous window so that you may select a different chart type. The preview of the chart is based on the information that is given in the data range. There are three ways to specify the data range. One is to highlight the data to be included in the chart before invoking the Chart Wizard. A second is to highlight the data once the second window has been selected and the Data range area has been selected. The third is to type the cell references directly into the data range area.

The second window also shows two tabs, one labeled Data Range and the other labeled Series. The important thing to know about the series tab is that this window provides an opportunity to specify the data that will serve as the labels for the X axis. The labels, Day 1, Day 2, and so on in Figure 2.16 were put in by specifying the range A4:A8 (from Figure 2.12) as the X axis series. Had this not been done, the X axis values would have simply read 1, 2, 3, and so on.

The third window in the Chart Wizard is shown as Figure 2.17. The third window provides the opportunity to format the finished chart in a number of different ways, including adding an overall chart title and names for the axes. It also provides tabs to other windows that allow modifications of the axes, gridlines, the legend (the box with Series in it on the right of the chart), data labels, and data tables (the possibility of showing the actual data values on the graph). Again, if you are not happy with the way the graph looks, it is possible to go back to earlier screens to change the chart configuration. Window four of the Chart Wizard provides you with the option of putting the graph in the spreadsheet that contains the data from which it is derived or on a separate graph sheet. If you prefer to have the graph on the spreadsheet with the data, it is possible to go directly to Finish from sheet three (or if you do not wish to put labels on the graph, it is possible to go to Finish from sheet two).

FIGURE 2.17. CHART WIZARD, SCREEN 3.

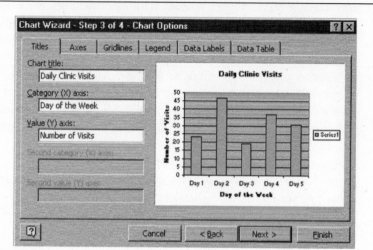

What has been discussed so far with respect to graphs is only an opening statement. A number of exercises in the book will employ the Excel graph capability, and further detail on the use of graphs will be given as specific uses of the graph capability are introduced. Some introductory exercises in creating graphs are given in the following.

Exercises for Section 2.5

1. At the well-baby clinic referred to in Exercise 1 of Section 2.3, a clerk tallied the number of infants who received care for the day into four weight categories. The weight categories and the number of infants in each is given below. Enter the data into an Excel spreadsheet and do the following:

Weight (lbs.)	Number
<=12	2
>12<16	5
>16<20	11
>20<24	3

a. Use the Excel Chart Wizard to construct a histogram (bar chart with vertical bars) of the number of infants in each weight category.

b. Insert the weight categories as labels for the X axis.

c. Use screen 3 of the Chart Wizard to give the chart an appropriate title.

d. Use screen 4 of the Chart Wizard to designate that the chart should go on a new worksheet.

2. The Mercy Hospital accounting office has produced the following average daily inpatient census data for each day of the week for a one-year period. Enter the data into an Excel spreadsheet and do the following:

Day of Week	Inpatient Average
Monday	98.6
Tuesday	107.5
Wednesday	102.2
Thursday	96.4
Friday	90.7
Saturday	89.1
Sunday	93.4

a. Use the Excel Chart Wizard to construct a histogram (bar chart with vertical bars) of the average inpatient census for each day of the week
b. Insert the days as labels for the X axis
c. Use screen 3 of the Chart Wizard to give the chart an appropriate title
d. Use screen 4 of the Chart Wizard to designate that the chart should go on a new worksheet
e. Does the chart suggest any kind of pattern in inpatient census for Mercy Hospital?

3. A dentist kept track of the time he spent with each patient over the course of six months, according to the major purpose of the visit. Below is recorded the average time of the visit by purpose. Enter the data into an Excel spreadsheet and do the following:

Purpose	Time
Orthodontic	25.2
Gum Related Problems	14.5
Filling/Crown	12.2
Extraction	10.1
Routine Check-up	4.3

a. Use the Excel Chart Wizard to construct a histogram (bar chart with vertical bars) of the time spent by the dentist with each type of visit
b. Insert the purpose of the visit as labels for the X axis
c. Use screen 3 of the Chart Wizard to give the chart an appropriate title
d. Use screen 4 of the Chart Wizard to designate that the chart should go on a new worksheet
e. What does the chart say about the dentist's time distribution?

Section 2.6 Sorting a String of Data

A very useful Excel capability, especially with regard to sample selection (discussed in detail in Chapter Three) is the ability to sort a data set. Figure 2.18 shows the first step in a data sort using the small data set introduced in Figure 2.3 with the edition of a column representing sex (column C). The entire data set is going to be sorted on two variables, Sex and Age. The first step is to choose Data/Sort, as shown in Figure 2.18. It might also be noted that the cursor has been positioned in cell C2. It doesn't matter what cell in the data set the cursor is positioned in, but it is important to have it inside the boundaries of the contiguous data set that is to be sorted.

On choosing Sort, two things happen, as is shown in Figure 2.19. The entire data set to be sorted is highlighted, and the Sort window appears. Since the cursor had been in the Sex column when Data/Sort was selected, the Sort window automatically opens with Sex indicated as the Sort by variable. That is what we desired. Also, it is possible to see that the sort can be done in ascending or descending order. We will leave the default, which is ascending. Finally, since we want to sort by both Sex and Age, we need to include Age as the Then by

FIGURE 2.18. FIRST STEP IN DATA SORT.

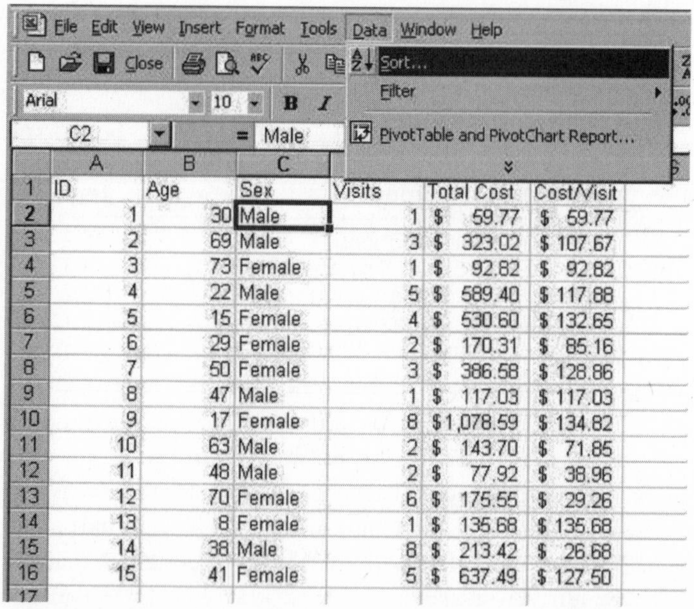

	A	B	C	D	E	F
1	ID	Age	Sex	Visits	Total Cost	Cost/Visit
2	1	30	Male	1	$ 59.77	$ 59.77
3	2	69	Male	3	$ 323.02	$ 107.67
4	3	73	Female	1	$ 92.82	$ 92.82
5	4	22	Male	5	$ 589.40	$ 117.88
6	5	15	Female	4	$ 530.60	$ 132.65
7	6	29	Female	2	$ 170.31	$ 85.16
8	7	50	Female	3	$ 386.58	$ 128.86
9	8	47	Male	1	$ 117.03	$ 117.03
10	9	17	Female	8	$1,078.59	$ 134.82
11	10	63	Male	2	$ 143.70	$ 71.85
12	11	48	Male	2	$ 77.92	$ 38.96
13	12	70	Female	6	$ 175.55	$ 29.26
14	13	8	Female	1	$ 135.68	$ 135.68
15	14	38	Male	8	$ 213.42	$ 26.68
16	15	41	Female	5	$ 637.49	$ 127.50
17						

FIGURE 2.19. SECOND STEP IN DATA SORT.

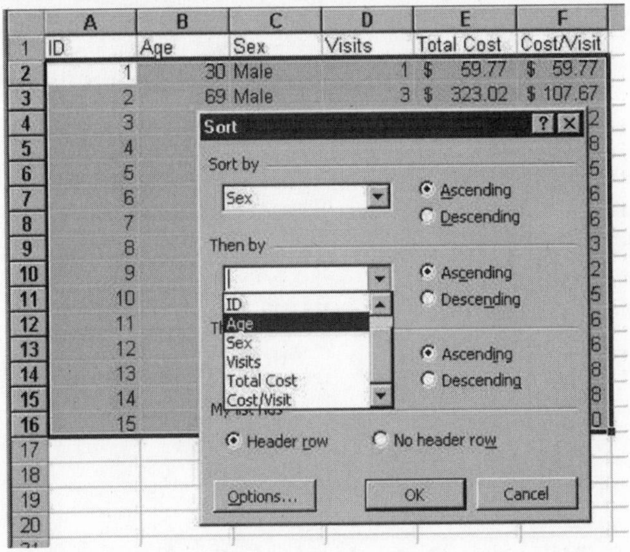

variable. To do this, we left-click the arrow in the Then by space and select Age. Again, we will sort in ascending order.

The black dot in Header row indicates that the data to be sorted has a set of titles in the first row above the data. If we had checked No header row, Excel would have sorted the column titles in with the rest of the data. Now if we select OK, the data will be sorted by both Sex and Age in that order, and the resulting data set can be seen in Figure 2.20. Looking at this figure, you can see that the data are ordered first into those who are female and those who are male, and within these two groupings by age from youngest to oldest. This sorting capability of Excel is very useful, especially for sampling.

Exercises for Section 2.6

1. Use the data for the exercises for Section 2.2 (data from Figure 2.3 or Chpt 2–1.xls) and do the following:
   a. Sort the data on the variable Age.
   b. Sort the data on the variable Visits.
   c. Sort the data on Visits first and Age second.
   d. Return the data to the original configuration by sorting on ID.

FIGURE 2.20. RESULT OF DATA SORT.

	A	B	C	D	E	F
1	ID	Age	Sex	Visits	Total Cost	Cost/Visit
2	13	8	Female	1	$ 135.68	$ 135.68
3	5	15	Female	4	$ 530.60	$ 132.65
4	9	17	Female	8	$1,078.59	$ 134.82
5	6	29	Female	2	$ 170.31	$ 85.16
6	15	41	Female	5	$ 637.49	$ 127.50
7	7	50	Female	3	$ 386.58	$ 128.86
8	12	70	Female	6	$ 175.55	$ 29.26
9	3	73	Female	1	$ 92.82	$ 92.82
10	4	22	Male	5	$ 589.40	$ 117.88
11	1	30	Male	1	$ 59.77	$ 59.77
12	14	38	Male	8	$ 213.42	$ 26.68
13	8	47	Male	1	$ 117.03	$ 117.03
14	11	48	Male	2	$ 77.92	$ 38.96
15	10	63	Male	2	$ 143.70	$ 71.85
16	2	69	Male	3	$ 323.02	$ 107.67
17						

Section 2.7 Excel's Data Analysis Pack

Microsoft Excel comes with a set of statistical analysis tools in addition to the functions available with the *fx* icon. These are contained in what is referred to by Excel as the Analysis ToolPak. The Analysis ToolPak is found under Tools/Data Analysis. Frequently, someone who is the first user of a particular Excel program will not be able to find the data analysis menu item under tools. If you cannot find the data analysis menu item, it means that the Analysis Tool-Pak has not been "added in" to the Excel program. To add in the Analysis ToolPak, it is necessary to left-click Tools/Add-Ins. This brings up the Add-Ins window. The second and third items in the Add-Ins window are Analysis Tool-Pak and Analysis ToolPak—VBA. It is necessary to check the box preceding both of these items for the data analysis options of Excel to be available. Once these have been checked, closing the Add-Ins window will allow you to bring up the first data analysis window with Tools/Data Analysis.

The first data analysis window is shown in Figure 2.21. Shown in that figure are only ten of the nineteen different analysis options available through the Analysis ToolPak. Selecting a specific analysis and right-clicking OK brings up an analysis window that will be tailored to the particular analysis requested. Specific analyses using the Analysis ToolPak are discussed as we move into the various categories of analysis available through this mechanism.

FIGURE 2.21. DATA ANALYSIS OPTIONS WINDOW.

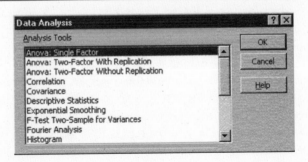

Section 2.8 Functions That Give Results in More Than One Cell

Excel incorporates several functions useful for statistical applications that produce results in more than one cell of the worksheet. One of the most important of these is the =FREQUENCY() function, which can be used to calculate frequency distributions for a set of data according to a set of categories. The =FREQUENCY() function takes two arguments—the data range and the range of categories into which the data are to be counted (called bins by Excel). The application of the =FREQUENCY() function is shown in Figure 2.22, and as the figure shows, there are two arguments included in an =FREQUENCY() function. These are

FIGURE 2.22. FREQUENCY CALCULATION.

D2		= {=FREQUENCY(B2:B13,C2:C4)}			
A	B	C	D	E	F
1	Data	Bins	Frequency		
2	2	3	2		
3	8	6	6		
4	4	9	4		
5	7				
6	9				
7	4				
8	3				
9	6				
10	5				
11	7				
12	5				
13	4				

the DATA range (in this case, B2:B13) and the BIN range (C2:C4). A comma separates the two ranges. The =FREQUENCY() function accumulates the number of observations that lie at or below the value of the bin but lie above the value of the next lower bin. So the bin values are actually the top of the bin range. You can confirm that the data range contains three numbers that are 3 or lower, six numbers that are 6 or lower, and four numbers that are 9 or lower.

In order for the =FREQUENCY() function to work properly, it is necessary first to highlight the entire area into which the resulting frequency distribution will be placed by Excel. Then, the =FREQUENCY() function is entered into the first of these cells, and the results are obtained by depressing CTRL/SHIFT, and, while holding these down, pressing ENTER. If this is not done, the correct results will not be obtained.

Excel also includes a function called =RAND(), which puts a random number into a single cell, or, if desired, into any number of cells. As mentioned earlier, =RAND() has no arguments. It is possible to highlight, for example, twenty cells in four rows and five columns. If the =RAND() function is then used, CTRL/SHIFT, and then ENTER, will put a random number between 0 and 1 into each of the twenty cells.

> IMPORTANT: To complete functions in Excel that put results into a single cell, it is necessary only to type the function into the appropriately highlighted cell and depress 'enter'. To complete a function that puts a result into more than one cell, it is necessary, first, to highlight all the cells into which the results are to go, enter the formula according to the convention for that formula and then simultaneously depress CNTL/SHIFT and then ENTER. If the CNTL/SHIFT/ENTER is not used, the right answer will not be obtained.

Excel also incorporates several functions with the ability to perform matrix math operations directly in the spreadsheet. While most statistical analyses can be carried out without any reference to matrix math, such statistical operations as multiple regression are much more easily understood by using matrix math. There are three matrix math capabilities of Excel that are most useful in statistical applications. These are =MMULT(), that multiplies two matrices together, =MINVERSE() that inverts a matrix, and =TRANSPOSE() that changes a vertical range of cells into a horizontal range and vice versa. =MMULT() and =MINVERSE() are found in the Math and Trig function category (see Figure 2.9); the =TRANSPOSE() function is found in the Lookup and Reference function category.

The matrix capabilities of Excel are demonstrated partially in Figure 2.23, which shows an example of matrix multiplication (=MMULT()). On the equation line, it is possible to see that the =MMULT() function is multiplying the matrix

FIGURE 2.23. MATRIX MATH EXAMPLE.

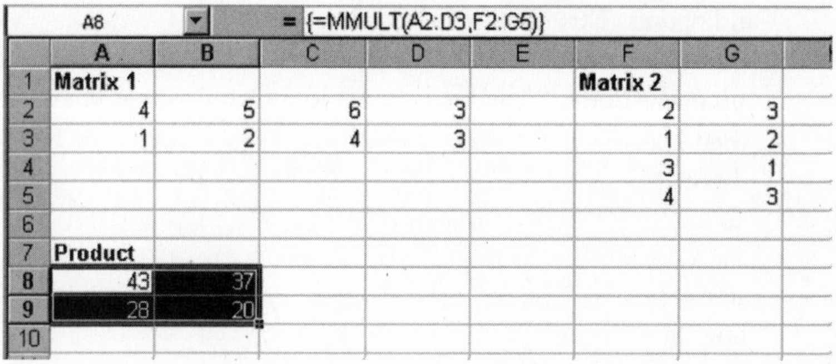

	A8	▼		= {=MMULT(A2:D3,F2:G5)}			
	A	B	C	D	E	F	G
1	Matrix 1					Matrix 2	
2	4	5	6	3		2	3
3	1	2	4	3		1	2
4						3	1
5						4	3
6							
7	Product						
8	43	37					
9	28	20					
10							

in A2:D3 times the matrix in F2:G5. The result, for those who are familiar with matrix math, will be a two-by-two matrix (because matrix 1 has two rows and matrix 2 has two columns). In order to complete a matrix operation with Excel, it is necessary to know the dimensions of the resulting matrix. The area of the resulting matrix is highlighted, and the =MMULT() formula is entered into the upper left-hand cell of the highlighted area. Then, the cell references of the two matrices to be multiplied are typed within the parentheses, or the cell ranges are highlighted, always with a comma separating them. To complete the matrix multiplication operation, it is necessary to use the convention CTRL/SHIFT/ENTER.

Exercises for Section 2.8

1. Use the data for the well-baby clinic from Exercise 1 of Section 2.3 (data from Chpt 2–2.xls, worksheet Infants). Create a frequency distribution with Excel using 14, 18, and 22 as the top of the bin ranges. Remember that you have to highlight three contiguous cells in a column, enter =FREQUENCY() into the first of the cells, and press CNTL/SHIFT/ENTER in order to produce the frequency distribution.
2. Use the data from Figure 2.3 (Chpt 2–1.xls).
   a. Create a frequency distribution for Total Cost using $400 as the first bin range and $400 increments thereafter.
   b. Create a frequency distribution for Age in ten-year age intervals.

3. Use the =RAND() function to fill the cells A2:B12 with random numbers. (Make sure that you first highlight the area A2:B12, enter =RAND() in A2, and depress Ctrl/Shift and Enter.)

4. Enter the data for matrix A and matrix B, below, into an Excel spreadsheet and perform the =MMULT() function. Confirm that the result is as given in matrix C.

	Matrix A	
2	3	5
3	3	4
5	4	5

	Matrix B
2	3
4	2
3	4

	Matrix C
31	32
30	31
41	43

Section 2.9 The Dollar Sign Convention for Cell References

The *dollar sign convention* for handling data in a spreadsheet is critical to understand for the maximum effectiveness of Excel operations. Dollar signs in any particular row or column reference indicate that the row or column designation preceded by the dollar sign is fixed.

In general, Excel uses what are known as relative references. For example, if you wished to average the clinic visits for Week 1 in Figure 2.12 (those in column B), the formula would be =AVERAGE(B4:B8). If this operation were carried out, the result would be the average of the five clinic visit totals for Week 1. To get the average for the clinic visit totals for Week 2, it is possible to copy the result in B9 and paste it into D9. If this is done, the formula in D9 will read =AVERAGE(D4:D8). This is what is meant by relative reference. When a formula is copied from one cell in an Excel spreadsheet to another cell, the cell references change to make the formula refer to the same *relative* area rather than to the same *actual* area.

FIGURE 2.24. CALCULATIONS OF PERCENTAGES.

	C4	▼	=	=B4/$B$9	
	A	**B**	**C**	**D**	
1					
2					
3	Day	Clinic Visits	Percent		
4	Day 1	23	15%		
5	Day 2	47	30%		
6	Day 3	19	12%		
7	Day 4	37	24%		
8	Day 5	31	20%		
9		157			
10					

When a dollar sign appears before any column or row reference, it means that the particular row or column is fixed. If the formula in B9 discussed earlier had been =AVERAGE($B4:$B9), and that formula had been copied into D9, the result would have been that the formula in D9 would still read =AVERAGE($B4:$B9). The value that appeared in cell D9 would be the average of the number of clinic visits in Week 1. Although in this case, a fixed reference would not have produced the result desired, a fixed reference is often critical for producing the expected result. For example, suppose you wished to know what proportion of all visits occurred on each day of Week 1. There are 157 visits to the clinic in Week 1. This is shown in B9 of Figure 2.24, which now contains the sum of clinic visits for Week 1. Column C shows the percentage of visits that took place in each day. In the formula line, it is also possible to see that the formula for the percentage in C4 is calculated as =B4/$B$9. The cell reference to B9 in the formula is fixed. This means that it is possible to copy the formula in C4 to each of the cells in C5 through C8, and the proper formula will be calculated for each of the cells in the C column. The numerator, being a relative reference, changes for each cell in the C column, whereas the denominator, which is an absolute reference, remains the same for each cell in the C column. For example, the formula in cell C5 is actually =B5/$B$9. Because the percentage values are always in the C column, it would have been equally feasible to use the formula =B4/B$9 to calculate the first percentage and then to copy that formula to each cell in column C. The results would have been the same.

Rather than go through the somewhat tedious process of putting dollar signs in front of each row and column reference when they are needed, the F4 function key can be used to select dollar sign status, and it is possible to toggle through all four possible combinations of dollar signs status for any cell reference. For example, if the cell reference B9 is entered into a formula, depressing F4 once will change that cell reference to $B$9. Depressing F4 a second time will change the cell reference to B$9. A third time will change the cell reference to $B9, and the fourth time will change it back to B9. The importance and versatility of the dollar sign convention—and the F4 function key—should become clearer as you proceed through the book.

CHAPTER THREE

DATA ACQUISITION: SAMPLING AND DATA PREPARATION

Most statistics texts take the facile approach to data, which is to assume that the data were all successfully collected and made ready for analysis before anyone with an interest in statistical analysis came along. The happy result of this is that the statistics text can usually ignore the thorny issues of where the data come from, how good they are, how they were collected, and how much confidence one can place in them. This text departs from that tradition—at least to the extent of talking a little about where data come from, how to get data, and what to do with data before analysis begins. This chapter is devoted to the acquisition of data: sampling and data collection.

Section 3.1 The Nature of Data

The first thing to be discussed in this chapter is simply the nature of data. Data are the fodder, the raw material of statistical analysis. There are two aspects of data that are essential to understand in any analysis setting. First, data are recorded in regard to or about cases or observations. Each case or observation represents a record in the data file. Second, data are made up of variables. Each case or observation—each data record—includes one or more measures on the case or record. These are the components of data that are subjected to analysis. For example, Figure 3.1 shows the Excel spreadsheet that was shown and discussed

FIGURE 3.1. A SMALL DATA FILE.

	A	B	C	D	E	F
1	ID	Age	Sex	Visits	Total Cost	Cost/Visit
2	1	30	Male	1	$ 59.77	$ 59.77
3	2	69	Male	3	$ 323.02	$ 107.67
4	3	73	Female	1	$ 92.82	$ 92.82
5	4	22	Male	5	$ 589.40	$ 117.88
6	5	15	Female	4	$ 530.60	$ 132.65
7	6	29	Female	2	$ 170.31	$ 85.16
8	7	50	Female	3	$ 386.58	$ 128.86
9	8	47	Male	1	$ 117.03	$ 117.03
10	9	17	Female	8	$1,078.59	$ 134.82
11	10	63	Male	2	$ 143.70	$ 71.85
12	11	48	Male	2	$ 77.92	$ 38.96
13	12	70	Female	6	$ 175.55	$ 29.26
14	13	8	Female	1	$ 135.68	$ 135.68
15	14	38	Male	8	$ 213.42	$ 26.68
16	15	41	Female	5	$ 637.49	$ 127.50
17						

in various ways in Chapter Two. This spreadsheet represents a small data set of fifteen observations and six variables.

The observations in Figure 3.1 represent fifteen people who may have come to an ambulatory clinic. Each observation appears on a different row of the spreadsheet. The variables in Figure 3.1 are in columns A through E. They include a unique identifier for each observation (ID in column A). The age of the person (Age), the sex of the person (Sex), the number of visits that the person has made to the clinic (Visits), a total cost for visits to the clinic for each person (Total Cost), and an average cost per visit (Cost/Visit).

Data are usually displayed and conceived of in the way that is pictured in Figure 3.1. That is to say that the observations are perceived as occupying rows and the variables are perceived as occupying columns. Observations, it should be pointed out, do not need to be persons. They could be organizations such as hospitals, health departments, or well-baby clinics. They could be political or geographic entities, such as states, counties, or hospital service areas. But variables always represent some attribute of the observation.

Types of Variables

A general characteristic of variables—at least as far as statistical analysis is concerned—is that they vary. In looking at the data set shown in Figure 3.1, it is easy to see that every variable takes on at least two values (Sex takes on two), and most take on a different value for each observation. In the unusual event that a variable does not vary—that is, it is a constant—it is useless for statistical analysis. Statistical analysis is almost universally about relating one variable to another. If a variable takes on only one value, it cannot statistically be related to other variables. This idea was discussed in some detail in Chapter One.

Also, as indicated in Chapter One, variables may be characterized as being two basic types—categorical and numerical. Sex in Figure 3.1 is a categorical variable, classifying each person in the file as male or female. ID is also a categorical variable, classifying each person in the file as a separate entity. Other types of categorical variables could include membership in an HMO, a coding for the seriousness of an emergency, such as yellow and red, the source of coverage for a hospital charge, or blood type.

The remaining variables in the file in Figure 3.1 are numerical data. Again, as introduced in Chapter One, there are two types of *numerical* data: discrete and continuous. *Discrete* numerical data are produced by a counting action and represent measures that can only be made in discrete individual units—never fractions of units. The number of visits to the clinic shown in Figure 3.1 is an example of discrete numerical data. Visits must always be in terms of whole units. Other discrete variables would include the number of persons in an emergency room, the number of unpaid accounts, or the number of immunizations received by a child.

Continuous numerical data are the result of a measurement or a mathematical operation. Age (a measure of the length of time from birth to the present moment) and cost per visit (the result of the division of total cost by the number of visits) are both continuous numerical variables. Other continuous numerical variables include waiting time in an ER or average waiting time, blood pressure, height, temperature, or drug dosage.

The total cost of all visits to the clinic is a little more difficult to classify. When cost is measured in dollars, fractions of dollars (such as pennies) might be considered to produce a continuous variable. When measured in pennies, however, each cost is a discrete measure—a result of counting—and cannot be expressed as fractions of pennies. But it is possible, as with height or age, to think of cost as an abstract notion that is approximated (as are height and age) by our measuring tool—in this case, dollars. From this perspective, cost is definitely a continuous variable. But, at the same time, it is possible to say that cost in the abstract is a meaningless concept, and that it only becomes meaningful when measured in some currency; thus, it is a discrete variable. Happily, although we may never resolve this issue, the type of statistics that applies to numerical variables tends to apply equally well to either discrete or continuous variables.

There is a second way—introduced in Chapter One—of distinguishing variables that refers to the scale upon which they are measured. Scale of measurement is classified as nominal, ordinal, interval, or ratio. The categorical variable, Sex, in Figure 3.1, is a nominal variable. It names each observation—each person in the file—as male or female. All nominal variables are categorical variables, but all categorical variables are not necessarily nominal variables. They may be ordinal variables, or even, possibly, interval variables.

Ordinal variables are nominal variables, the values of which establish some logical order. For example, young, middle-aged, and old, assigned to three age groups based on the data in Age in Figure 3.1, could be an ordinal variable. An assignment to the young age group might include all three people under twenty (persons with ID 5, 9, and 13). The middle-aged group might include all eight persons from twenty to fifty (persons with ID 1, 4, 6, 7, 8, 11, 14, and 15). Finally, the old group might include the remaining four persons (ID 2, 3, 10, and 12). This variable would be ordered in the sense that there is a logical order assumed by the young, middle-aged, and old. However, there is no assumption that the intervals are equal in any way.

The variable ID in Figure 3.1 is not an ordinal variable. There is no underlying logic to the assignment of 1 to the first person, 2 to the second, and so on. It would be equally possible to distinguish one person from another, to assign C to the first person, 231 to the second, Ralph to the third, and 17 to the fourth. As long as we assign a different code to each, we can keep them separated in our analysis, which is the primary function of an ID. ID, whether it is a number, a letter, or a sequence of nonsense syllables, is a nominal variable.

Interval variables are ordinal variables that have equal intervals. The categories young, middle-aged, and old are ordinal variables without equal intervals. It would, however, be feasible to create a set of age groupings that contained equal intervals. Suppose we were concerned with a population of Medicare patients and divided their ages into five-year categories, beginning at age sixty-five. If we assign 1 to the first group (ages sixty-five to sixty-nine), 2 to the second group (ages seventy to seventy-four), and so on, we would have created an interval variable.

Ratio variables are interval variables with a true zero point. In the interval measure assigned to the ages of Medicare patients mentioned earlier, there is no true zero point as the scale is given, because a 0 would simply mean the age group sixty to sixty-four. It would be possible to create a ratio variable for age in five-year-age intervals by beginning with 1 as the ages birth to four. Of course, age measured in one-year intervals is a ratio measure. In Figure 3.1, in addition to Age, Visits, Total Cost, and Cost/Visit are all ratio variables. Each of these variables has equal intervals and each has a true zero point.

Independent and Dependent Variables

In most statistical analysis there is a basic assumption that variables are either independent or dependent. Independent variables may often be termed causal variables, whereas dependent variables are considered caused variables. The term *causal variable* is quite commonly employed in statistics and research, but the term *'caused variable'* is rarely used. Independent variables are typically perceived as variables that are not affected or changed by the other variables under analysis, whereas dependent variables are, as the name implies, assumed to be dependent on or affected by the other variables in the analysis. Independent variables may also be termed predictor variables, because they are perceived to predict the performance of the dependent variables.

The distinction between independent and dependent variables is not always completely black and white, but with regard to data that is of interest to the health world, there are some clear types. For example, Figure 3.1 includes two variables—Age and Sex, which are always considered independent variables. It is generally true that age and sex are determined (rather predetermined) independent of any other variables in a data set. They are also generally perceived as independent of one another.

Conversely, the number of visits to the clinic (Visits) might be determined by age or sex or both. In this context, visits would be a dependent variable. Total cost might also be seen as dependent on age or sex or both, but it is also likely to be dependent on visits. So visits may be dependent relative to age or sex, but they may also be independent relative to total cost. Cost per visit (Cost/Visit) might be seen as dependent on age or sex, but not on visits or total cost. A statistical analysis might show that there is a relationship between either visits or total cost and cost per visit, but because cost per visit is a composite of visits and total cost (in fact dependent on both because it was created from both), there is no appropriate way to apply statistics to the relationship.

In the first chapter, we suggested that the big picture was that statistics was used to determine whether a value found in a sample could be assumed, on the basis of a statistical analysis, to have come from a population with certain characteristics. Another way of viewing statistical analysis is to think of it as a means of establishing whether a variable assumed to be dependent on another (assumed independent) can be shown from the data to be so. Although these two views may seem incompatible, or at least not obviously compatible, the discussion of various statistical analyses will attempt to show how the analysis addresses both questions.

Statistics That Apply to Different Types of Variables

As indicated in Chapter One, this book includes sections on five different basic types of statistical analysis: chi-square statistics, *t* tests, the analysis of variance (ANOVA), regression, and Logit. The chi-square statistic is designed specifically for data analysis that is limited to categorical data. A chi-square could be used in the case of the data shown in Figure 3.1 to determine, for example, whether there was a relationship, for this data set, between age and sex. However, in order to do this, age would have to be collapsed into two or a few categories. The categories young, middle-aged, and old that were developed earlier in this chapter could be an example of such an operation. This would result in a new variable that could be used for the chi-square analysis.

The *t test* can be thought of as a special case of a single dependent variable and a single independent variable. The dependent variable must be numerical and can be measured either on an interval or a ratio scale. The single independent variable can take on only two values and must be categorical. It can be either nominal or ordinal. Thus, a *t* test could compare, for example, cost per visit for males and females. In this case, cost per visit is the dependent, continuous numerical ratio variable, whereas sex is the single two-value independent variable.

Analysis of variance (ANOVA) can be thought of as a direct extension of the *t* test to a single categorical, either nominal or ordinal independent variable, that may take on several different values, as opposed to simply two. But analysis of variance may also be extended to include more than one independent variable. In general, however, all independent variables would be categorical and measured either on nominal or ordinal scales. Again, as with the *t* test, the dependent variable must be numerical—either discrete or continuous—and hence must be measured either on an interval or a ratio scale.

Regression analysis may be thought of as an extension of analysis of variance to numerical independent variables. At the same time, regression analysis does allow the inclusion of categorical variables that take on only two values. The ability to code categorical variables with more than two values as multiple two-value categorical variables also extends the utility of regression to encompass almost the entire range of capabilities of analysis of variance. But as with the *t* test and with analysis of variance, the dependent variable in regression must remain a numerical (discrete or continuous) variable.

Finally, *Logit analysis* is one of a family of techniques designed specifically to analyze data where the dependent variable is a two-level categorical variable (for example, the presence or absence of health insurance coverage), whereas the independent variable may be either categorical or numerical.

Much of what has been discussed in the preceding paragraphs will probably not be clear at this time. One of the things this book tries to do is to make these points clear and show how they are important in the use of statistics.

Exercises for Section 3.1

Figure 3.2 represents constructed data (made-up data) for an imaginary clinic. There is an ID for each of the twenty people who are included in the data set, along with eight variables. The variable Age is coded as expected, in years of life.

FIGURE 3.2. CONSTRUCTED DATA FROM A CLINIC.

	A	B	C	D	E	F	G	H	I
1	ID	Age	Sex	Opinion 1	Opinion 2	Charges	Visit Time	Insurance	Prior
2	1	33	F	5	3	$ 58.00	40	Self Pay	5
3	2	21	F	2	3	$ 59.00	44	Medicaid	1
4	3	56	F	1	3	$ 78.00	51	Medicaid	5
5	4	53	M	2	4	$ 24.00	36	BCBS	2
6	5	51	F	5	4	$ 46.00	55	Private	5
7	6	22	F	1	5	$ 30.00	21	BCBS	2
8	7	62	F	4	1	$114.00	33	BCBS	0
9	8	39	F	1	2	$ 51.00	43	BCBS	4
10	9	60	F	5	5	$100.00	34	Private	4
11	10	61	F	3	4	$ 45.00	59	Private	6
12	11	65	M	1	3	$ 55.00	24	Private	2
13	12	60	F	1	2	$ 36.00	53	Medicaid	6
14	13	61	M	3	2	$ 62.00	31	Self Pay	4
15	14	28	F	4	3	$100.00	25	Self Pay	3
16	15	54	F	4	3	$111.00	48	Self Pay	3
17	16	64	F	2	4	$ 59.00	44	Medicaid	3
18	17	44	F	3	2	$ 45.00	57	BCBS	4
19	18	25	F	2	3	$ 58.00	43	Private	1
20	19	35	M	1	1	$ 95.00	45	Private	3
21	20	32	F	5	3	$ 92.00	33	Private	4
22									

Sex is coded as F or M for female or male. The variable Opinion 1 is the answers to the question (asked on a patient questionnaire) "Do you feel this clinic meets your medical service needs: all the time, most of the time, about as often as not, some of the time, never?" An answer of never was coded 1, some of the time was coded 2, and so on. Opinion 2 is the answer to the statement "The service here is better than I would get at a hospital emergency room." The answers were Strongly agree—coded 5, Agree—coded 4, Undecided—coded 3, Disagree—coded 2, and Strongly disagree—coded 1. Charges represents the charge for the most recent clinic visit for each person. Visit Time represents the amount of time the person was at the clinic, from sign-in to departure. Insurance represents the type of insurance held by the patient and Prior represents the number of previous times the patient has come to the clinic.

1. Using the data given in Figure 3.2 (or the data in Chpt 3–1.xls), tell whether each of the variables in the figure is categorical or numerical, and if numerical, whether continuous or discrete, and give your reason for saying so.
2. Using the data given in Figure 3.2, do the following:
   a. Using the =IF(), transform Sex into a 1 if Sex is F and a 0 if Sex is M. Call this Sex1. Show the results in an Excel spreadsheet. What type of variable is the resulting variable and why?

b. Using nested =IF(), transform age to another variable that combines age into ten-year age groups, beginning with the youngest age among the patients listed. Assign 1 to the youngest group. Call this Age1. Show the results in an Excel spreadsheet. What type of variable is the resulting variable and why?

c. Using nested =IF(), transform age to another variable that combines age into ten-year age groups, beginning at birth. Assign 1 to the youngest age group. Call this Age2. Show the results in an Excel spreadsheet. What type of variable is the resulting variable and why?

d. Using nested =IF(), transform the variable Insurance into a new variable called Insurance1—that is, 1 if the insurance type is Medicaid, 2 if the insurance type is BCBS, 3 if the insurance type is Private, and 4 for Self-Pay. Show the results in an Excel spreadsheet. What type of variable is the resulting variable and why?

e. Using nested =IF(), transform the variable Prior into a variable called Prior1, where no prior visits is coded None, 1 to 2 prior visits is coded Low, 3 to 4 prior visits is coded Medium, and 5 or 6 prior visits is coded High. Show the results in an Excel spreadsheet. What type of variable is the resulting variable and why?

Section 3.2 Sampling

All statistical analysis assumes that a sample of some type is under study. Thus the subject of sampling is central to the study of statistics.

Samples and Populations

The term *statistics* is generally used to refer to the subject of this book—that is, the set of calculations that can be used to draw inferences about the relationships between variables and make inferences about populations from samples. Statistics is also frequently used as simply the plural of statistic. The affinity between these two meanings should be made clear. Statistics is the study of samples and characteristics of samples and the ways in which inferences about populations may be drawn from those samples. A statistic is a value derived from a sample that can be used to infer something about a population.

Imagine that the data shown in Figure 3.1 represent a fifteen-person sample from some much larger population of all persons who have come to the health center or clinic from which the data had been taken. We can calculate the mean or average of, for example, the number of visits to the clinic for this sample, which comes out to about 3.47 visits per person. This number is a statistic because it came from a sample, and we would designate the number $\bar{x}$, pronounced *x-bar*, because it was a statistic. The corresponding mean or average for the population from which the sample came would be called not a statistic but a parameter, and it would be designated μ, which is pronounced *mu* and represents the lowercase Greek letter m. This leads to a generally applicable statement. Statistics refer to samples and are designated by lowercase Roman letters; parameters refer to populations and are designated by lowercase Greek letters. As you proceed through this book, you will encounter other measures for both samples and populations that have similar distinctions.

The one important contradiction to this general statement about the designation of sample and population values is the designation of size. Sample sizes are universally designated n for number. Population sizes are universally designated N for number. So in the case of the data in Figure 3.1, n is fifteen, but since we do not know the size of the population from which the data were drawn, N is unknown.

Drawing a Random Sample from a Population

There are complete books devoted to the subject of sampling, so this treatment will necessarily be only an introduction. But all of the statistics discussed in this text assume at some point that a sample has been taken. Furthermore, as was suggested in the first chapter, the statistics discussed in this book also assume that the sample selected was either a simple random sample, or it was perhaps a systematic sample. This section will discuss sampling and sample selection with specific reference to simple random sampling.

It is generally accepted that a person, without some resources other than his or her own intellect, cannot draw a true random sample. No matter how hard we might try, any sample we might draw would be very likely to be nonrandom. For example, suppose we wished to draw a random sample of five persons from a group of twenty people that was equally divided into four groups by gender and age at, for example, age thirty, so that within the overall group there was a group of five young men, five young women, five older men, and five older women. The basic premise of a simple random sample is that each possible sample that may be selected must have an equal probability of selection as the actual sample.

If we were to try to draw a simple random sample of five from this group of twenty, we would almost unconsciously end up with a sample that included two men and two women and two older persons and two younger persons. Filling out the five-person sample would be a problem for us because we would be concerned that adding a fifth person would not make the sample representative of the entire group. And herein lies the problem of trying to draw a random sample with no form of external aid. Random samples are not representative; they are random. Human beings seek to be representative when they try to extract a smaller group from a larger. This inevitably results in the exclusion of many possible combinations of samples that a truly random selection would allow. For example, a person would be very likely not to select five young men as the sample, because it would not be perceived to be representative of the group of twenty as a whole. But random sampling allows for the selection of the five young men. It is unlikely that it would occur in a random sample, but all statistical analysis is based on the premise that it might happen.

Because the basic assumption of statistics is that a random sample has been selected (and for the purposes of this book, a simple random sample), it is essential to have some mechanism to make this sample selection. One way to do this would be to assign a number to each member of a population from which a sample is to be drawn. Next, write each number on a slip of paper. Then put each slip of paper into a large box, shake it up very well, and draw out (without looking at the numbers on the paper slips) the number needed. However, this could be both time-consuming and very boring. For years, prior to the common availability of computers, statisticians used a modification of this slip-of-paper technique to draw random samples. They did this by using tables of random numbers, which were published in book form for the specific purpose of drawing random samples. Excerpts from these tables of random numbers—usually two to four pages—are often reproduced in the back of statistics texts, occasionally with instructions on how to use the tables to draw true random samples. Typically, the use of these tables involved the time-consuming task of associating each observation in the population with an entry in the random number table. If that entry was smaller than some predetermined value, the observation in the population would become a member of the sample. For example, if the random number table was divided into three-digit sequences and the population consisted of a thousand observations, to select a 5 percent sample, any observation in the population associated with a three-digit sequence less than 050 would be included in the sample. If the observation was associated with a three-digit sequence larger than 050—for example, 274, that population observation would not be included in the sample.

The advent of computers made tables of random numbers obsolete. Even though tables of random numbers continue to be published, it is now many years since anyone has used them to draw random samples. The computer can generate sequences of random numbers and associate them with population observations far faster than we could from a random number table. Excel, as a computer program, is able to generate random numbers in a variety of different ways. This capability allows the Excel user to draw random samples in a variety of different ways, with a great deal of ease and efficiency. Perhaps the simplest of these mechanisms is the =RAND( ) Method.

To employ the =RAND( ) Method of selecting a random sample, it is necessary to have a worksheet reference for each observation in the population. If a researcher desired to draw a random sample from among all the people who work for a state department of health, for example, it would be necessary to have some reference to each of these persons in an Excel spreadsheet. This might be each employee's name on the spreadsheet or, at a very minimum, a number associated with each employee. To continue with the example, suppose names were not on a spreadsheet but were only in an alphabetical hard copy list. Suppose that there are 3,427 employees on the list and we wish to draw a random sample of a hundred. To draw this sample, we can begin by listing the numbers 1 through 3,427 in column A of a spreadsheet. *Do not type each number into 3,427 subsequent cells in column A.* Listing the numbers might be done in a couple different ways, but the simplest procedure is probably to put 1 in Cell A1 and 2 in Cell A2. Then highlight both cells—A1 and A2, and, with the cursor on the lower right corner of the highlighted area (the cursor should appear as a small black cross rather than a large white cross), drag the cursor down to cell A3427. This probably takes thirty seconds or less.

Now go back to the top of the spreadsheet and type =RAND( ) in cell B1. As was indicated previously, it is not necessary to type an Excel function such as =RAND( ) in caps; lowercase will work just as well. With =RAND( ) in cell B1, put the cursor on the lower right corner of the cell (the cursor becomes a small black cross) and double-click the left button. This will fill cells B1 to B3427 with random numbers in the range 0 to 1. Figure 3.3 shows the appearance of the spreadsheet just prior to the double-click that fills column B with random numbers. Column A in Figure 3.3 is the beginning eight entries in a list that runs to 3,427. When cell B1 is double-left-clicked with the small black cross on the lower right

FIGURE 3.3. BEGINNING OF RANDOM NUMBER GENERATION.

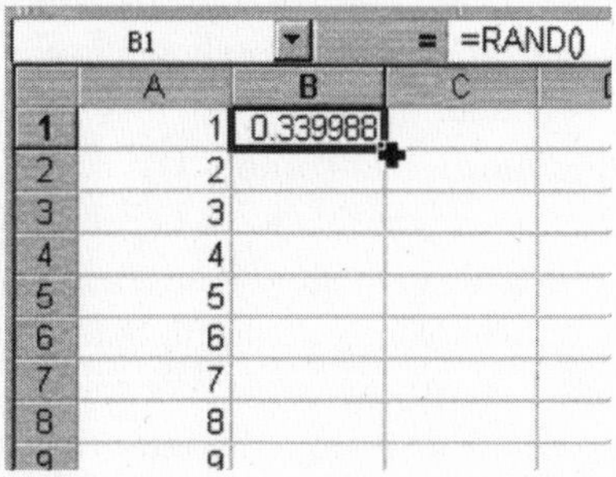

corner of the cell, the random number represented by the entry in B1 will be copied to the first 3,427 cells in column B.

Now we have a random number associated with each entry in cells A1 through A3427. We could now go down the list of random numbers and include in the sample any entry in cell A associated with a random number equal to or less than .02918 (100/3427 = .02918). But this has two disadvantages. First, it is still quite time-consuming to look at all 3,427 entries. Second, because the generated numbers are random, it is likely that there will be more or fewer than exactly one hundred random numbers with values of .02918 or less. A more efficient strategy will be to sort the data in column A and column B (the first 3,427 cells in each column) by column B. This will order the data in column A by column B, after which the first one hundred cases (or any hundred cases determined a priori) can be selected as the sample. This will not only make the sample selection fast and efficient but will also ensure for us a sample of exactly one hundred observations.

There is one important additional piece of information that is needed before you can proceed, however. When the =RAND() function is used to enter values in the cells B1 through B3427, what is actually entered into the cells is not a random number but, rather, the random number *function*. The random number function is regenerated every time the worksheet recalculates. The function also regenerates if an operation, such as sorting, is applied to the worksheet. Consequently, if you sort the data on the column containing the =RAND() function, you will have the unsatisfying result of not seeing the entries in column B appear ordered from lowest to highest, or in any other apparent order, because as soon as the sort occurs, the random number function is regenerated. Hence, the sequence in B will never appear ordered.

There is an easy way to get around the problem of recalculation, however, and to feel a little more secure in the result of the sort. After the random numbers have been copied to the first 3,427 cells in column B, while the entire 3,427 cells are still highlighted, select Edit/Copy, followed by Edit/Paste Special. In the Paste Special window, check the box marked Values. Figure 3.4 shows the Paste Special window with the Values box checked. When you click on OK, the formulas in column B, which to this point all show =RAND() in the formula line if you highlight them, will change to the actual number shown in the cell. Now both columns A and B can be sorted on column B.

The Excel Sort routine is found under Data/Sort. When you invoke the Sort command, you will see a window that looks like that shown in Figure 3.5. The sort window allows for sorting on up to three columns at a time. As shown in Figure 3.5, the sort will be only on one column (column B) and it will be in ascending order. Because there is no label on either column A or column B, the circle in front of "No header row" is checked (this is done by left-clicking on the circle in front of

FIGURE 3.4. PASTE SPECIAL WINDOW.

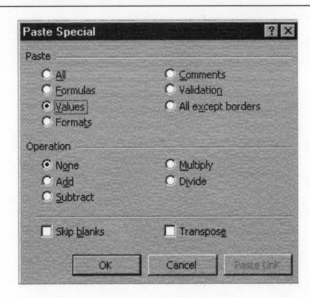

FIGURE 3.5. SORT WINDOW.

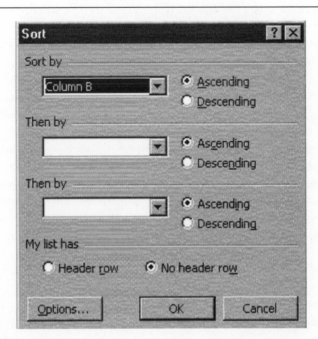

FIGURE 3.6. SORTED SAMPLE.

	B1	▼	=	0.000151695338435953	
	A	B	C	D	E
1	777	0.000152			
2	1966	0.000288			
3	1415	0.000802			
4	953	0.001047			
5	2063	0.001391			
6	190	0.001846			
7	1999	0.00198			
8	878	0.002364			
9	3378	0.003274			
10	2976	0.004237			
11	616	0.004636			
12	1513	0.005061			
13	13	0.005577			
14	2648	0.005616			

"No header row"). By left-clicking OK in the sort window, the 3,427 numbers in column A will be sorted by column B. The result of this sort is shown in Figure 3.6. Figure 3.6 shows the first fourteen rows of the spreadsheet that contain the 3,427 numbers in column A, now sorted on column B. The entry in row 1 of column A is observation 777. This is associated with the smallest random number in column B—.000152—and is the first observation to be included in the sample of one hundred. The second observation included is number 1,966, which is associated with the next smallest random number, .000288. The last observation in the sample (not shown in Figure 3.6) is the observation numbered 3,066, which is associated with the random number .030386.

Having carried out the steps previously discussed, a random set of one hundred observations has been selected from among the original 3,427 observations. It remains to the researcher to go to the files and select the employee records corresponding to each of the first one hundred numbers in the sample. But the task of selecting the random sample is completed. This random sample of employees can now be used to calculate any estimates of the total population of employees that one would normally calculate from a random sample.

A Random Sample of Home Health Agency Records

Chapter One introduced the problem of the home health agency that wished to do an audit of 10 percent of its eight hundred records each quarter. The agency had been selecting the records for audit by taking the first record and every tenth record thereafter. It was suggested that perhaps a better way would be to select a simple random sample of records for review. A simple random sample can be selected easily by following the process described previously, in the second subsection of Section 3.2. Assuming that the records can be put into some consecutive list, each of the files can be given a number from one to eight hundred, which can be listed in column A of an Excel spreadsheet. Having listed the numbers, each can be assigned a randomly generated number between 0 and 1 using =RAND(). The list can then be sorted on the random number, and the first eighty records can be selected for audit.

Selecting a Sample of Women to Receive a Cancer Education Intervention

Chapter One also introduced an example of the use of statistics in which a resident was expected to develop a study in which a sample of women received one type of breast cancer education—a pamphlet, whereas another sample of women experienced a short talk on breast cancer from a physician, as well as receiving the pamphlet. The question was whether the women who had experienced the talk would show greater knowledge of breast cancer on a brief questionnaire administered after the fact.

For such a study to be effective, it is essential that the women who receive the two different interventions be randomly assigned to the two groups. Suppose the resident hopes to have thirty women in each of the two groups at the completion of the study, but she does not know who these sixty women are because they are women who will be coming to the clinic in the future.

The easiest way to assign the sixty women randomly to either of the two interventions would be to begin by listing the numbers 1 through 60 in column A of an Excel spreadsheet. Then each of the sixty numbers is assigned a random number using =RAND() in column B, and after Copy and Paste Special/Values, the sixty numbers can be sorted by the random numbers. Now the first thirty numbers in the list (those in rows A1:A30) represent the women who will receive one intervention (the pamphlet only, for example), and the second thirty numbers (those in A31:A60) represent the women who receive the other intervention (both pamphlet and the talk).

Having randomly assigned the numbers 1 through 60 to two groups, the list of those assigned to each group can now be sorted so that they are easier to track. The results of such a sort might be as those shown in Figure 3.7. The figure shows the first fifteen women in each of the two groups—those receiving the pamphlet only and those receiving the pamphlet plus the talk. As the figure shows, at the initiation of the study, the first two women seen in the clinic will receive both the pamphlet and the talk. The third woman will receive only the pamphlet, the

FIGURE 3.7. PARTIAL LIST OF THOSE WHO WILL RECEIVE EACH INTERVENTION.

	A	B	
1	**Pamphlet**	**Talk**	
2	3	1	
3	6	2	
4	7	4	
5	8	5	
6	9	12	
7	10	13	
8	11	14	
9	15	21	
10	16	22	
11	17	24	
12	18	25	
13	19	26	
14	20	28	
15	23	32	
16	27	33	
17	29	39	

fourth and fifth women will receive both interventions, and so on. This assignment can be used for the next sixty women coming to the clinic who meet the other study criteria.

There is an important point to be made from Figure 3.7 beyond that of a way to display the women who will be selected for each group. It might be noted that the sixth through the eleventh woman arriving at the clinic will be given only the pamphlet. Readers might be tempted to ask how this can be a random ordering if six people in a row are assigned to the same group. However, that is precisely why humans cannot carry out random selections. We are put off by a sequence of six in a row. But random numbers don't care. And in this case, the sequence of six from six to eleven was the result of random selection.

Other Random Sampling Mechanisms

Excel provides a number of different ways to draw random samples. The simplest is the =RAND() method discussed earlier. A similar way is to use the =RAND-BETWEEN (first, second) function that returns a random integer between the two numbers specified as first and second. If the =RANDBETWEEN() function is to

FIGURE 3.8. RANDOM NUMBER GENERATION WINDOW.

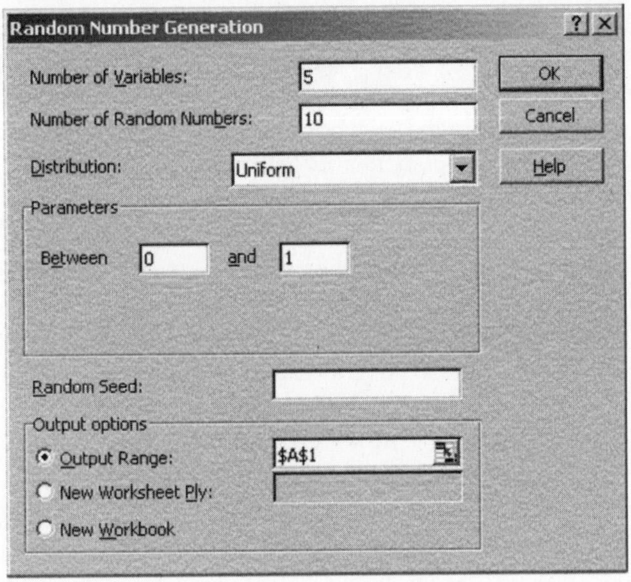

be used, it should be realized that the random numbers selected may be repeated if the range between the two numbers selected as first and second is small. This function recalculates just as =RAND() does, so it is necessary to use the Copy/Paste Special/Values sequence prior to sorting if the satisfaction of seeing a sorted list is important.

Several other methods of selecting random samples can be found in the data analysis add-in under Tools/Data Analysis/Random Number Generation. If the Tools/Data Analysis/Random Number Generation option is invoked, the window that appears on the spreadsheet screen looks like that shown in Figure 3.8. The Number of Variables box indicates the number of sets of random numbers that are to be generated. In the case shown in Figure 3.8, there will be five sets. The Number of Random Number box indicates the number of random numbers each set will contain. In this case, there will be ten numbers in each set. The Distribution box indicates the type of distribution that will be generated. Seven different distributions of random numbers can be generated using this add-in. They are Uniform, Normal, Bernoulli, Binomial, Poisson, Patterned, and Discrete. More will be said of these later.

For each different type of distribution, there are corresponding parameters that must be specified. For the Uniform distribution, as shown in Figure 3.8, the parameters are the two numbers between which the random number will be generated. In the case shown, the numbers will be between 0 and 1, just as generated by the =RAND() function. Any real numbers can be used as the numbers between which random numbers will be generated, but the numbers generated will not be integer values, even if integers such as 5 and 25 are the numbers chosen for the range. Every distribution that can be generated has a separate set of parameters, which will be pointed out as each distribution type is discussed.

Each of the random number generation windows allows for the inclusion of a random seed. To understand the random seed, it is necessary to realize that no computer-driven random generating scheme can actually produce true random numbers. Computers can produce what are generally termed pseudorandom numbers. Any pseudorandom number generating scheme takes some part of the last random number generated and uses that as a *seed* to begin the generation of the next random number. But in order for this to work, the computer has to have some number to work with as the first seed. Typically, the seed is taken from some source that is constantly changing in no predictable way. In the case of the =RAND() function, the seed is taken from the last several digits of the computer's time clock. These change so rapidly that it is impossible to predict what value they will have when the =RAND() function is invoked. But the random number generating schemes in the Tools/Data Analysis/Random Number Generation add-in all begin with a fixed seed by default. This means that *every time Excel is started anew, these random number generating schemes will produce exactly the same string of numbers.* This is true for every one of the seven different random number generating schemes, Uniform, Normal, Bernoulli, Binomial, Poisson, Patterned, and Discrete.

If the random number generating schemes produced the same set of random numbers every time Excel was started anew, they would not seem to be producing very random numbers. But this problem has a relatively simple solution. Each of the seven random number generating schemes allows for the specification of a random seed. Before using any of these random number generators, it would be best to use the =RAND() function to generate at least one random number. The first four digits of the result of =RAND() can then be used as an integer (that is, without the decimal point) and as a random seed in whatever random number generation add-in is being used. Only the first four digits should be used because the random seed value cannot exceed 9999. This strategy will produce a distinct and different set of random numbers each time the random number generating schemes are invoked.

The random number generation window in Figure 3.8 will produce a set of random numbers, as shown in Figure 3.9. The five in the Number of Variables box has produced five columns of numbers, and the ten in the Number of Random Numbers box has produced ten rows of numbers. It can be seen that all these numbers are between 0 and 1. It should be further noted that the uniform

FIGURE 3.9. FIVE SETS OF TEN RANDOM NUMBERS.

	A	B	C	D	E
1	0.673757	0.557695	0.681936	0.914029	0.103977
2	0.273385	0.853511	0.429579	0.507523	0.089206
3	0.695853	0.92584	0.27131	0.073336	0.817316
4	0.638661	0.004639	0.947264	0.905637	0.448714
5	0.734123	0.125706	0.732475	0.492782	0.19425
6	0.470077	0.019074	0.191382	0.870235	0.785211
7	0.070009	0.973388	0.948454	0.592303	0.580065
8	0.479324	0.832057	0.207923	0.521836	0.52443
9	0.376659	0.661275	0.519242	0.602527	0.503525
10	0.48027	0.61388	0.212531	0.345408	0.878414
11					

distribution generates what are essentially continuous random numbers—that is, the numbers are generated to nine decimal places.

The *Uniform* distribution is discussed earlier. The *Normal* distribution window looks exactly like that shown in Figure 3.8, except that in the parameters box the user is asked to supply the mean and the standard deviation of the distribution. These terms will be discussed in detail in Chapter Six, but for the present, it is sufficient to note that the normal distribution option generates numbers that have no limit but will most likely be close to the mean value and will vary from the mean value as a function of the value of the standard deviation. The normal distribution also generates continuous random numbers up to nine decimal places.

The *Bernoulli* distribution window also matches the uniform window, except for the parameters box. For the Bernoulli distribution, only one parameter, p, is requested. The p stands for probability and must be between 0 and 1. The Bernoulli distribution option will generate a random sequence of ones and zeros, with the average number of ones being equal to p. So if you were to generate ten random ones and zeros using the Bernoulli option with a p of .5, it would be like flipping a coin ten times. You would expect to get five heads (ones) and five tails (zeros), but you would not be surprised if you got four ones and six zeros, or three zeros and seven ones. Because the Bernoulli option generates only 0 or 1, it can be considered as generating discrete random numbers.

The *Binomial* distribution window requests two parameters—the p value and the Number of trials. Again, as with the Bernoulli distribution, the p value refers to the probability of an occurrence. Number of trials refers to the number of times the probability will be applied. In the coin-flipping example of the Bernoulli distribution mentioned previously, the number of trials was 10. Rather than generate a series of ones and zeros, the Binomial distribution generates a single number between 0 and the number of trials (for example, 10) that represents the number of ones that would result from applying p for the number of trials times. In the case of flipping a coin ten times, the binomial distribution result would be a number between 0 and 10. Since the probability of a head or a tail is equal, the random numbers generated by the binomial distribution will be predominantly fours, fives, and sixes. The binomial distribution option generates only integer values, so it generates discrete random numbers.

The *Poisson* distribution window requests a single parameter: Lambda. Lambda refers to the mean value of the distribution, or the average number that will be generated by the distribution over a large number of trials. In a Poisson distribution, the value of lambda is also the variance of the distribution. The Poisson distribution will be discussed further in Chapter Five. The Poisson distribution also generates only integer values, so it, too, generates discrete random numbers.

The *Patterned* distribution is not actually a random number generator at all, but, rather, it generates a list of numbers that repeat as many times as desired in a pattern that is set by the parameters box. In terms of the materials in this book, the patterned distribution is not relevant.

The *Discrete* distribution requests two parameters: the Value and the Probability Input Range. The discrete distribution generates random numbers from a prespecified set of numbers (the value range), according to the probabilities assigned to these numbers (the probability range). So, for example, if the value range was as that shown in A1:A10 of Figure 3.10, and the probability range was as shown in B1:B10, the discrete random number generator would generate values

FIGURE 3.10. EXAMPLE VALUE AND PROBABILITY INPUT RANGE.

	A	B
1	1	0.30
2	2	0.20
3	3	0.10
4	4	0.10
5	5	0.05
6	6	0.05
7	7	0.05
8	8	0.05
9	9	0.05
10	10	0.05
11		

of 1 to 10 according to the probabilities shown in column B. It should also be pointed out that the probability range must sum to 1. So if you wanted to generate a random series of, for example, twenty numbers from the list in A1:A10, you would expect, on average, that the random number generation would result in six ones, four twos, two each of three and four, and one each of five through ten. Of course, since this is a random number generation process, it is likely that the result will not be exactly as indicated in the previous sentence. But, in general, the result will be similar to this.

One point must be made about the random seed in the discrete distribution generator. For some reason, the space following the random seed will be grayed out so that it cannot be used in many instances. The solution is to change to another type of distribution, put in the desired random seed, and then go back to the discrete distribution. The random number generator will pick up the random seed as specified.

Although it is useful to know of these random number generation capabilities of Excel, in general, the material in this book will rely either on the =RAND() method of selecting random samples or, in some examples with regard to the consequences of selection of random samples, on the discrete sampling capability of the random number add-in. However, in order to provide some familiarity with sampling in general, and these options in particular, the following exercises are offered.

Exercises for Section 3.2

1. Use the data set from Figure 3.2 (Chpt 3–1.xls) and do the following:
   a. Use the =RAND() function to draw a random sample of five patients from the twenty patients given in the file.
   b. Use the Uniform option in the Tools/Data Analysis add-in to generate random numbers between 0 and 1 and use these numbers to select a simple random sample of seven patients from the twenty in the file. Specify a random seed of 1,325.
   c. Use the Normal option in the Tools/Data Analysis add-in to generate random numbers with a mean of 0 and a standard deviation of 1 and use these numbers to select a simple random sample of ten patients from the twenty in the file. Specify a random seed of 7936.

2. The file Chpt 3–2.xls contains data from the State and Metropolitan Area Data book for 1998 on nurses and health insurance coverage by state, including the District of Columbia. Use the data from this file and do the following:
   a. Use the =RAND() function to draw a random sample of ten states (including D.C.) from among all the states.

b. Use the Uniform option in the Tools/Data Analysis add-in to generate random numbers between 1 and 100, and use these to select a random sample of fifteen states (including D.C.) from among all the states. Specify a random seed of 1359.

c. Use the Normal option in the Tools/Data Analysis add-in to generate random numbers with a mean of 20 and a standard deviation of 4, and use these numbers to select a simple random sample of ten states (including D.C.) from among all the states. Specify a random seed of 8109.

3. Staff members at a prenatal clinic, who see many women who smoke, have decided to assess the effectiveness of a video on the dangers of smoking during pregnancy. They have decided to divide the women who come to the clinic—the ones who smoke—into two groups: one that receives the normal warnings about the dangers of smoking and one that is asked to view the video. Over the next six months, the clinic expects to see about forty women who are smokers.

   Use =RAND() to select a sample of twenty women who will view the film and twenty who will not—out of the next forty women to arrive at the clinic.

4. Use the Bernoulli option in the Tools/Data Analysis add-in to simulate the flip of a coin fifty times. Generate a random seed using =RAND(). If you consider a value of one to be a head, use the =SUM() function to determine the number of heads and tails flipped.

5. Use the Binomial option in the Tools/Data Analysis add-in to simulate the distribution of men and women among the next ten arrivals at an emergency room, assuming that on average, six people out of ten who arrive are men. Generate a random seed using =RAND(). Simulate the arrival of fifty sets of ten people. Use the =COUNTIF() function to determine how many of the fifty sets of ten people will be all men and how many will be nine men and one woman.

6. Use the Discrete option in the Tools/Data Analysis add-in to simulate the role of a six-sided die fifty times. Generate a random seed using =RAND(). Use the =COUNTIF() function to determine how many of the fifty roles will produce a six.

Section 3.3 Data Access and Preparation

Data access can be the subject, just as sampling can, of an entire book. This section provides only a basic introduction to the issues involved. Essentially, data can be accessed and acquired in only two ways; it can be collected directly by the investigator (the user of this statistics text, for example) or it can be obtained as secondary data. If it is to be collected by the investigator, the options available for collection include questionnaires that are filled out by respondents themselves (patients or hospital CEOs, for example) or interview schedules to which answers are given by respondents. Direct data collection can also include observation in which the researcher observes and records these specific details on a predetermined schedule.

Secondary data are data that have been collected for some purpose other than the study of interest to the researcher but can be accessed by the investigator for study purposes. Secondary data could include such information, for example, as patients' records (when appropriate clearances for use and informed consent have been obtained), operating data from a hospital or other health care organization, or data in the public domain, such as county by county statistics on median income, percent below poverty, low birth weight rates, and so on.

A major advantage of the use of directly collected data is that data can be collected in a way that is specific to the needs of the investigator. To take a relatively simple example, if the interest is in a patient's age, the investigator can ask the patient for his or her age (although this question may not always result in the true age). However, if secondary data are used to get a patient's age, the data actually available may not be age but, rather, date of birth. This leads to the general issue of how one takes data that may be collected in a form convenient to the act of collection, or appropriate to use for purposes other than the investigation in question, and then turn it into data that can be used in the application of other statistical analysis. Happily, Excel is a very useful tool in this process.

An Examination of Data Preparation Using Secondary Data

This section describes an example of the use of Excel in the preparation of some secondary data for analysis. The secondary data to be examined is actual data, but it is data from which all identifying information has been deleted. The data file represents information for one hundred hospital discharges for Medicare-eligible persons randomly selected from a much larger file of discharges. There are nine different pieces of information included in the file. These are sex, date of birth, date of hospital admission, date of discharge, DRG code, total hospital charges, actual Medicare payment, number of diagnoses for the hospital stay, and admitting ICD-9 code. (The ICD-9 code is one digit. Normally, ICD-9 codes are three digits or more, but this is the way the data were actually coded and made available, because the institution from which the data came was having trouble coding the ICD-9. Problems such as this are not uncommon in using secondary data.)

FIGURE 3.11. TEXT IMPORT WIZARD, STEP 1.

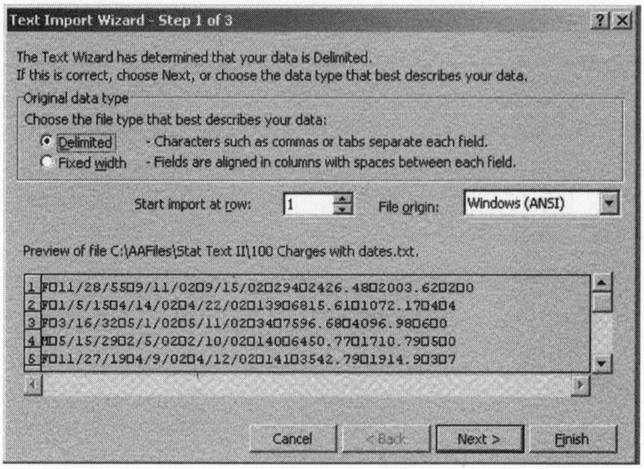

The data file is initially in a simple text format, and it must be put into Excel format to be used by Excel. This is not unusual. It is not uncommon to find data in a format other than the Excel format. Excel provides a Text Import Wizard with three steps to import text data into Excel. The Text Import Wizard will automatically come up in the Excel screen whenever Excel recognizes that the user is trying to open a text file. The first step of the Text Import Wizard is shown in Figure 3.11.

The Text Import Wizard will assume that the text file to be imported is a data file. It will also assume that each line of the text file represents a separate observation and that individual data elements (the variables) for any observation are all contained on the same line. It will first attempt to determine the way in which each data element is distinguished from every other data element. There are two ways that data elements may be separated: by using a delimiter or by using a fixed width field. A delimiter is a character (such as a tab or an ampersand) that generally will not be used to represent data but will simply be included in the text file to separate one variable from another. Data may also be stored in a text file in fixed width. Fixed width means that every variable will take up exactly the same number of spaces-for example, ten spaces-in the text file. Delimited data is the most common format, because a fixed length file requires a certain number of spaces for each variable, even though there may be no data in a particular field, or the actual data may be much shorter than the number of spaces allocated. The delimited data file takes up only as much space as is required for each data element.

The Text Import Wizard has correctly determined-in the case of the data in the text file referenced here (see Figure 3.11)—that the data are delimited, and it has indicated this with the dot in the Delimited circle and the dotted line around the word *delimited*. It further indicates that the importing of data to the Excel spreadsheet will begin in row 1 and that the text file is actually contained in a Windows (ANSI) format. The other formats that can appear in the file origin window are Macintosh and MS-DOS. The preview screen shows the data that will be imported by Excel with the delimiter (in this case, actually a tab character), indicated by a square box. Line 1 of the preview screen shows "F" as the first code (representing Female for sex), 11/28/55 representing the date of birth, 9/11/02 and 9/15/02 representing the date of admission and discharge respectively, and 294 representing the DRG code. The remaining information on the first line includes 2,426.48 representing the total dollar charges for the stay, 2,003.62 representing what Medicare actually paid, 2 indicating two separate diagnoses for the stay, and 0 indicating no admitting ICD-9 code.

Figure 3.12 shows the second step of the Text Import Wizard. This step allows the user to select the character that is actually used to delimit the data and see the result of the selection of this delimiter in the data preview box. The check before Tab indicates that Excel correctly determined on its own that the text file was delimited with tab characters.

The final step in the Text Import Wizard is shown in Figure 3.13. This window provides an opportunity to do several things. These include setting the format of each imported column and indicating whether a column should not be imported. The highlighted first column will be acted upon by anything checked in the Column data format box. Each successive column in the data can be

FIGURE 3.12. TEXT IMPORT WIZARD, STEP 2.

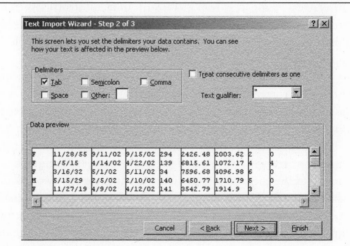

FIGURE 3.13. TEXT IMPORT WIZARD, STEP 3.

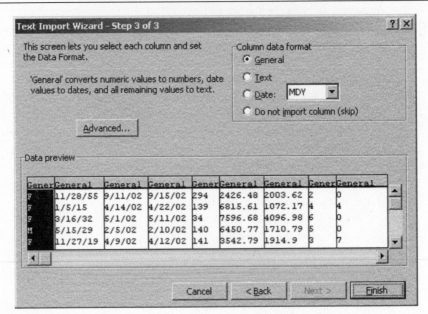

highlighted in turn and its format can be set to General, Text, or Date. General is the most versatile format, as it treats numeric values as numbers, treats text values as text, and treats data in date format (that is, 11/28/55) as dates.

In general, if Excel correctly recognizes that the data file is delimited (or fixed length) and there is no desire to change the format of the actual data elements, or to delete some variables on entry, it is usually not necessary to go beyond the first screen of the Text Import Wizard. In fact, the first screen is all that is necessary to convert the file under discussion here to an Excel file. If the Finish button is selected in step 1 of the Text Import Wizard, the text file will automatically appear as an Excel spreadsheet.

The data as imported into the Excel spreadsheet is shown, as initially imported, in Figure 3.14. Only the first ten records in the file are shown, although, as mentioned earlier, the data file actually contains one hundred records. On looking at the file as shown in Figure 3.14, several things are immediately apparent. First, columns B, C, and D contain several cells with number signs (#######) instead of recognizable data. This can be corrected simply by widening the column (put the cursor between the letters heading any two columns and drag it to the right or double-left-click). A second thing that is immediately apparent as one looks at column B is that several of the dates (5/15/2029, in row 4, for example) have not even occurred yet. But this is the date of birth column. Obviously, Excel

FIGURE 3.14. DATA AS INITIALLY IMPORTED FROM A TEXT FILE.

	A	B	C	D	E	F	G	H	I
1	F	#######	9/11/2002	9/15/2002	294	2426.48	2003.62	2	0
2	F	1/5/2015	4/14/2002	4/22/2002	139	6815.61	1072.17	4	4
3	F	3/16/1932	5/1/2002	5/11/2002	34	7596.68	4096.98	6	0
4	M	5/15/2029	2/5/2002	2/10/2002	140	6450.77	1710.79	5	0
5	F	#######	4/9/2002	4/12/2002	141	3542.79	1914.9	3	7
6	F	#######	1/13/2002	1/15/2002	15	2590.86	2601.14	5	4
7	F	6/23/2028	2/9/2002	2/14/2002	294	5082.83	2035.31	7	2
8	M	#######	9/11/2002	9/17/2002	241	3580.55	2320.42	6	0
9	M	8/7/2029	#######	11/6/2002	335	11045.79	4184.26	1	0
10	F	1/3/2008	#######	#######	148	19708.11	12158.49	4	0
11	F	7/2/2007	6/1/2002	6/12/2002	89	8953.38	4345.84	4	0

has misinterpreted the date 5/15/1929 and has made it a complete century later. This problem is one that should be anticipated when using date data that is for a date prior to 1930. Any date prior to that time that is not given as the entire date (that is, is given only as the last two digits of the year) is treated by Excel on being imported as a date in 20xx rather than a date in 19xx. But since we know that this is date of birth, it is obvious that we will have to change any dates shown in the imported file as 20xx to dates in the form 19xx.

The solution to this problem is a little tricky, but it depends on the fact that Excel stores dates as a number beginning with 1/1/1900 as 1. The number that corresponds to 1/1/2000 is 36526. In order to convert the dates in column B in Figure 3.14 that are given as 20xx to numbers in the form 19xx, it will be necessary to subtract 36525 from each of the dates that are in the form 20xx. Figure 3.15 shows the data shown in Figure 3.14. The columns containing dates have been widened to show all the dates (no ######). In addition, a column has been inserted between B and C, as shown in Figure 3.14, in which the corrected date of birth has been calculated.

In order to insert a column or a row between two other columns or rows, left click the cursor on the letter (column) or number (row) where you wish to make the insert. Then right click the cursor while it is still on the letter or number and select insert from the menu. A column will be moved to the left and a new one inserted. A row will be moved down and a new one inserted.

The =IF() statement that was used to produce the correct date is shown in the formula line of Figure 3.15. The =IF() statement says that if the date given in column B is <36526 (that is, if it is a date prior to 1/1/2000), it should remain as in column B. But if not, it should be changed to whatever is in column B

FIGURE 3.15. MAKING IMPORTED DATES CENTURY-CORRECT.

C1	▼	=	=IF(B1<36526,B1,B1-36525)							
	A	B	C	D	E	F	G	H	I	J
1	F	11/28/1955	11/28/1955	9/11/2002	9/15/2002	294	2426.48	2003.62	2	0
2	F	1/5/2015	1/5/1915	4/14/2002	4/22/2002	139	6815.61	1072.17	4	4
3	F	3/16/1932	3/16/1932	5/1/2002	5/11/2002	34	7596.68	4096.98	6	0
4	M	5/15/2029	5/15/1929	2/5/2002	2/10/2002	140	6450.77	1710.79	5	0
5	F	11/27/2019	11/27/1919	4/9/2002	4/12/2002	141	3542.79	1914.9	3	7
6	F	11/22/2016	11/22/1916	1/13/2002	1/15/2002	15	2590.86	2601.14	5	4
7	F	6/23/2028	6/23/1928	2/9/2002	2/14/2002	294	5082.83	2035.31	7	2
8	M	12/27/1936	12/27/1936	9/11/2002	9/17/2002	241	3580.55	2320.42	6	0
9	M	8/7/2029	8/7/1929	10/31/2002	11/6/2002	335	11045.79	4184.26	1	0
10	F	1/3/2008	1/3/1908	11/11/2002	11/25/2002	148	19708.11	12158.49	4	0
11	F	7/2/2007	7/2/1907	6/1/2002	6/12/2002	89	8953.38	4345.84	4	0

minus 36525 (a century of days). There is one small drawback to this strategy. In the unlikely event that a person was actually born in the 1800s rather than in the 1900s, this would change his or her date of birth to a date near the end of the 1900s. This can possibly be checked for these data, however, because anyone who had a birth date in the late 1900s would quite likely not be eligible for Medicare. With other types of data, it might be more difficult to determine if a date of birth should be prior to 1900.

Having corrected the date of birth in column C, several other modifications should be made to the imported data set. First, the current column C, which gives the corrected date of birth, should be changed from a formula dependent on column B to the value shown in column C. This can be done by using the sequence Copy/Paste Special/Values for the data in column C (and it can be done while the data are still highlighted, as shown in Figure 3.15). Having done this, it is a good idea to eliminate column B by left-clicking on the B at the top of the column, and then right-clicking and selecting Delete. This will put the corrected date of birth in column B. A new first row (row 1) should be added as a place to put an identifier for each variable. A new first column (column A) should be added as a place to put a unique identifier for each hospital stay (an ID number). Finally, the formatting for the hospital charges and actual Medicare payments can be changed from general to dollar format to clearly appear as dollar amounts. This can be done by first highlighting the cells that should be in dollar format and then selecting Format/Cells/Currency. The completed transformation of the data is shown (again, for the first ten observations) in Figure 3.16. At this point the data should be saved as an Excel file.

The ID number given in Figure 3.16 may not seem important, since each record is in a different row and it is not likely that one row will be confused with another. But the ID number can be used to return the data set to the original order

FIGURE 3.16. DATA FILE IMPORTED TO EXCEL WITH ID AND VARIABLE LABELS.

	A	B	C	D	E	F	G	H	I	J
1	ID	Sex	DOB	DOA	DOD	DRG	Charges	Medicare	Diag	ICD-9
2	1	F	11/28/1955	9/11/2002	9/15/2002	294	$ 2,426.48	$ 2,003.62	2	0
3	2	F	1/5/1915	4/14/2002	4/22/2002	139	$ 6,815.61	$ 1,072.17	4	4
4	3	F	3/16/1932	5/1/2002	5/11/2002	34	$ 7,596.68	$ 4,096.98	6	0
5	4	M	5/15/1929	2/5/2002	2/10/2002	140	$ 6,450.77	$ 1,710.79	5	0
6	5	F	11/27/1919	4/9/2002	4/12/2002	141	$ 3,542.79	$ 1,914.90	3	7
7	6	F	11/22/1916	1/13/2002	1/15/2002	15	$ 2,590.86	$ 2,601.14	5	4
8	7	F	6/23/1928	2/9/2002	2/14/2002	294	$ 5,082.83	$ 2,035.31	7	2
9	8	M	12/27/1936	9/11/2002	9/17/2002	241	$ 3,580.55	$ 2,320.42	6	0
10	9	M	8/7/1929	10/31/2002	11/6/2002	335	$11,045.79	$ 4,184.26	1	0
11	10	F	1/3/1908	11/11/2002	11/25/2002	148	$19,708.11	$12,158.49	4	0

if it is sorted on some variable, such as hospital charges or Medicare payments. It can be used to ensure that data stay with the right observation if a subset of observations and variables is moved to another spreadsheet. In general, it is good practice to include an ID number. It takes up little space in a file, and if you do not include it, you will wish you had.

Usually, importing any data set to Excel and getting it into a format that looks like an Excel spreadsheet (and ensuring that such things as date of birth look reasonable) is not the last step in getting data ready for analysis. In certain cases (such as date of birth), it might be desirable to perform some data checks to see if the data are all within a reasonable range. It was mentioned earlier that in the unlikely event that someone represented in the data file was born before 1900, the method used here to give the correct date of birth would give a date incorrectly recorded as 19xx rather than 18xx. But this would show up in the data file as a date in the 1990s (assuming that no one is over 112 years of age). So one way to ensure that no one has been incorrectly shown as having been born in the 1990s, when they were actually born in the 1890s, is to check the date of birth column (DOB) for a date in the 1990s.

A date in the 1990s in the date of birth column can be found simply by looking at each individual entry in column C. But even with only one hundred records, this is unnecessarily time-consuming. A better choice is to use the =IF() statement as shown in Equation 3.1.

$$=IF(C2<32874,1,0) \tag{3.1}$$

where C2 references the first data cell in column C (date of birth) and 32874 is the number corresponding to the date, 1/1/1990.

This =IF() statement will record a 1 for dates of birth prior to 1990 and a zero for any dates of birth shown as after 1990. The =IF() statement should be put into an unused column in the spreadsheet (for example, column K). It should then be copied to the end of the data file (in this case, the first 101 rows in the spreadsheet). An easy way to determine if any of the dates are in the 1990s is to sum the column containing the =IF() statement. If the sum is one hundred, then it is likely that no dates of birth should have been recorded as in the 1800s. If the sum is less than one hundred, it is easy to find the records for which date of birth should probably have been recorded as 18xx by sorting the entire data set on the column containing the =IF() statement.

In the case of the hospital data being discussed here, none of the dates of birth are recorded as being in the 1990s, so it is probably unlikely that there are any records in the data file with true date of birth prior to 1900. Once the =IF() statement has done its job to determine if the data in the date of birth column are correct, the column containing the =IF() statement can be deleted.

Other logical checks might be made on the data as initially imported. For example, it might be useful to be certain that every entry in the column representing sex is coded either M or F. This can be done by using either the =IF() statement (in this case, a nested =IF() statement) or an =OR() statement. The two statements that can check for either an M or an F in column B are as those shown in Equation 3.2.

$$=IF(B2="F",1,IF(B2="M",1,0))$$
$$\text{or} \tag{3.2}$$
$$=OR(B2="F",B2="M")$$

where B2 references the first data cell in column B.

In the case of the =IF() statement in Equation 3.2, Excel first checks to see if the entry in B2 (or whatever cell is being referenced) is an "F". The quote marks are necessary for Excel to recognize a text character. It will not recognize any text character without quote marks. If Excel finds an "F", it will put a 1 in the cell in which the =IF() statement appears. If the entry in the referenced cell is not an "F", Excel then checks to see if it is an "M". If it finds an "M", it will record a 1. If Excel finds neither an "F" nor an "M", it will record a 0. The entries in the column in which =IF() is invoked can then be summed to determine if the sum is equal to the number of observations. If not, the whole date file can be sorted on the =IF() column to find the anomalous data entries in column B. It should be pointed out that "F" and "f" are the same character to Excel, as they are in general to you and me. Excel sees both capital letters and small letters as the same in function applications. So the statement in Equation 3.2 will also find an "f".

The =OR() statement operates much the same way as =IF(). But it checks both "F" and "M" and if it finds either, it records a TRUE in the column in which it is invoked. If it finds neither "F" nor "M", it records FALSE. Whether there are any entries that are not "F" or "M" in the column, recording sex can be determined by counting the number of TRUE entries in the column in which the =OR() statement was invoked. If this is equal to the number of observations, then sex is recorded as "F" or "M" (or "f" or "m") for each observation. Counting the number of TRUE entries is easier than looking at each entry in the column in which =OR() is invoked. It can be done with the =COUNTIF() function, as shown in Equation 3.3.

$$=COUNTIF(K2:K101,TRUE) \quad\quad (3.3)$$

where K2:K101 references the data cells in which the =OR() function has been invoked.

Again, once the data checks indicated here have been made, the column in which the check has been carried out can be deleted from the data set. This helps keep the data set from becoming cluttered with unneeded information.

There are a number of other data checks that might be carried out. These would depend entirely on whether it is possible to specify what codes should appear in given cells. For example, it could be possible to see if date of discharge (in column E) is always later than date of admission (column D). It might be possible to determine if the code given for DRG was, in fact, a legitimate DRG code. But that could require a large number of nested =IF() statements and it still might not work. Incidentally, it is possible to nest up to sixteen =IF() statements together. Excel will not deal with more than sixteen nested =IF() statements.

Having checked for data errors, it is time to think about the kind of analysis that will be done with the data. As an initial step, it is likely that at some point in any analysis involving this data set, length of hospital stay will be important information. Similarly, it is quite possible that the age of the patient at the time of hospitalization will be of interest. So, at a minimum, these two pieces of information should be developed from what is already in the data.

Length of hospital stay (LOS) can be determined simply by subtracting the date of discharge (DOD) from the date of admission (DOA). Just as Excel can deal with addition or subtraction in regard to a date and a number, it can also deal with addition and subtraction in regard to two dates. Figure 3.17 shows the calculation of the length of stay in days by subtracting the date in column D from the date in column E (see the equation line in the figure). A new column was first inserted between DOD and DRG, and then the subtraction was carried out in the new column F, labeled LOS. When the calculation was made, the initial result was not 4 (for cell F2) but rather 1/4/1900. It was necessary to

FIGURE 3.17. CALCULATION OF LENGTH OF STAY.

	F2		=	=E2-D2		
	B	C	D	E	F	G
1	Sex	DOB	DOA	DOD	LOS	DRG	Cha
2	F	11/28/1955	9/11/2002	9/15/2002	4	294	$ 2
3	F	1/5/1915	4/14/2002	4/22/2002	8	139	$ 6
4	F	3/16/1932	5/1/2002	5/11/2002	10	34	$ 7
5	M	5/15/1929	2/5/2002	2/10/2002	5	140	$ 6
6	F	11/27/1919	4/9/2002	4/12/2002	3	141	$ 3
7	F	11/22/1916	1/13/2002	1/15/2002	2	15	$ 2
8	F	6/23/1928	2/9/2002	2/14/2002	5	294	$ 5
9	M	12/27/1936	9/11/2002	9/17/2002	6	241	$ 3
10	M	8/7/1929	10/31/2002	11/6/2002	6	335	$11
11	F	1/3/1908	11/11/2002	11/25/2002	14	148	$10

reformat the data in column F from date to general in order for it to appear as days of stay.

Calculation of age at admission by subtracting the date of birth from the date of admission would work, in general, but would be a little more complicated. First, it would be necessary to make the subtraction; then convert the resulting age in days from a date format to general format. Finally, it would be necessary to divide the resulting age in days by 365 (or 365.25, allowing for leap years). This would still not give exactly the right age in years and fractions of years, because the number of leap years one has lived through will not always be exactly one fourth of the years lived. An easier way to find the age is to use the Excel function, =YEARFRAC() which will give the number of years and fractions of years between two dates.

The use of =YEARFRAC() is shown in Figure 3.18. A new column has been inserted between DOB and DOA and given the title "Age." Age has been calculated as is shown in the formula line of the spreadsheet depicted in the table. It does not matter in what order the two columns are referenced in the =YEARFRAC() function, the function calculates the number of years between the two dates in either order. An additional function is included in the calculation of age and shows how function statements in Excel can be used together to accomplish a desired data goal. The function =TRUNC() truncates (that is, cuts off) a number at a specified number of decimal digits. If no number of decimal digits is specified (as in this case), the number is assumed to be zero. After about three years, we cease to refer to people as being a certain number of years old and fractions of years, and refer to them only as the number of years they have attained. So even though the first person on the list (who was born on November 28, 1955, and entered the hospital on September 11, 2002) was actually 46.786 years old at the time of admission, we would refer to her as being forty-six years old.

FIGURE 3.18. CALCULATION OF AGE.

	D2	▼		=	=TRUNC(YEARFRAC(E2,C2))	
	A	B	C	D	E	F	
1	ID	Sex	DOB	Age	DOA	DOD	LO
2	1	F	11/28/1955	46	9/11/2002	9/15/2002	
3	2	F	1/5/1915	87	4/14/2002	4/22/2002	
4	3	F	3/16/1932	70	5/1/2002	5/11/2002	
5	4	M	5/15/1929	72	2/5/2002	2/10/2002	
6	5	F	11/27/1919	82	4/9/2002	4/12/2002	
7	6	F	11/22/1916	85	1/13/2002	1/15/2002	
8	7	F	6/23/1928	73	2/9/2002	2/14/2002	
9	8	M	12/27/1936	65	9/11/2002	9/17/2002	
10	9	M	8/7/1929	73	10/31/2002	11/6/2002	
11	10	F	1/3/1908	94	11/11/2002	11/25/2002	

Now that the age at admission and length of stay have been calculated, it is reasonable to assume that we will not need DOB, DOA, or DOD (date of birth, date of admission, and data of discharge, respectively) any further in our data analysis. So we can now create a spreadsheet that does not include these variables. To do this, we insert a new spreadsheet in the existing Excel workbook with Insert/Worksheet. We then highlight the entire original worksheet (containing the data as originally imported to Excel) by right-clicking on the box in the extreme upper left-hand corner of the spreadsheet (the intersection of the letters designating the columns and the numbers designating the rows) and select Edit/Copy. And then we move to the new spreadsheet (which is probably labeled "Sheet1") and left-click in cell A1. Finally, we select Edit/Paste. The entire data set will now be copied to the new spreadsheet.

Having copied the data set to the new spreadsheet, it is now possible to delete the columns DOB, DOA, and DOD. But before doing that, it is necessary to convert the two variables—Age and LOS—from formulas depending on DOB, DOA, and DOD to actual numbers. To do this, first highlight the entire Age column, and while the column is highlighted select Edit/Copy/Edit/Paste Special/Values. This will change the entries in the Age column from a formula depending on DOB and DOA to actual numbers. Repeat the process for LOS. Now you can delete DOB, DOA, and DOD by clicking on the appropriate column letter (C for DOB in Figure 3.18) and selecting Edit/Delete.

One last data modification should be discussed before leaving the topic of importing data and making it ready for analysis. This is the transformation of categorical variables to numeric variables. Certain data analysis techniques to be discussed later in the book—such as cross-tabulations and chi-square statistics, *t* tests, or analysis of variance—can accept categorical variables in the form—for

FIGURE 3.19. IMPORTED FILE READY FOR ANALYSIS.

	C2		▼		=	=IF(B2="F",1,0)			
	A	B	C	D	E	F	G	H	I	J
1	ID	Sex	Sex1	Age	LOS	DRG	Charges	Medicare	Diag	ICD-9
2	1	F	1	46	4	294	$ 2,426.48	$ 2,003.62	2	0
3	2	F	1	87	8	139	$ 6,815.61	$ 1,072.17	4	4
4	3	F	1	70	10	34	$ 7,596.68	$ 4,096.98	6	0
5	4	M	0	72	5	140	$ 6,450.77	$ 1,710.79	5	0
6	5	F	1	82	3	141	$ 3,542.79	$ 1,914.90	3	7
7	6	F	1	85	2	15	$ 2,590.86	$ 2,601.14	5	4
8	7	F	1	73	5	294	$ 5,082.83	$ 2,035.31	7	2
9	8	M	0	65	6	241	$ 3,580.55	$ 2,320.42	6	0
10	9	M	0	73	6	335	$11,045.79	$ 4,184.26	1	0
11	10	F	1	84	11	148	$12,708.11	$12,158.48	4	0

example, of sex as "F" or "M". Other techniques, particularly regression, cannot accept categorical variables. But a variable such as sex can be included as an independent variable in regression if it is recoded as what is called a *dummy variable*. A dummy variable is a variable that takes on two values (as does sex) but is coded 1 for one of the values and 0 for the other.

The result of the import process with the data modified for analysis might be as that shown in Figure 3.19. That figure shows Sex1 as modified to a 1/0 variable (with the =IF() statement that produces that change shown in the formula bar). It also shows the ID number and the other variables—Sex, Age, LOS, DRG, Charges, Medicare (payments), Diag (diagnosis), and ICD-9. This working file no longer contains any dates. But if the dates become important at some time during the analysis, it will always be possible to recover them from the original imported worksheet by matching the ID numbers on both worksheets.

Exercises for Section 3.3

1. Use the data in Chpt 3–3.txt (this is the data set discussed in Section 3.3).
   a. Import the data to an Excel spreadsheet by using the Excel Import Wizard.
   b. Make the data century correct as discussed in relation to Figure 3.15.
   c. Provide a label line above the data (it will become row 1) and label the data, as shown in Figure 3.16.
   d. Insert a column after DOD, as shown in Figure 3.17, and calculate a length of stay for each observation.
   e. Insert a column after DOB and calculate Age for each person, as shown in Figure 3.18.

f. Insert a column after Sex and create a variable Sex1, as shown in Figure 3.19.

g. Save the resulting file as an Excel file.

2. Chpt 3–4.txt is a data file for fifty people from which the first twenty were selected, as shown in Figure 3.2. Import the data to an Excel spreadsheet by using the Import Wizard and do the following:

a. Insert a column at A and give every observation an ID number.

b. Insert a column at B and, using Date of Birth and Date of Visit, calculate an Age for each person.

c. Insert a column at D and, using Opinion 1, convert the words to numbers, with All of the time being 5, Some of the time being 4, and so on. Name this variable Opinion 1a.

d. Insert a column at E and, using Opinion 2, convert the words to numbers, with Strongly agree being 5, Agree being 4, and so on. Name this variable Opinion 2a.

e. Insert a column at F, name it Charges, and accumulate the costs for Procedure 1 through Procedure 4 in that column.

f. Insert a column at G, name it Visit Time, and, using Arrival time and Departure time, calculate the number of minutes for each visit. (Hint: format Visit time using the first format option under Time.)

g. Use Copy and Paste Special/Values to fix all the calculations and save the result as a .xls file.

Section 3.4　Missing Data

One thing that has not yet been discussed in regard to the use of data—either collected by the investigator or taken from an existing source—is missing data. The term *missing data* refers to the situation in which some of the observations have no data at all for some or all of the variables under study. In the example given in Section 3.3, the missing data issue was not considered because it was known that there were no data missing at the outset. But in most real applications, it is likely that some of the observations will have missing data. The question then is, what to do about this?

First, it is important to recognize that virtually all statistical techniques assume complete data. If one wished to use a statistic to determine, for example, if males had greater or lesser hospital charges than females, based on the data discussed in the previous section, it would be assumed that complete data were available for sex and hospital charges for all one hundred observations. But let us now assume that complete data were not available for all one hundred observations. Let us assume that some of the data for charges are missing—specifically, that there are no charge data for nine of the one hundred observations. How might we deal with that situation?

The simplest way to deal with the missing charges in this case would be to delete those observations from the data set and base the analysis on ninety-one rather than one hundred observations. There are difficulties with this strategy, however. The first and, in this case, the least important is that dropping the observations with no charge data from the data set reduces the number of observations under consideration and, consequently, the likelihood of finding a statistically significant difference between males and females, if one exists. In general, the more observations one has made, the more likely it is that statistical significance, if it exists, will be found. But going from one hundred to ninety-one cases is likely to have little effect on statistical outcomes, because it is a proportionally small decrease in an already relatively large number for statistical purposes. However, going from one hundred cases to thirty or from thirty cases to twenty would have a substantial effect on the ability to find statistically significant results.

Dropping observations can become even more of a problem if there are missing values in more than one of the variables that are to be considered in statistical analysis. Perhaps there might be nine missing values for charges and five for sex. Unless all the missing values for sex are also missing for charges, there will be more than nine total cases with missing values. All hypothesis testing requires at least two variables, so the number of nonoverlapping missing values in the two variables will determine the number of cases without data. In regression analysis there may be a number of variables involved. The total number of missing values will be the total of nonoverlapping missing values for all variables. In some cases, this will act to reduce the total data set to unacceptable levels. In such a case, there are two strategies. The first is to try to go back to the original source to obtain data for the missing values. But this is often impossible.

The second strategy is to impute values for those that are missing. There are a number of ways that this may be done, none of which gets high marks from statisticians but which are nevertheless used. The simplest and least time-consuming is to use the mean of the available data to fill in the missing values. So if there are nine missing values for charges and the mean value for charge for the ninety-one other observations is $5676.24, then that value could be assigned to the observations with missing values. There are a number of other strategies that can be used to assign missing values, all of which provide somewhat more sophisticated ways of assigning values than does using the simple mean. In general, this text will not cover these techniques in any detail.

There is a significant problem to assigning any type of imputed value to data that are missing. Regardless of how it is done, assigning a value to a missing data element will inevitably reduce the variance in that variable and will be more likely to produce statistically significant results than if the missing values were simply deleted from the data. With this fact in mind, some investigators have used what is known as a Monte Carlo technique to randomly assign values within reasonable ranges to the missing elements and see how these assigned values affect the statistical results over a large number of trials. While this is probably the ideal method for assigning missing values, it is both time-consuming and costly in terms of data analysis.

The bottom line with regard to missing data, then, is that it is probably best to drop cases with missing values if fewer than 10 percent of cases will be dropped and the overall sample size remains relatively large—for example, over thirty. If these circumstances do not prevail, randomly assigning reasonable values to the missing elements is probably the best strategy.

CHAPTER FOUR

DATA DISPLAY: DESCRIPTIVE PRESENTATION, EXCEL GRAPHING CAPABILITY

One of the most important aspects of statistical analysis is to be able to present the results of the analysis in a way that is easily accessible to your audience. Excel provides several useful tools to accomplish accessible presentations. These include, in particular, the Excel frequency function, the Excel pivot table report capabilities and the Excel graphing capability.

Section 4.1 The Excel Frequency Function for the Display of Numerical Data

One of the recurring needs in statistical analysis is to be able to summarize quickly and efficiently the data that are under analysis. Later sections of the book, particularly Chapter Six, discuss measures of central tendency and dispersion (the mean and the standard deviation), which are useful devises for summarizing numerical data. This section discusses the Excel =FREQUENCY() function that was introduced in Chapter Two.

Recall the data file that was imported to Excel in Chapter Three. When the import process was finished, that file contained an ID number for each record and nine variables. The variables were Sex (as indicated by "F" and "M"), Sex1 (the Sex variable recoded to 1 and 0), Age, LOS (length of hospital stay), DRG, Charges, Medicare (payments), Diag (number of diagnoses), and ICD-9 (the admitting ICD-9 code). Although the file was only one hundred records selected from a much larger set of records, it was still impossible in the original presentation of the data import discussion to show more than a few of the records in the figures that were presented. Those figures gave some indication of what the data were like. For example, age tended to be above the average age of the general population, which is not surprising, since this is a Medicare-eligible population. Charges—for the records that were visible in the tables—were in the thousands of dollars. Length of stay ranged from two days to more than ten. But viewing the small portion of the records shown in the tables does not give a very good idea of what the data actually look like.

Of course, if one has access to the Excel data file, it is possible to view all one hundred observations to get a better idea of the nature of the data. But an alternative to viewing all the data as one hundred separate observations is to use the =FREQUENCY() function to summarize the data. To see the use of the =FREQUENCY() function for summarizing data, consider the variable age. We are going to generate a frequency distribution for the variable age that groups the ages into a small number of categories and that includes all the ages in the one hundred observations. The first step in creating the frequency distribution is to determine the minimum and maximum ages represented in the data. To do this, we can use the Excel =MIN() and =MAX() functions, as seen in Figure 4.1.

The =MIN() and =MAX() functions are a way of determining the minimum and maximum values in any set of data. In Figure 4.1, it can be seen that the minimum age is thirty-nine (cell C2) and the maximum age is ninety-six (cell C3). The way in which the =MIN() and =MAX() functions are written is shown for =MIN() in the formula line. Basically, the =MIN() and =MAX() functions each

FIGURE 4.1. =MIN() AND =MAX() FUNCTIONS.

C2	▼	=	=MIN(B2:B101)		
	A	B	C	D	E
1	ID	Age			
2	1	46	39		
3	2	87	96		
4	3	70			
5	4	72			
6	5	82			
7	6	85			
8	7	73			
9	8	65			
10	9	73			
11	10	94			

take a single argument, but this argument represents a data range. In Excel, data ranges are indicated by the two cell references that define the range separated by a colon.

In developing a frequency distribution, it is important to have few enough categories to ensure that there will be observations in each category but enough to get a view of how the data are actually distributed. In general, five to eight categories are probably useful in developing a frequency distribution. Fewer than five will not give enough categories to show a meaningful picture of the data, and many more than eight is difficult to conceptualize in a single look. Having determined that the minimum age in the one hundred records is thirty-nine and the maximum is ninety-six, it is necessary to decide how many categories the frequency distribution will contain. In this case, we will develop a frequency distribution with six categories.

Figure 4.2 shows the completed frequency distribution with six categories. The individual cells contain the following information. Cell C4 contains the difference between ninety-six and thirty-nine. This age separation (fifty-seven years) will be divided into six categories for the frequency distribution. Cell C5 is 57 divided by 6. Each category for the frequency distribution will include 9.5 years of age. Column D represents what Excel refers to as *Bins*, Bins are the categories that define the frequency distributions. The first bin value is the minimum age (cell C2) plus the size of the first frequency category (9.5 years in cell C5). Each observation with an age of 48.5 years or less (actually, forty-eight years, since the years are given only in whole numbers) will be recorded in cell E2 to represent that it is in that age category.

FIGURE 4.2. FREQUENCY DISTRIBUTION OF AGE.

E2	▼		= {=FREQUENCY(B2:B101,D2:D7)}		
	A	B	C	D	E	F
1	ID	Age		Bins	Freq	
2	1	46	39	48.5	2	
3	2	87	96	58.0	4	
4	3	70	57	67.5	5	
5	4	72	9.5	77.0	36	
6	5	82		86.5	33	
7	6	85		96.0	20	
8	7	73				
9	8	65				
10	9	73				
11	10	94				

FIGURE 4.3. FORMULAS FOR FREQUENCY DISTRIBUTION OF AGE.

	A	B	C	D	E
1	ID	Age		Bins	Freq
2	1	46	=MIN(B2:B101)	=C2+C5	=FREQUENCY(B2:B101,D2:D7)
3	2	87	=MAX(B2:B101)	=D2+$C$5	=FREQUENCY(B2:B101,D2:D7)
4	3	70	=C3-C2	=D3+$C$5	=FREQUENCY(B2:B101,D2:D7)
5	4	72	=C4/6	=D4+$C$5	=FREQUENCY(B2:B101,D2:D7)
6	5	82		=D5+$C$5	=FREQUENCY(B2:B101,D2:D7)
7	6	85		=D6+$C$5	=FREQUENCY(B2:B101,D2:D7)
8	7	73			
9	8	65			
10	9	73			
11	10	94			

Cell D2 is simply cell C2 plus cell C5. However, the additional bin values make use of the F4 function key and the dollar sign convention so that the formula for these bins need to be written only once (in cell D3) and copied into the remaining four cells by dragging or double-left-clicking the lower right corner of cell D3. Figure 4.3 shows the formulas that have been used to create the frequency distribution shown in Figure 4.2. Essentially, the bin range (9.5 years) has been added successively to each of the previous bin values. When the =FREQUENCY() function is invoked, Excel looks at each data value and compares it with each Bin value. If the data value is equal to or less than any bin value but larger than any other bin value, Excel adds one to the total for that bin. It is important to remember that the value of a bin that appears on the Excel spreadsheet is the largest value that will be recorded in any specific bin. The =FREQUENCY() function is shown in the formula line of Figure 4.2 and in the cells E2 to E7 of Figure 4.3. The format of the =FREQUENCY() function can be seen in either view. The function takes two arguments, the first being the data range (in this case, B2:B101 representing the Age data) and the second being the bin range (in this case, D2:D7). In the formula line of Figure 4.2, the two curly brackets that surround the =FREQUENCY() function indicate that it is an Excel function that is invoked by holding down Ctrl/Shift and then hitting Enter.

The formulas view of the spreadsheet is available at any time by clicking Tools/Options, selecting the View screen, and checking the Formulas box, then clicking OK. The same process can return the standard view by removing the check in the Formulas box.

FIGURE 4.4. CHART OF THE AGE FREQUENCY DISTRIBUTION.

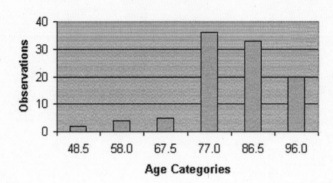

The view of the data in Figure 4.4 clearly shows the tail to the left that makes these data skewed to the left. It also shows that the largest single category is the

Using the Chart Function of Excel to Graph a Frequency Distribution

The frequency distribution shown in cells E2:E7 of Figure 4.2 show a distribution that has only a few observations in the lower ages and many more in the upper ages. This type of distribution is said to be *skewed* to the left because it seems to tail off to the left. The fact that most people in the data set are in the older ages is not surprising, as this is a Medicare-eligible population. But the actual numbers in a frequency distribution are only one way of picturing (and hence understanding) the data. An additional valuable tool for viewing a frequency distribution that is provided by Excel is the chart function or graphing capability of Excel, which was also introduced in Chapter Two. If we use the Chart Wizard to construct a column chart of the data in cells E2:E7, it produces the result shown in Figure 4.4.

The Y axis in the chart—labeled Observations—was supplied automatically by Excel from the number of observations in each age group. The numbers in the X axis represent the bin values in cells D2:D7. These were included in the chart by selecting the Series tab in step 2 of the Chart Wizard-Chart Source Data—and then selecting Category (X) axis labels and highlighting the bin value range, D2:D7. The titles Graph of Age, Observations, and Age Categories were included on step 3 of the Chart Wizard—Chart Options-on the Titles tab.

In any chart, such as the one shown in Figure 4.4, the Y axis is always considered to be the vertical axis on the left and the X axis is always considered to be the horizontal axis on the bottom.

The view of the data in Figure 4.4 clearly shows the tail to the left that makes these data skewed to the left. It also shows that the largest single category is the

FIGURE 4.5. CHART OF AGE SHOWING BIN RANGES.

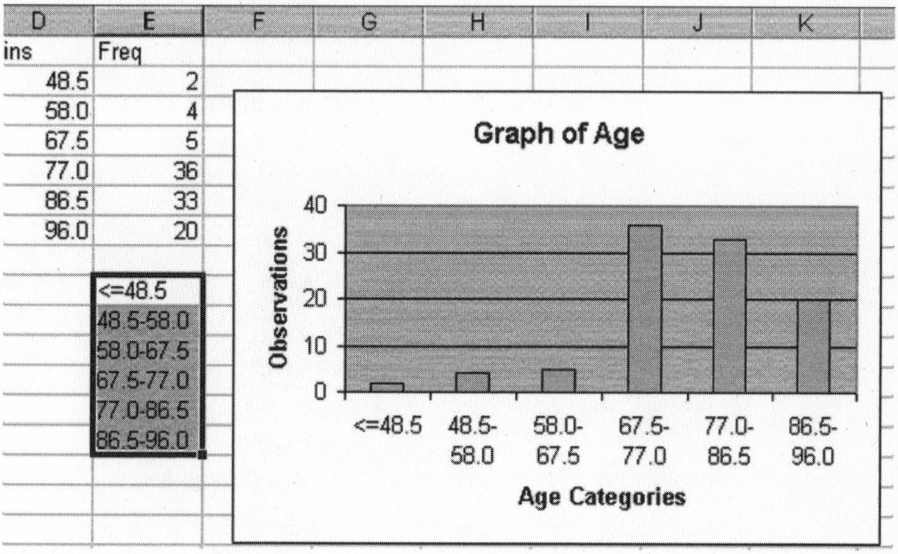

D	E	F	G	H	I	J	K
ins	Freq						
48.5	2						
58.0	4						
67.5	5						
77.0	36						
86.5	33						
96.0	20						
	<=48.5						
	48.5-58.0						
	58.0-67.5						
	67.5-77.0						
	77.0-86.5						
	86.5-96.0						

Graph of Age — a bar chart titled "Graph of Age" with Y axis "Observations" (0 to 40) and X axis "Age Categories" with labels <=48.5, 48.5-58.0, 58.0-67.5, 67.5-77.0, 77.0-86.5, 86.5-96.0.

age group with the X axis value of 77.0. It should be remembered that the X axis designation 77.0 actually refers to all observations with ages between 67.5 years and 77.0 years. This characteristic of Excel, to use the largest value in a frequency as the bin value, can be confusing when displayed in a chart such as that shown in Figure 4.4. Since the X axis values are supplied by the creator of the chart, it is possible to make the X axis titles more descriptive.

Figure 4.5 shows part of the spreadsheet for the age frequency distribution, which includes the graph of the frequency distribution with new X axis designations. These are put into the chart by first entering them as a set of categories in cells E9:E14. Then the X axis in the chart is changed by first left-clicking the chart and then selecting Chart/Source Data from the menu bar, picking the Series tab, and changing the Category (X) axis labels to cells E9:E14. This makes the X axis labels much more descriptive of what is actually in those categories and what the bars in the graph actually represent. It is worth mentioning that the chart shown in Figure 4.5 is the same chart (in the original spreadsheet) as that shown in Figure 4.4. This demonstrates an extremely useful and important characteristic of the chart function. When data or labels that make up the chart are changed, either by selecting different data or labels, or by changing the actual data or labels themselves, the comparable changes appear in the Excel chart.

It is important to mention that the categories shown in Figure 4.5 are still not exactly right. The range shown, for example, 48.5 to 58.0, is actually any age

FIGURE 4.6. LINE CHART DEPICTION OF AGE FREQUENCIES.

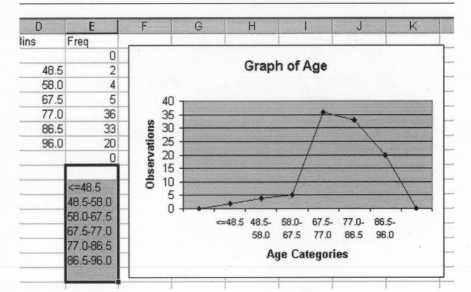

greater than 48.5 to 58.0, because if there were an age recorded as 48.5, it would be in the <=48.5 category. This is true in every other age category as well.

There are a number of other ways that data can be displayed using the Excel chart function. In fact, the Chart Wizard offers fourteen standard types of graphs and twenty of what Excel calls custom types. All of the standard types have a number of subtypes. For most of the work in this book, the simple column chart (frequently called a *histogram*) is all that will be used. It is useful to look at four other of the charts that Excel can produce, however.

The first alternative chart type is the line chart. The line chart is a column chart where the presentation is made with a single line rather than a number of columns. The data charted in Figure 4.6 are the same as the data charted in Figure 4.4 and Figure 4.5, but the columns have been changed to a single line. This is done by selecting the chart in Figure 4.5 and then Chart/Chart Type, and then choosing the line chart option. It is not uncommon to make the addition to the line chart by dropping the line to the X axis at each end. This was done by inserting a zero cell at both ends of the frequency distribution and a blank cell at each end of the age categories that form the X axis values. Then, both the zero values and the blank cells were included as part of the chart. The result is the data depiction in Figure 4.6.

A second chart of interest is the bar chart, as shown in Figure 4.7. The bar chart shows exactly the same information as that shown in the column chart, but

FIGURE 4.7. BAR CHART DEPICTION OF AGE FREQUENCIES.

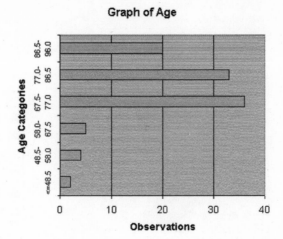

it shows it in a different orientation. To put the data into this chart, it was necessary only to select the chart in Figure 4.5, choose Chart/Chart Type, and then select the bar chart option from the Standard Types tab. Notice that with the bar chart the smallest charted value is always at the lower end of the vertical column.

A third chart that is useful to consider is the pie chart. The pie chart presents data as the pieces of a pie, each piece representing its proportional part of the whole. The notion that each piece represents its proportional part of the whole is a significant factor in the use of a pie chart. The pie chart assumes that the material depicted represents the entire set of information and, furthermore, that all the pieces accumulate to the total. This is true with the Age data. Each frequency category represents a part of the entire frequency distribution, and all taken together add to all hundred observations. The pie chart can be created from the original chart shown in Figure 4.5 by selecting the chart again, choosing Chart/Chart Types, and selecting Pie from the Standard Types tab. The result, after some manipulation of labels and axes, is shown in Figure 4.8.

It is important to reiterate that the pie chart, by its very nature, implies that 100 percent of observations of any type are being included in the graph. This is further depicted by the percentages that are shown in the chart in Figure 4.8. These percentages add to 100 percent. A pie chart should never be used to depict a total amount and its subcomponents together, or part of a total amount.

To this point, the discussion has focused on looking at the frequency distribution of a single variable at a time. Excel offers an entirely different type of chart that will be very useful in examining the relationship between two separate variables at the same time. This is what Excel calls the XY(Scatter) chart. The XY chart

FIGURE 4.8. PIE CHART DEPICTION OF AGE FREQUENCIES.

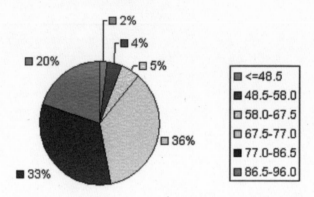

Graph of Age

FIGURE 4.9. XY(SCATTER) CHART OF AGE AND LOS.

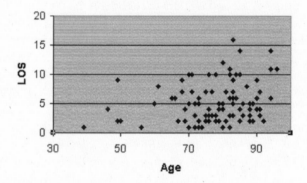

Graph of Age and LOS

requires two separate variables. The XY chart of Age and LOS (length of stay) is shown in Figure 4.9. Several points about this chart should be mentioned. First, this chart is based not on frequencies in categories, as the other charts discussed here have been, but on the actual values of the two variables. The horizontal axis, or X axis, represents the values of the variable Age. The lowest value of Age in the data set is thirty-nine and the highest value of Age is ninety-nine. The vertical axis, or Y axis, represents the values of the variable LOS (length of stay). LOS ranges, from the shortest length of stay of one day to the longest stay of sixteen days.

Excel always treats the left-most variable in the spreadsheet as the X axis variable when constructing an XY chart and the right-most variable as the Y axis variable. The variables do not have to be in contiguous columns to construct the XY chart, but the data must begin in the same row in order to successfully construct an XY chart. Each four pointed star in the XY chart represents one observation. For example, the left-most star in the chart represents the single person who was thirty-nine years of age and had a hospital stay of one day. The only star above the line marked 15 on the vertical axis is the single person who had a sixteen-day hospital stay and, from the horizontal axis, appears to have been eighty-three years old. Each of the other points in the chart is interpreted in the same way, although one would not count on the chart to know the actual values. The chart works more to provide a general view of what the entire data *distribution* looks like. This information is valuable, particularly, in deciding whether regression analysis (discussed in Chapters Eleven to Thirteen) will be appropriate to the data.

Cumulative Frequencies and Percentage Distributions

Obtaining a frequency distribution of a numerical variable is one way to understand the nature of the data. It is often useful to look also at the cumulative frequency distribution and the percentage distributions and cumulative percentage distributions. This section considers these three distributions.

A cumulative frequency distribution begins with the smallest bin value and accumulates observations so that the first category contains only the observations in that bin, the second category contains observations in both the first and second bins, the third contains observations in the first three bins, and so on. Figure 4.10 shows a cumulative frequency distribution for the variable Age in cells F2:F7. The cumulative frequency was calculated by making cell F2 equal to cell E2 and then adding each successive cell in column E to the current total in column F. For example, cell F3 is F2+E3 and cell F4 is F3+E4.

FIGURE 4.10. CUMULATIVE FREQUENCY AND PERCENTAGE DISTRIBUTIONS.

	D	E	F	G	H
1	Bins	Freq	Cum Freq	Perc	Cum Perc
2	48.5	2	2	2%	2%
3	58.0	4	6	4%	6%
4	67.5	5	11	5%	11%
5	77.0	36	47	36%	47%
6	86.5	33	80	33%	80%
7	96.0	20	100	20%	100%

FIGURE 4.11. FORMULA VIEW OF FIGURE 4.10.

	D	E	F	G	H
1	Bins	Freq	Cum Freq	Perc	Cum Perc
2	=C2+C5	=FREQUENCY(B2:B101,D2:D7)	=E2	=E2/$F$7	=G2
3	=D2+$C$5	=FREQUENCY(B2:B101,D2:D7)	=F2+E3	=E3/$F$7	=H2+G3
4	=D3+$C$5	=FREQUENCY(B2:B101,D2:D7)	=F3+E4	=E4/$F$7	=H3+G4
5	=D4+$C$5	=FREQUENCY(B2:B101,D2:D7)	=F4+E5	=E5/$F$7	=H4+G5
6	=D5+$C$5	=FREQUENCY(B2:B101,D2:D7)	=F5+E6	=E6/$F$7	=H5+G6
7	=D6+$C$5	=FREQUENCY(B2:B101,D2:D7)	=F6+E7	=E7/$F$7	=H6+G7
8					

The formulas used to construct the cumulative frequency are shown in the formula view of Figure 4.10, which is given in Figure 4.11. Cell F2 in this view shows that it is simply equal to E2. Cell F3 shows that the number in that cell was developed with the Excel formula =F2+E3. Once the =F2+E3 has been entered into cell F3, the remainder of the cells in column F can be entered by placing the cursor in the lower right corner of cell F3 and either dragging the cell references down to cell F7 or double-clicking the lower right corner of cell F3. As the formula moves down each cell, it becomes the correct formula for that cell by virtue of the relative cell referencing of Excel. *It is extremely important to remember that, in general, you need enter any formula into Excel only once. You are doing way too much work if you enter the formulas for cells F3:F7 separately in each cell.*

Cells G2:G7 and H2:H7 in both Figure 4.10 and Figure 4.11 show the percentage distribution and the cumulative percentage distribution for the Age frequency data. Because the original data involved exactly one hundred observations, the percentage values are the same as the actual frequencies. In general, this will not be the case. In any event, the formulas for the percentage distribution are clearly different from the formulas for the actual frequencies (cells E2:E7), which rely on the =FREQUENCY() function. The formulas for the percentage distribution (column G) rely on the dollar sign convention (cycle through with function key F4) to fix cell F7 as the cell by which each value in column E is divided. Again, it is necessary only to enter the formula =E2/$F$7 (F7 is the cumulative total value) into cell G2. Then the formula can be copied into each of the other five cells in G. The relative reference to each cell in E in the numerator changes as the formula is copied down column G, but because of the dollar signs before the F and before the 7 in the denominator, that reference does not change.

The formulas for the cumulative percentage distribution (H2:H7) are the same as the formulas for the cumulative frequency distribution. Because of this, it is only necessary to copy the range F2:F7 and paste the copy in cell H2. That will enter all the values for the cumulative percentage distribution in H2:H7. It should be

FIGURE 4.12. GRAPH OF AGE SHOWING ACTUAL AND CUMULATIVE VALUES.

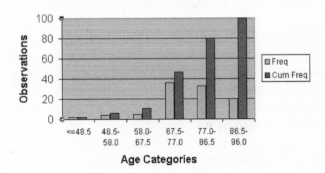

mentioned that the actual values that will appear in both G2:G7 and H2:H7 will be decimal values until they are reformatted to percentages. This can be done by highlighting G2:H7 and selecting Format/Cells and choosing Percentage on the Number tab, or by highlighting G2:H7 and left-clicking the % icon on the Formatting menu bar.

It may be useful to look at a graph that includes both the actual frequency and the cumulative frequency. Figure 4.12 shows such a graph. The actual frequency is in light grey and the cumulative frequency is shown in dark grey. It should be mentioned that there were a number of things done to this graph to make it look as it does (and almost all graphs need some modifications to make them look good when they are first created).

When a graph is first generated, it frequently is too narrow vertically to get a very good view of the comparative length of the columns, so this graph was stretched out both vertically and horizontally. (After left-clicking the chart, grab one of the black squares on the chart border to resize it.) The data labels, Freq and Cum Freq, were initially given as Series 1 and Series 2. These were changed by going to Chart/Source Data, selecting the Series tab, and renaming Series 1 as Freq in the Name box on the right of the series box on that tab. Once the name has been changed, the new name will appear in the Series window. Series 2 was renamed Cum Freq in the same way.

The age categories shown in Figure 4.12 were originally given in too large a font to be displayed entirely in the graph. They were also displayed at an angle because of their larger size. To put them into the form in which they now appear, it was first necessary to right-click anywhere in the set of numbers that appeared as the Age categories (the horizontal scale) for a Format Axis menu. After selecting that menu, the Font tab was selected and the font size changed to 9. Then the Alignment tab was selected and the cursor was used to move the diamond on that tab from the horizontal and back again. That produced the age category format, as shown in the figure.

The initial graph, before reformatting, also had a vertical scale that went to 120. As there are only a hundred total observations, and in order to indicate that the last dark grey column represented all of the observations, the vertical scale was changed so that it would go only to 100. This was done by right-clicking anywhere in the numbers on the vertical scale to get the Format Axis menu for the vertical axis, and then, after left-clicking that menu, selecting the Scale tab and changing the maximum to 100. The graph as it appears in Figure 4.12 is the result of all these operations.

The total number of changes and modifications that can be made to a graph to serve the purposes desired is extremely large—far beyond what can be described in this text. The plot area itself can be reformatted in a number of ways, the colors of the columns can be changed, and many other modifications can be made. The only way to get a good notion of the modifications that can be made in an Excel graph is to create a graph and try out the various options. Sooner or later, you will hit on a series of style changes that will best serve your purposes.

Types of Distributions

Frequency distributions can take on many different shapes, but four different distribution configurations deserve mention. These are *skewed left, skewed right, normal,* and *uniform distributions.* Figure 4.13 shows examples of these four types of distributions. The distribution that is skewed left appears to have a tail that moves off to the left side of the distribution while the bulk of the observations is to the right. The distribution that is skewed right appears to have a tail to the right while the bulk of the observations is to the left. The distribution that is generally referred to as normal will be discussed in detail in Chapters Five and Six, but it essentially has tails of equal length, and the bulk of the observations is in the center of the distribution. The uniform distribution (sometimes called a *flat* distribution) has equal numbers of observations at each point in the distribution.

The graph of Age shown in Figure 4.4, as well as subsequent graphs, is skewed to the left because the distribution shows the characteristic tail on the left side of the distribution. Data distributions may also be skewed to the right. In the data file under discussion thus far in this chapter, LOS (length of stay), Charges (total hospital charges), and Medicare (Medicare payments) are all skewed to the right.

Figure 4.14 shows the distribution of Medicare payments in six categories. It is clear that this distribution has a tail that moves off to the right, thus making

FIGURE 4.13. FOUR DISTRIBUTION TYPES.

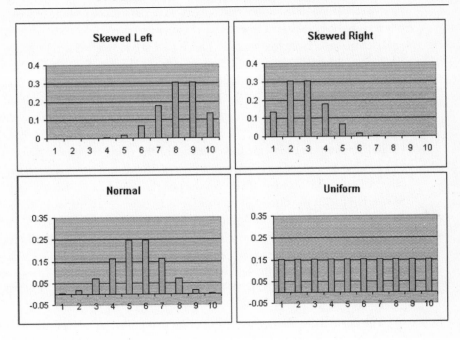

FIGURE 4.14. GRAPH OF MEDICARE PAYMENTS.

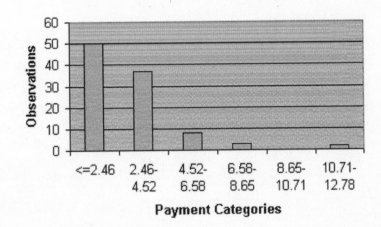

it right-skewed. In general, it is more common to encounter distributions that are right-skewed than distributions that are left-skewed. Costs of health services—either office visits, hospital stays, emergency room visits, or any other categories of cost—are likely to be skewed to the right. This is because most costs will be more or less similar, but there will be a few encounters with very high costs. This produces a distribution that is skewed to the right. Disease or morbidity patterns are similar.

The State of the World's Children 2001 (2000) provides one example of a distribution that is skewed to the right. UNICEF reports data on infant mortality for countries of the world (http://www.unicef.org/sowc01/tables/#). According to UNICEF, infant mortality for 149 countries of the world with more than one million inhabitants ranged in 1999 from a high of 182 deaths per thousand live births (Sierra Leone) to a low of three deaths per thousand live births (Sweden and Switzerland). But the distribution of infant mortality by countries of the world is skewed to the right, as demonstrated in Figure 4.15.

As Figure 4.15 shows, more than seventy countries of the World have infant mortality rates of thirty-three or less. The number of countries with infant mortality rates in each of the higher categories decreases monotonically to the 153 to 183 deaths category, where there are exactly five countries. This distribution is decidedly skewed to the right.

The normal distribution is a distribution that is skewed neither to the right nor to the left but, rather, has tails of approximately equal length. Exact characteristics

FIGURE 4.15. INFANT MORTALITY FOR 149 COUNTRIES OF THE WORLD.

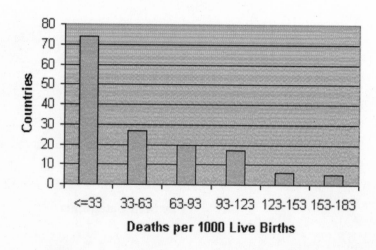

of normal distributions will be discussed in Chapters Five and Six. But for the current presentation, the notion that the normal distribution is skewed in neither direction is sufficient. Approximately normal distributions are found in many health-related types of data. The body temperature of healthy human beings, for example, is probably normally distributed around 98.6 degrees. Not every person's body temperature is exactly 98.6 degrees; body temperature varies from that *normal* temperature by a fraction of a degree or more. This variance is probably as likely to be below 98.6 as it is likely to be above 98.6 degrees. Average height of adults is another example of data that is generally normally distributed with a more or less equal number of persons on each side of the distribution.

Data on infant mortality for the world is skewed to the right. But data on infant mortality for the United States by state more closely approximates a normal distribution. Infant mortality in the United States ranged in 1998 from a low of 4.4 deaths per thousand live births (New Hampshire) to 10.2 deaths per thousand live births (Alabama) (U.S. National Center for Health Statistics, Table 125, 2000 Statistical Abstracts of the United States).

The graph of infant mortality by state in the United States is shown in Figure 4.16. This graph clearly shows that the bulk of states have infant mortality rates in the center of the distribution rather than at the left side. The number of states that have infant mortality rates at each end of the continuum is, while not exactly equal, certainly in the same order of magnitude. The infant

FIGURE 4.16. INFANT MORTALITY FOR STATES OF THE UNITED STATES.

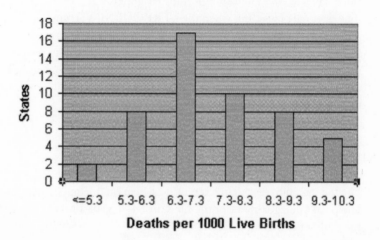

FIGURE 4.17. SIMULATION OF THE ROLL OF A FAIR DIE ONE HUNDRED TIMES.

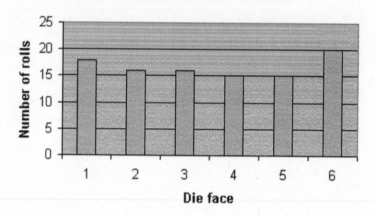

mortality rate by state in the United States is much closer to normal than that for the same measure by country of the world.

Uniform distributions are not often found in health statistics, but it is still useful for comparative purposes to show an example of a uniform distribution. A uniform distribution is one that has approximately equal numbers at each interval. To give an example of a uniform distribution, the Random Number Generation selection in the Data Analysis add-in was used and the Uniform distribution option was selected. This option allows one to generate a random number between any upper and lower limits. One hundred random numbers were generated in the range zero to six. The random number generation add-in produces numbers to nine decimal places, but when the =FREQUENCY() function is used to put these numbers into the six categories—1, 2, 3, 4, 5, and 6, a reasonable simulation of the roll of a fair die one hundred times is produced. The result is shown in Figure 4.17. An actual uniform distribution (or a simulated one as in Figure 4.17) will not look exactly like the example in Figure 4.13, but it will look approximately like that example.

Exercises for Section 4.1

Use the data file created in Exercise 1 of Section 3.3 (in Chapter Three) (or use the Hospital Charges sheet in the file Chpt 4–1.xls). This data set corresponds to the data set discussed in Section 4.1.

1. Select the variable Age and do the following:
   a. Using the =MIN(), =MAX(), and =FREQUENCY() functions, replicate Figure 4.2.
   b. Using the results of a, generate the chart shown in Figure 4.5 and put in the relevant labels as shown in that chart. Show this chart on the spreadsheet.
   c. Modifying the data as shown in Figure 4.6, generate a line chart as shown in that figure and show this chart on the spreadsheet.
   d. Create a bar chart as shown in Figure 4.7 and show this chart on the spreadsheet.
   e. Create a pie chart as shown in Figure 4.8 and modify the chart to look as much like that figure as possible and show this chart on the spreadsheet.
   f. Replicate the chart of Age and LOS as shown in Figure 4.9. Show this chart on the spreadsheet.
   g. Generate a cumulative frequency for the variable Age as well as percentage and cumulative percentage distributions as shown in Figure 4.10.
   h. Create a chart showing the actual and cumulative values of Age as given in Figure 4.12 and show this chart on the spreadsheet.

2. Select the variable Charges and do the following:
   a. Using the =MIN(), =MAX() and =FREQUENCY() functions, create a frequency distribution with seven categories.
   b. Using the results of a, generate a column chart for the data and put in relevant labels and show this chart on the spreadsheet.
   c. Transform the chart to a line chart and include the necessary additions to make the line drop to the horizontal axis at each end and show this chart on the spreadsheet.
   d. Create a bar chart from the data and show this chart on the spreadsheet.
   e. Create a pie chart from the data and put in appropriate labels and show this chart on the spreadsheet.
   f. Create a scatterplot for LOS and Charges and show this chart on the spreadsheet.
   g. Generate a cumulative frequency for the variable Charges as well as percentage and cumulative percentage distributions.
   h. Create a chart showing the actual and cumulative values of Charges and show this chart on the spreadsheet.

3. Use the SWC sheet in the file Chpt 4–1.xls and do the following:
   a. Generate the appropriate frequency distribution for infant mortality (IMR), and with it, replicate Figure 4.15.
   b. Generate a frequency distribution of five bins for under-five mortality (U5MR) and produce a column graph for that variable. Is it normal, flat, or skewed, and if skewed, in which direction?

   c. Generate a frequency distribution of eight bins for life expectancy at birth (LEB) and produce a column graph for that variable. Is it normal, flat, or skewed, and if skewed, in which direction?

4. Use the US IMR sheet in the file Chpt 4–1.xls and do the following:
   a. Generate the appropriate frequency distribution to replicate Figure 4.16 and replicate the figure.
   b. Generate a frequency distribution with twelve bin categories and use the column chart option to graph that frequency distribution.
   c. Which of a or b seems to you to provide the most useful information about the distribution?

5. Use the data from the Hospital Charges worksheet in Chpt 4–1.xls.
   a. Generate an XY chart for Age and LOS and show this chart on a spreadsheet.
   b. What conclusions might you draw from this chart about any possible relationship between Age and LOS?
   c. Generate an XY chart for LOS and Charges and show this chart on a spreadsheet.
   d. What conclusions might you draw from this chart about any possible relationship between LOS and Charges?

6. Use the data from the SWC worksheet in Chpt 4–1.xls.
   a. Generate an XY chart for IMR and LEB and show this chart on a spreadsheet.
   b. What conclusions might you draw from this chart about any possible relationship between IMR and LEB?

Section 4.2 Using the Pivot Table to Generate Frequencies of Categorical Variables

Thus far, the data discussed in this chapter have been numerical data. We are going to turn now to the discussion of frequency distributions for categorical data. There are actually three categorical variables in the data on hospital charges that have been discussed thus far in this chapter. These are Sex, DRG, and ICD-9. In the original data, Sex was given as F or M and was later converted to 1 and 0. But DRG and the ICD-9 code were given as numbers. But despite the fact that they are given as numbers, DRG and ICD-9 remain categorical variables. The numbers simply represent a category rather than having meaning as a number.

FIGURE 4.18. PIVOT TABLE WINDOW 1.

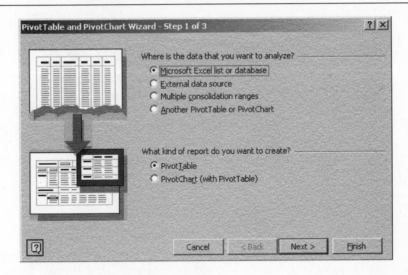

Using the categorical variable Sex1 in the data set to create a frequency distribution is fairly easy with the =FREQUENCY() function. Because that variable is coded 0 and 1, it is necessary only to create two bin values—0 and 1, and use the =FREQUENCY() function to accumulate all one hundred observations into these two bins. But categorical data are not always that easy to work with. If the data were left with the sex variable coded only "F" and "M", the =FREQUENCY() function could not be used. The alternative, for most categorical data, would be to use what Excel calls the Pivot Table. The Pivot Table is accessed from the Menu bar with Data/Pivot Table and Pivot Chart Report. When Pivot Table and Pivot Chart Report is selected, the first window that appears is as shown in Figure 4.18. Several things in Figure 4.18 deserve mention.

First, the window is, as it says, the first of three. This is a little misleading, because you actually have to access four windows to produce a pivot table, but more on that later. Second, this window provides several sources from which to access data. In general, when the Pivot Table is used in this book, the data will be in an Excel spreadsheet, so the first circle is selected. The other possibilities are not discussed in this text, but the directions for accessing data from other sources are fairly easy to follow. Also, the first window provides the opportunity to specify whether the result desired is a pivot table only or a pivot table and a chart based on the pivot table. In general, this book limits itself to the pivot table only option, with charts being created later.

The checked circles in the window in Figure 4.18 are OK, so the button Next can be selected, which then generates the window shown in Figure 4.19.

FIGURE 4.19. PIVOT TABLE WINDOW 2.

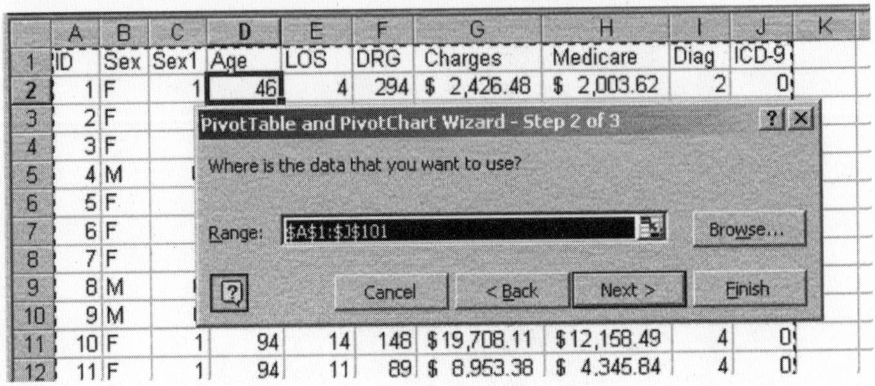

	A	B	C	D	E	F	G	H	I	J	K
1	ID	Sex	Sex1	Age	LOS	DRG	Charges	Medicare	Diag	ICD-9	
2	1	F	1	46	4	294	$ 2,426.48	$ 2,003.62	2	0	
3	2	F									
4	3	F									
5	4	M									
6	5	F									
7	6	F									
8	7	F									
9	8	M									
10	9	M									
11	10	F	1	94	14	148	$19,708.11	$12,158.49	4	0	
12	11	F	1	94	11	89	$ 8,953.38	$ 4,345.84	4	0	

PivotTable and PivotChart Wizard – Step 2 of 3

Where is the data that you want to use?

Range: $A$1:$J$101

Browse...

Cancel | < Back | Next > | Finish

Figure 4.19 also shows the first ten observations in the data set, along with step 2 of 3 of the Pivot Table. The spreadsheet is included in Figure 4.19 to show something about how data are selected for the Pivot Table. Before entering the Pivot Table sequence, cell D2 had already been selected. When the Pivot Table window 2 came up, Excel automatically assumed that all data contiguous to cell D2 were to be included as data to be used in the Pivot Table construction. That is indicated in two ways. First, Excel puts a dashed line around all the data (visible as the line above the data, to the left of column A, and to the right of column J). Excel also puts the cell references for the entire data set in the area marked Range. Although only column B will be used, there is no disadvantage to allowing Excel to select the entire data set.

Had no cell been selected when the Pivot Table sequence was initiated, it would be necessary to select the data for the pivot table in step 2. This could be done by putting the cursor in the area marked Range and then selecting the appropriate data, or by typing the data range into the Range area. It is important to note that the column labels are included as part of the data range. The Pivot Table requires that the data to be included in the table have labels in the first row. Without the labels, the Pivot Table process will assume that the first data values are labels and will treat them as such.

When the appropriate data range is selected for the Pivot Table, the selection of Next will produce the window shown in Figure 4.20. This window asks whether the Pivot Table should be on a new worksheet or the existing worksheet. If the existing worksheet is selected, it is necessary to include the cell where the upper left corner of the Pivot Table will be placed. This area cannot overlap existing data. But before the pivot table can be generated it is necessary to select Layout from this window. (In earlier versions of Excel, the Layout window was step 3 of 4,

FIGURE 4.20. PIVOT TABLE WINDOW 3.

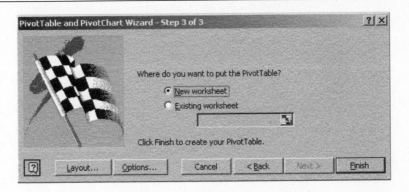

FIGURE 4.21. PIVOT TABLE LAYOUT.

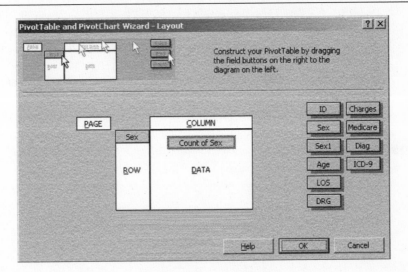

but with Excel 2000, the process was streamlined and made more difficult at the same time.)

When the layout button is selected, with the data that were specified in Window 2, the Layout window comes up. The Layout window is the place where the pivot table is actually created. The Layout table with the necessary changes to create a frequency distribution by Sex is shown in Figure 4.21.

When the Layout window comes up, there is nothing in the area marked Row nor in the area marked Data. The label Sex, representing the variable that is coded

"F" and "M", was dragged from the list on the right side of the Layout table to the area marked Row by left-clicking on the label on the right and dragging it to the area marked Row, as indicated in the instructions at the top of the window. By doing this, the resulting Pivot Table will have two rows, one labeled "F" for females and the other labeled "M" for males. But a frequency distribution must also have data. To provide data, the label marked Sex on the right was again left-clicked and dragged into the area marked Data.

Because the variable Sex is not only categorical but also coded as a letter, when it was dragged into the Data area, it automatically changed to Count of Sex. This means that the data for the table will be the count of the number of times Sex is coded "F" and the number of times it is coded "M".

It is not necessary to select the same variable for the Data area as that selected for the row area. Any other variable would work. All Excel requires is that something be there to be counted. But if we had selected, for example, Sex1 to put in the Data area, it would have been shown as Sum of Sex1 as soon as we dragged it into the data area, because Sex1 is coded as numbers, even though it is a categorical variable. Sum of Sex1 is not what we want, because since Sex1 is coded 1 for females and 0 for males, the pivot table would have totaled only to the total of all females. In order to correct this, it is necessary to double-left-click the object in the Data area, which will generate a window, as shown in Figure 4.22. In that Window it is possible to select any one of eleven different presentations of the data that are given in the Row area. For the present purposes, Count should be selected, which will change the designation Sum of Sex1 to Count of Sex1 and will add one to the total for "F" and "M" each time these values are encountered in the variable Sex.

FIGURE 4.22. SELECTION OF DATA FIELD.

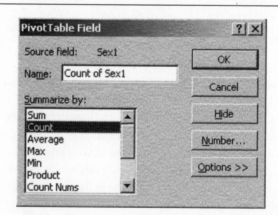

FIGURE 4.23. FINISHED PIVOT TABLE FOR SEX.

	A	B	C	D	E	F	G	H
1	Drop Page Fields Here							
2								
3	Count of Sex							
4	Sex ▾	Total						
5	F	64						
6	M	36						
7	Grand Total	100						
8								
9								
10								
11								
12								
13								
14								
15								

PivotTable

PivotTable ▾

ID	Sex	Sex1	Age	LOS
DRG	Charges	Medicare	Diag	ICD-9

Going back to Figure 4.21, when OK is selected, Excel returns to the window in Figure 4.20. Selecting Finish in that window will produce the frequency distribution shown in Figure 4.23. Figure 4.23 is a copy of the new spreadsheet that is created by the Pivot Table option. The actual frequency distribution for sex is in cells B5 and B6. As can be seen there, there are sixty-four women and thirty-six men in this sample of a hundred hospital discharges. But the initial result of the Pivot Table option is to produce an additional window, along with the frequency distribution.

This additional window, designated Pivot Table, shows all the variables that made up the original set when the Pivot Table was initiated. It is possible to drag and drop any of the variables into the area where Sex appears now (cell A4) or where Count of Sex appears (cell A3) or into the area of cell B3. This will change the data in the pivot table and, consequently, the way the pivot table appears. It is equally possible to drag Sex and Count of Sex back into the Pivot Table window, which would delete those from the table. It is also possible to drag and drop any variable into the area in cells A1 and B1 labeled Drop Page Fields Here. It is then possible to select only one level of a variable that is in this area for display in the table. So, for example, if LOS, which indicates the length of stay, were dragged into that area, it would be possible to show the distribution by sex for only those stays of one day or two days, and so on. If you try a different option in the Pivot Table window and find that you do not like the results, you can always click on the undo button on the Standard toolbar.

The Pivot Table window also allows you to do some other things with the Pivot Table. You can format the table into any of several standard formats, you can create a chart automatically by clicking the chart icon, and you can refresh the data. If you are interested in all the things this window provides, try it out. You can only learn. Clicking the **X** in the upper right corner will close the Pivot Table window. If you want to retrieve it, right-click anywhere in the Pivot Table, select Wizard from the pop-up menu, and Finish on the next window. The Pivot Table window is back.

But the discussion now focuses on the Pivot Table itself rather than on the options. The Pivot Table now represents a frequency distribution for Sex for the data for a hundred hospital discharges. It is a frequency distribution for a categorical variable. It can be used to create a graph, just as can data for a numerical variable. An easy way to create such a graph is to left-click anywhere in the Pivot Table and then left-click the Chart Wizard icon on the Standard Toolbar. This automatically creates a graph of the Pivot Table on a new sheet called a Chart sheet. The result of automatically generating a chart from the Pivot Table in Figure 4.23 is the graph shown in Figure 4.24. As long as the Pivot Table window is open in the original Pivot Table spreadsheet (as it is in Figure 4.23), it will be open in the Chart sheet. Changes can be made directly to the chart by dragging

FIGURE 4.24. CHART AUTOMATICALLY GENERATED BY THE PIVOT TABLE.

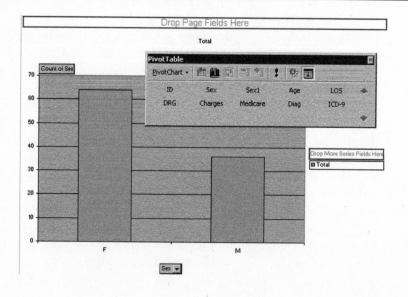

and dropping variables from the list into any of the designated places or to places where variables already appear. Any changes made to either the chart or the Pivot Table will change both. The Pivot Table window can be closed from either place. However, closing it does not delete the areas "Drop Page Fields Here" and "Drop More Series Fields Here" from the chart. Happily, though, these areas do not print with the chart, so they can be ignored.

The automatic chart option from a Pivot Table is OK in many instances, but not in all. The variable DRG in the data under discussion here is also a categorical variable. The numbers stand for charge categories for Medicare. The DRG categories appear as three numerical codes up to three digits and there are about five hundred separate categories, so a frequency distribution of the five hundred categories would not be very informative. But these categories can be collapsed into a much smaller set of categories that are generally defined by an area of the body or a body system or by a condition. For the data under discussion, which are primarily Medicare data, the general categories into which the DRG codes can be collapsed are the following:

- Digestive tract disorders
- Endrocine and nutritional disorders
- Female reproductive disorders
- Heart and circulatory disorders
- Injuries and poisoning
- Kidney and urinary disorders
- Liver and pancreas disorders
- Male reproductive disorders
- Mental illness
- Musculoskeletal and connective tissue disorders
- Nervous system disorders
- Rehabilitation and aftercare
- Respiratory disorders
- Skin disorders

Figure 4.25 shows the first ten records in the data file. It shows only the ID number for the record, the DRG number code, and the DRG Category into which the number code can be collapsed. A Pivot Table can be constructed with the DRG Category data (column K). If a cell in the spreadsheet shown in Figure 4.25 is clicked and the Pivot Table option is chosen from Data on the menu bar, Excel will automatically assume that the data to be included in the Pivot Table consist of all the data in the contiguous area on the spreadsheet. So even though columns B to E and G to I are hidden in the view shown in Figure 4.25, the variables in those columns will be included as options for the Pivot Table.

FIGURE 4.25. FIRST TEN RECORDS SHOWING BROAD DRG CATEGORIES.

	A	F	K	L	M
1	ID	DRG	DRG Categ		
2	1	294	Endrocine and Nutritional		
3	2	139	Heart and Circulatory		
4	3	34	Nervous System		
5	4	140	Heart and Circulatory		
6	5	141	Heart and Circulatory		
7	6	15	Nervous System		
8	7	294	Endrocine and Nutritional		
9	8	241	Musculoskeletal and Connective		
10	9	335	Male Reproductive		
11	10	148	Digestive Tract		
12	11	89	Respiratory		

FIGURE 4.26. LAYOUT WINDOW FOR DRG CATEGORIES.

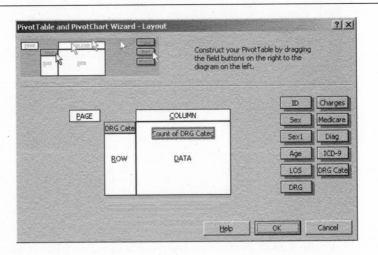

By moving through the Pivot Table windows for the data shown in Figure 4.25, the Layout window can be accessed from step 3 of 3. The Layout window for a frequency distribution of the DRG categories is shown in Figure 4.26. In that figure it is possible to see all the variables in the data set on the right side of the window. The variable DRG Categ has been dragged into the Row area and also into the Data area. Because the DRG Categ variable is text rather than numbers, Excel automatically assumes it will count the variable.

FIGURE 4.27. PIVOT TABLE FOR DRG CATEGORIES.

	A	B
1		
2		
3	Count of DRG Categ	
4	DRG Categ ▼	Total
5	Alcohol, Drugs	2
6	Digestive Tract	11
7	Endrocine and Nutritional	8
8	Female Reproductive	2
9	Heart and Circulatory	31
10	Injuries and Poisoning	2
11	Kidney and Urinary	4
12	Liver and Pancreas	5
13	Male Reproductive	3
14	Mental Illness	1
15	Musculoskelatal and Connective	6
16	Nervous System	5
17	Rehab and Aftercare	1
18	Respiratory	17
19	Skin Disorders	2
20	Grand Total	100
21		

When the Pivot Table is completed, the result is a frequency distribution, as shown in Figure 4.27. As the figure shows, Excel orders the frequency distribution output by the alphabetical order of the variable that has been used to construct the table. So there is no particular order for the frequencies themselves. But in the presentation of a frequency distribution based on categorical data, it is often common to order the data by size of the frequency from the largest category to the smallest. This can be done by sorting the Pivot Table result on the frequency column. To carry out this sort, first click on any cell in the frequencies in column B in Figure 4.27 (cells B5:B19) and then select Data/Sort from the Menu bar. When the sort window comes up, change Ascending to Descending and click OK. Both columns A and B in the table will be automatically sorted from largest to smallest by frequency of occurrence.

With the data in Figure 4.27 sorted into frequency of occurrence from most frequent to least frequent, a chart representing the frequency distribution of the DRG categories can be created by clicking anywhere in the sorted Pivot Table and clicking the Chart icon on the standard menu. A chart will be generated that will look like that shown in Figure 4.28.

If the active nature of the chart is not desirable for your purposes, it is possible to get rid of the blue outlined areas and the buttons by going back to the original

FIGURE 4.28. CHART OF DRG CATEGORIES BY SIZE.

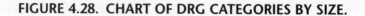

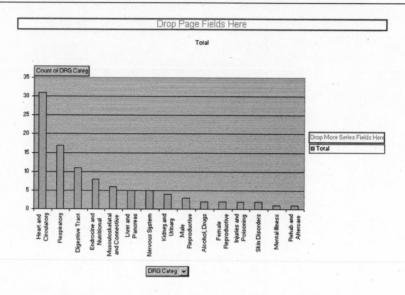

Pivot Table, copying the entire table (begin selection at the lower right corner), and then pasting special/values in the same spot. That will remove the blue outlined areas and the buttons from the chart and will allow you to carry out other formatting activities on the chart.

A Pareto Chart

One chart that may be interesting to look at, based on the data pictured in Figure 4.28, is what is known as a Pareto chart. A Pareto chart is a way of looking at both the individual frequencies and the cumulative frequencies at the same time, and it is typically confined to categorical data. The Pareto chart is often used in quality assurance efforts to see where the major problems in some process may lie, but it can also be used to look at major classes of hospital admission, for example. A Pareto chart combines the actually frequency distribution with the cumulative frequency distribution, as was the case in Figure 4.12. But with a Pareto chart, the categorical data are always arranged in order, from the most frequent to the least frequent (as shown in Figure 4.28), and the cumulative frequency is always shown as a line graph. A Pareto chart for the data in Figure 4.28 is given in Figure 4.29.

The easiest way to construct this Pareto chart is, first, to copy the Pivot Table and past it somewhere else on the spreadsheet, using Edit/Paste Special/Values. This eliminates the active nature of the Pivot Table and allows the inclusion of the cumulative line. Then calculate a set of cumulative frequency values, as was

FIGURE 4.29. PARETO CHART OF DRG CATEGORIES.

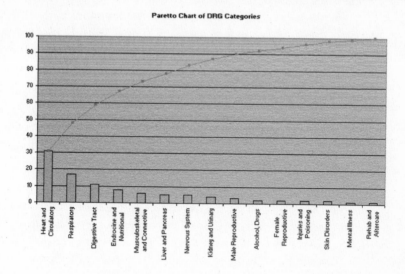

done in Figure 4.10 and Figure 4.11. With both the actual and the cumulative frequencies selected, click on the chart icon to create a new chart. This new chart will be created in the same spreadsheet as the data. In step 1 of 4 of the Chart Wizard, select Custom Types and then select Line-Column. In step 2 of 4 select the Series tab and then click in the area marked Category (X) axis labels. Now highlight the list of conditions and select Finish. A fair amount of reformatting of the X and Y axes will produce the chart shown in Figure 4.29.

A Pareto chart is typically used in situations where it is desirable to be able to see the major problems easily and quickly at the left side of the chart. Of course, with hospital admissions, it is not surprising to see that the major problems are heart and circulatory and respiratory disorders. In other cases, the major problems may not be so obvious until the chart is constructed. The cumulative line indicates that all observations are included in the chart, and, as there are a hundred observations, the cumulative line ends at one hundred.

Exercises for Section 4.2

1. Use the variable Sex on the Hospital Charges sheet in Chpt 4–1.xls.
   a. Create a frequency distribution using the Pivot Table that replicates the one in Figure 4.23, using Count of Sex in the DATA field.
   b. Create a frequency distribution using the Pivot Table that replicates the one in Figure 4.23, using Count of Age in the DATA field.
   c. Is there any difference between these two tables? Why or why not?

2. Use the variable LOS on the Hospital Charges sheet in Chpt 4–1.xls.
   a. Using a nested =IF() function, create a new variable, LOS1, which will take on the value "Short" when LOS is less than four days, "Medium" when LOS is four days to nine days, and "Long" when LOS is ten days or more.
   b. Create a frequency distribution of LOS1 using the Pivot Table.

3. Use the DRG worksheet in Chpt 4–2.xls.
   a. Replicate the frequency distribution shown in Figure 4.27.
   b. Sort the data in the pivot table by the frequency of each DRG category and replicate the chart shown in Figure 4.28.
   c. Generate a cumulative distribution for the DRG data from a and replicate the Pareto chart shown in Figure 4.29.

4. Use the Late Delivery worksheet in Chpt 4–2.xls. This worksheet is adapted from Figure 4.8, on page 84 of Veney and Kaluzny's *Evaluation and Decision Making for Health Services* (1998). The data in the worksheet show the reason for late delivery of the noon meal for 475 patients on three hospital wards.
   a. Use the Pivot Table to develop a frequency distribution for reasons for late delivery of the meal.
   b. Sort the frequency distribution so that the reason with the most instances is first, the second next, and so on, and create a chart showing the reasons from most to least.
   c. Generate a cumulative frequency for the data in a and construct a Pareto chart of the result.

Section 4.3 A Logical Extension of the Pivot Table: Two Variables

The last topic to consider in this chapter is the logical extension of the Pivot Table to two variables. A frequency distribution of DRG categories is interesting, but it might also be interesting to know how males and females compare on DRG categories. Of course, certain categories, such as Female reproductive and Male reproductive, will be limited to one sex only. But how are the admissions in the other categories distributed? The Pivot Table can provide this information.

Figure 4.30 shows the Pivot Table Layout window that will produce a Pivot Table for two variables. This figure is the same as Figure 4.26, except that Sex has now been dragged into the Column area. When the Pivot Table is created, the variable Sex will produce a table with two columns instead of the one column that was created in Figure 4.27. The Pivot Table generated by Excel with the configuration shown in Figure 4.30 is given in Figure 4.31. The table in Figure 4.31 is called a

FIGURE 4.30. PIVOT TABLE LAYOUT WINDOW FOR TWO VARIABLES.

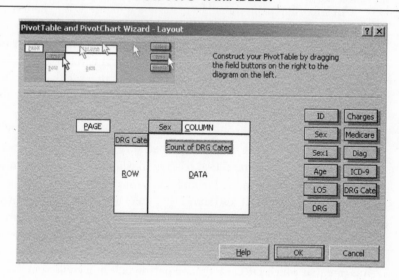

FIGURE 4.31. PIVOT TABLE FOR SEX AND DRG CATEGORY.

	A	B	C	D
1				
2				
3	Count of DRG Categ	Sex ▾		
4	DRG Categ ▾	F	M	Grand Total
5	Alcohol, Drugs		2	2
6	Digestive Tract	7	4	11
7	Endrocine and Nutritional	6	2	8
8	Female Reproductive	2		2
9	Heart and Circulatory	24	7	31
10	Injuries and Poisoning	2		2
11	Kidney and Urinary	3	1	4
12	Liver and Pancreas	3	2	5
13	Male Reproductive		3	3
14	Mental Illness	1		1
15	Musculoskeletal and Connective	3	3	6
16	Nervous System	4	1	5
17	Rehab and Aftercare	1		1
18	Respiratory	8	9	17
19	Skin Disorders		2	2
20	Grand Total	64	36	100

Pivot Table by Excel. In statistical parlance, the table is more likely to be called a *contingency table* or a *cross-tab* (short for cross-tabulation).

An important point should be made about Figure 4.31. There is a reason that Sex is the column heading rather than the row heading, and it goes beyond the fact that DRG was the row heading in the original frequency distribution. This reason has to do with the notion of causality. In general, if one variable may be the cause of the level of another variable, in a table such as that shown in Figure 4.31, the variable that may be a cause is typically used to define the columns. The other variable is typically used to define the rows.

What is meant by the idea that one variable may be the cause of the level of another variable? In the case of DRG category and Sex, there is every reason to expect that Sex has some causal relation to who is characterized in which DRG category. Female reproductive disorders, for example can only be relevant to women. But Figure 4.31 also shows that there are many more women than men with Heart and Circulatory disorders (there are also twice as many women as men in the sample), but there are more men in the Respiratory disorder category. These differences can be attributed to Sex. However, it would be unreasonable to imagine that which DRG category a person falls into could somehow determine the person's sex. In all but very rare instances, this would not be likely.

Exercises for Section 4.3

1. Use the data on the DRG worksheet in Chpt 4–2.xls and use the Pivot Table capability to replicate Figure 4.31.
2. Use the data on the Late Delivery worksheet in Chpt 4–2.
   a. Generate a cross tabulation using the Pivot Table capability with Ward as the column heading and Reason as the row heading.
   b. Add a new variable, Reason1, to the Late Delivery worksheet, assigning Other as the label for all but the two most common reasons for late delivery, and generate a cross-tabulation with Ward as the column headings and the reasons in Reason1.

3. Use the data on the SWC worksheet in Chpt 4–1.xls
   Create a new variable—IMR1, where IMR1 is 0 if IMR is less than 25, 1 if IMR is 25 to 74, and 2 if IMR is greater than 74.
   a. Create a new variable LEB1, where LEB1 is 0 if LEB is less than 50, 1 if LEB is 50 to 69, and 2 if LEB is greater than 69.
   b. Use the Pivot Table capability to produce a cross-tabulation for IMR1 and LEB1, with IMR1 as the column variable and LEB1 as the row variable. (Be sure to Count the Data field rather than summing it.)

References

The State of the World's Children 2001, UNICEF, New York, Dec. 2000.
    [http://www.unicef.org/sowc01/tables/#].
United States Bureau of the Census. [http://www.census.gov/statab/ranks/rank04.txt]. 2000.
Veney, J. E., and Kaluzny, A. D. *Evaluation and Decision Making for Health Services.* Chicago:
    Health Administration Press, 1998.

CHAPTER FIVE

BASIC CONCEPTS OF PROBABILITY

All statistics are based on probability. Probability is just a formal way of talking about chance. If, for example, we are to flip a coin, we know that there is some chance that it will come up heads and some chance that it will come up tails. We know, in general, that this chance is fifty-fifty for either heads or tails occurring. But we also know that there is no certainty at all to the way the coin will come up. If the coin is flipped in what any one of us would think of as the normally appropriate way, we are pretty sure that the resulting head or tail will have come up totally by chance or, in statistical terms, randomly. This random occurrence of heads or tails makes the result of a coin flip conform to what statisticians would call a *stochastic process*. Simply put, a stochastic process is one for which any result has a certain probability of occurrence. In this case, the probability of any result of the flip of a single coin (either heads or tails) is .5.

Section 5.1 Some Initial Concepts and Definitions

Any discussion of probability requires agreement on some initial concepts and definitions. The following sections provide working definitions for probability concepts.

Events, Independent Events, Outcomes, and Sample Space

An observation to which a probability can be assigned is often referred to as an *event*. If we flip a coin, we might reasonably think of that as an event (that is, the flip). But in this chapter we will actually think of the event as the viewing of the results of the flip. To understand how we will consider this, think of the story of the three umpires—the traditionalist, the pragmatist, and the existentialist. The traditionalist umpire, in calling balls and strikes, says, "I call 'em as they are." The pragmatist says, "I call 'em as I see 'em." The existentialist says, "They ain't nothin' till I call 'em." We will take the existentialist view. The result of a coin flip is nothing until we view it and "call" the result.

If we flip a coin twice, it is generally assumed that the outcome of the first flip will have no bearing on the outcome of the second flip. The first event does not influence the second event in any way. In statistical terms, it is said that the two events (flip one and flip two) are *independent* of one another. When we flip the coin the first time, the probability of either a head or a tail is .5. When we flip the coin the second time the probability of either a head or a tail is again .5. There are four possible *outcomes* of the flip of two coins: HH, HT, TH, or TT. The probability of any one of these four outcomes is .25, because each is equally likely and one divided by four is .25. But we can also arrive at the probability of any one of these four outcomes by the rule that says the probability of any outcome of two independent events is the multiplication of the probability of each separate event. Thus, the probability of the outcome HH, is .5 times .5, which is .25, which is also the probability of the outcome, TH, HT, or TT.

In general we will talk of individual observations as events and the accumulation of those observations as outcomes. However, a single event—the flip of a coin that results in a Tail—may also be considered an outcome if there is only one coin flip.

Just in passing, it might be interesting to think about what the multiplication of probabilities of independent events may mean for long sequences of coin flips. If we were told that a person had flipped a coin five times and gotten the sequence HTTHT, we would not be particularly surprised. But if we were told that they had gotten the sequence HHHHH, we would perhaps question the accuracy of reporting or the honesty of the reporter. But the probability of either of these two outcomes as the result of five flips of a coin is exactly the same: $.5 \times .5 \times .5 \times .5 \times .5$, or $.5^5$, or .03125. Why then are we not surprised by the first outcome but are surprised by the second? The answer lies in the fact that we would expect the result of five flips of a coin to include some heads and some tails, even though we would not necessarily expect any particular order of heads and tails. When we see a specific ordering that includes both heads and tails, our expectation is confirmed without recognizing that the specific ordering we see is no more likely than five heads in a row.

The two possible outcomes from the flip of a coin—heads or tails—are frequently called the *sample space* for this process. The sample space refers to all the possible outcomes of a particular process. The sample space for two flips of a coin includes the outcomes HH, HT, TH, and TT. For five flips of a coin, the sample space includes 2^5, or thirty-two, separate outcomes. As we have seen, each one of these individual outcomes has the same probability (.03125) of occurring. But it is often less the specific outcome than the mix of heads and tails that would interest us in the flip of five coins. From the perspective of the mix of heads and tails, the outcomes of five flips of a coin include five heads, four heads and one tail, three heads and two tails, two heads and three tails, one head and four tails, and five tails. There is only one way that an outcome of five heads can occur; that is, each flip is a head. The outcome of four heads and one tail can occur five ways. The first four flips could come up heads and the last a tail, the next to the last could be a tail, the third could be a tail, and so on. There are actually ten ways that the results could be three heads and two tails, ten ways to get two heads and three tails, five ways to get one head, and one way to get no heads (all tails).

Mutually Exclusive Outcomes

Figure 5.1 shows the thirty-two ways that the five flips of a coin can come out in terms of the number of heads realized. As the table shows, there is one way to obtain five heads, five ways to obtain four heads, and so on. In five flips of a coin, each of the thirty-two outcomes is *mutually exclusive* of all others. Being mutually exclusive means, for example, that the result HHHHH and the result HTTHT cannot both occur. One can occur or the other can occur, but the occurrence of

FIGURE 5.1. POSSIBLE COMBINATIONS OF FIVE COIN FLIPS.

	C8	=	=SUM(C2:C7)
	A	**B**	**C**
1	Outcome	Ways	Probability
2	Five Heads	1	0.03125
3	Four Heads	5	0.15625
4	Three Heads	10	0.3125
5	Two Heads	10	0.3125
6	One Head	5	0.15625
7	No Heads	1	0.03125
8		32	1

one rules out the occurrence of the other (and, similarly, all other outcomes). When outcomes are mutually exclusive, their probabilities can be summed. For example, there are five ways in which four heads can occur, each of the ways having a probability of .03125. The sum of these five ways is the total probability of getting four heads in any one of the five ways, which is shown in Figure 5.1 as .15625. The probability of getting three heads or two heads is given in Figure 5.1 as .31250, which is the sum of the probability of getting any combination of either three or two heads. The probabilities of all mutually exclusive outcomes in the sample space must add to 1.

The discussion of Figure 5.1 allows us to better understand why we would probably not be surprised by a sequence of HTTHT from the flip of five coins, whereas we would be surprised by the sequence HHHHH. The probability of seeing two heads and three tails from five flips of a coin is .31250—almost one third. In looking at the sequence HTTHT, we ignore the specific pattern and think only of the combination of heads and tails. The probability of seeing five heads, however, is only .03125, or about three chances out of a hundred. Consequently, we would be much more surprised to see that result.

A Priori Probability and Empirical Probability

There are two types of probability to consider. The first of these is the probability associated with the flip of a coin or, for example, with the roll of a die or the draw of a card from a deck of cards. The nature of the object or objects upon which the random process is based determines the probability of the outcome. The probability of the outcome of a head after the flip of a coin is .5 by the nature of the coin. The probability that a two will come up on the roll of a fair six-sided die is approximately .1667 (1/6) by the nature of the die. The probability of drawing an ace from the top of a well-shuffled deck is approximately .0769 (4/52) by the nature of the deck of cards (four aces in fifty-two cards). This type of probability is called a priori probability. Virtually all games of chance are based on a priori probabilities.

The second type of probability is probability associated with a set of objects about which we do not have the necessary knowledge to specify a probability a priori. For example, if we were to consider people arriving for treatment at a hospital emergency room, these people could be divided into two types: those who are coming for true emergencies, however defined, and those coming for non-emergency conditions. If we are interested in the probability that the next person arriving at the emergency room will be a true emergency, we cannot generally call upon some a priori knowledge of the people arriving and their propensity to be emergencies or nonemergencies in determining that probability.

What we can rely on, however, is some historical record of persons arriving at the emergency room. Suppose we have a record of all the arrivals at the emergency room for the last six months, during which time there were 7,320 total emergency room visits (about forty a day). We also have information about whether the visit was for a true emergency as assessed by the attending physician, physician's assistant, or nurse. Suppose the record indicates that 4,729 of the visits were true emergencies. Now we can say that for the last six months, the probability that a person coming to the emergency room came for a true emergency was .646 (4729/7320). Based on this, and assuming that the future is like the past, we could predict that when the next person arrives at the clinic, that person has about a .65 probability of being a true emergency and about a .35 probability of having a nonemergent problem. This type of probability is known as *empirical* probability.

To consider another example of empirical probability, suppose we have records on 2,556 married women, and for each of these women we have recorded the number of children born to that woman. Thinking back to the definition of *event* that was given earlier, in the first subsection of Section 5.1, the recording of the number of children born to each woman is the event. The distribution of women by number of children born might look something like Figure 5.2. This table shows that 256 of the women have had no children born, 682 have had one child, 796 have had two children, and so on. Among these 2,556 women, no woman has had more than seven children born.

Figure 5.2 also shows the proportion of women with no children, one child, two children, and so on. This proportion also represents an empirical probability. In this case, it is the empirical probability that any woman drawn at random from

FIGURE 5.2. CHILDREN EVER BORN TO 2,556 WOMEN.

	A	B	C	
1	Children Born	# Women	Proportion	
2	0	256	0.1001	
3	1	682	0.2670	
4	2	796	0.3115	
5	3	531	0.2076	
6	4	221	0.0865	
7	5	59	0.0231	
8	6	10	0.0038	
9	7	1	0.0004	
10		2556		

our group of 2,556 will have no children, or one child, and so on. For example, the empirical probability that a woman drawn at random from among the 2,556 would have four children is .0865. The probability that a woman drawn at random would have no children is .1001. The other probabilities follow similarly.

If our 2,556 women had been a random sample from some larger population, we would also be able to ascribe the probabilities associated with numbers of children to that larger population as well. In particular, if we were to select another woman from that larger population, we would be able to anticipate that the probability was about .0004 that the woman selected would have seven children, based on the empirical probabilities for our 2,556 women. Similarly, we would be able to say that the probability was about .2076 that she would have three children, again based on the empirical probabilities.

Empirical probabilities work just like a priori probabilities in regard to what may be said about them. For example, if we looked at the record of the sequential arrival of any two people at the emergency room, we would see four possible events. If we classify true emergencies as E and nonemergent conditions as O (other), then the results of the arrival of two sequential people could be EE, EO, OE, and OO. Now, however, despite the fact that there are four possible outcomes, the probability of each outcome is not .25. If we do assume for the moment that the outcome of the arrival the first person (that is, E or O) does not influence the outcome of the arrival of the second person, then we can say that the arrival outcomes are independent of one another. Under the assumption of independence, the probability that the outcome will be EE is .65 $\times$ .65, or .42. The probability of EO is .65 $\times$ .35, or .23. The probability of the outcome OE is the same as EO, and the probability of the outcome OO is .35 $\times$ .35, or .12. Since these four mutually exclusive outcomes represent the entire sample space, the reader can confirm that the probabilities for the four sum to 1.

With empirical probabilities, though, unlike the case with a priori probabilities, we may not always be justified to view many events as independent. It is not unlikely that several persons arriving at an emergency room in a sequential manner might not be independent of one another in regard to their emergency or nonemergent status. If, for example, there occurred a large highway accident that sent a number of persons to emergency rooms, several persons arriving at the same time might all be related (and hence not independent) emergencies. In fact, one of the most important capabilities of statistics—one that we will return to over and over in the course of this book—is the ability to assess whether events are independent of one another or not.

In many instances, it will seem that data of interest to health workers can be viewed only from the standpoint of empirical probability. Whether an arrival at an emergency room is an emergency or not can be understood only as an empirical probability. But, interestingly, once we know what the overall probability of being an emergency is, and if we assume that the arrival of an emergency is independent of whether the last person arriving was an emergency, we can apply a priori probability assumptions to the arrival of several people at a time. The a priori assumption we can apply is the binomial distribution, which is discussed later in this chapter. Similarly, there are other underlying probability assumptions that may be made about data, depending on the specific character of the data. One of the most important assumptions for statistics is that both discrete numerical data and continuous numerical data will somehow follow a priori, a normal distribution. This is discussed further in this chapter, and also in Chapter Six.

Exercises for Section 5.1

1. Calculate the probability of the following:
   a. The sequential role of the die faces 2, 4, and 3
   b. The sequence of coin flips HTHH
   c. Assuming a probability of any arrival at an emergency room being an emergency as .646, and assuming that arrivals are independent, the probability of the next four arrivals being all emergencies
   d. Assuming c (preceding), the probability of the next five arrivals being all nonemergencies
   e. Assuming c (preceding), the probability of the next four arrivals being two emergencies and two nonemergencies, in that order
   f. Assuming a probability of .5 that any child born will be a boy, the probability of any family of five children having no girls

2. Lay out on an Excel spreadsheet the possible outcomes of two rolls of a fair die and calculate the following:
   a. The probability that the two faces of the dice will equal 7
   b. The probability that the two faces of the dice will equal 11
   c. The probability that the two faces of the dice will equal 8 or more

3. Lay out on an Excel spreadsheet the possible outcomes of a visit by three persons to an emergency room. Assuming that the visits are independent, with a probability of .646 of being an emergency, calculate the following:
   a. The probability of two emergencies out of three arrivals
   b. The probability of no emergencies out of three arrivals
   c. The probability of at least two emergencies out of three arrivals

Section 5.2 Marginal Probabilities, Joint Probabilities, and Conditional Probabilities

To continue with the discussion of probability, it will be useful to distinguish three different types of probabilities: marginal probabilities, joint probabilities, and conditional probabilities. Marginal probabilities refer to the probabilities associated with a single event. Joint probabilities and conditional probabilities refer to the outcomes of two different types of events that may or may not be independent of one another.

Marginal Probability

The probability (proportion) shown in Figure 5.2 is often referred to as *marginal probability*. Marginal probability is the probability of the occurrence of a single outcome. The probability that any single woman selected at random from among the 2,556 women will have no children is the number of women with no children divided by the total number of women. Marginal probability refers to the probability of occurrence of any single outcome. By the same token, whether the next person appearing at the emergency room arrives with a true emergency or a nonemergent condition is also a single outcome (or event if we are counting only that one person). The marginal probability for true emergencies, according to the discussion earlier in this chapter, is .65, and for nonemergent conditions, it is .35.

Marginal probabilities refer to outcomes that are mutually exclusive of one another. For example, a woman cannot at the same time have no children and three children. These categories are mutually exclusive. Those arriving at an emergency room can be coming either for a true emergency or for a nonemergent condition. In this context, they would not be coming for both. As was noted earlier, the probabilities of mutually exclusive events can be added together. Furthermore, the sum of the probabilities of *all* possible mutually exclusive marginal probabilities will always be 1. To see the consequences of these two points, consider again Figure 5.2. If we wished to know the probability that a woman would have at least four children, we could add together the probability of having four, five, six, and seven children. The resulting probability, .1138, is the probability that a woman will have at least four children. In regard to the second point, it is relatively easy to verify that the sum of all probabilities in Figure 5.2 is 1.

Joint Probability

Marginal probability refers to the outcome of a single event or type of event (the birth of children, the arrival at an emergency room). *Joint probability* refers to

FIGURE 5.3. FIRST TWENTY OBSERVATIONS IN AN EMERGENCY ROOM VISIT FILE.

	A	B	C
1	Visit	Shift	Emergency Status
2	1	3rd	Emergency
3	2	1st	Emergency
4	3	2nd	Emergency
5	4	2nd	Emergency
6	5	3rd	Emergency
7	6	1st	Other
8	7	1st	Emergency
9	8	1st	Other
10	9	1st	Other
11	10	2nd	Emergency
12	11	2nd	Emergency
13	12	1st	Other
14	13	1st	Emergency
15	14	1st	Emergency
16	15	2nd	Other
17	16	2nd	Emergency
18	17	2nd	Emergency
19	18	1st	Other
20	19	3rd	Emergency
21	20	2nd	Emergency
22	21	2nd	Emergency

the simultaneous occurrence of two or more types of events. Return to the example of persons arriving at an emergency room. Figure 5.3 shows the first twenty observations in a file that contains records of 7,320 emergency room visits. Column C shows whether the visit was for an emergency or not. Column B is labeled Shift. The first shift (labeled 1st) is from 7 A.M. to 3 P.M. The second shift (2nd) is from 3 P.M. to midnight, and the third shift (3rd) is from midnight to 7 A.M.

In this example, we might, in addition to determining whether the visit was for a true emergency or a nonemergent condition, determine when during the day the arrival took place. The Pivot Table option in Excel was used to produce Figure 5.4, which shows the joint occurrence of a true emergency or a nonemergent condition and the shift during which the visit took place. It should be easy to recognize that Figure 5.4 is an example of a *contingency table*. If a contingency table is a table that shows the simultaneous occurrence of two or more events, then, in this case, the events are whether the arrival at the emergency room is or is not an emergency and the shift during which the arrival occurred.

FIGURE 5.4. CONTINGENCY TABLE OF SHIFT AND EMERGENCY STATUS.

	A	B	C	D	E
1					
2					
3	Count of Shift	Shift ▾			
4	Emergency Status ▾	1st	2nd	3rd	Grand Total
5	Emergency	1504	1852	1373	4729
6	Other	1148	980	463	2591
7	Grand Total	2652	2832	1836	7320
8					

FIGURE 5.5. JOINT PROBABILITIES FOR SHIFT AND EMERGENCY STATUS.

B11 ▾	= =B5/$E$7				
	A	B	C	D	E
1					
2					
3	Count of Shift	Shift ▾			
4	Emergency Status ▾	1st	2nd	3rd	Grand Total
5	Emergency	1504	1852	1373	4729
6	Other	1148	980	463	2591
7	Grand Total	2652	2832	1836	7320
8					
9	Count of Shift	Shift			
10	Emergency Status	1st	2nd	3rd	Grand Total
11	Emergency	0.205	0.253	0.188	0.646
12	Other	0.157	0.134	0.063	0.354
13	Grand Total	0.362	0.387	0.251	1.000

Figure 5.4 shows that of the 4,729 visits that were true emergencies, 1,504 occurred during the first shift, 1,852 occurred during the second shift, and 1,373 occurred during the third shift. Similarly, for visits to the emergency room that were not for true emergencies (the Other category), 1,148 occurred during the first shift, 980 occurred during the second shift and 463 occurred during the third. The probability that, for example, a visit took place during the first shift and was for a true emergency is a joint probability. The joint probability for the simultaneous occurrence of a visit during the first shift and for a true emergency is 1,504/7,320, or .205.

Figure 5.5 shows the contingency table for all the joint probability combinations as well as the marginal probabilities for both reason for visit (true emergency or other) and time of day. The calculation of the joint probability is shown in the formula line at the top of the figure. Notice that the $ convention is used to fix the divisor as cell E7 for every internal cell.

The probabilities shown in Figure 5.5 can also be obtained directly from the Pivot Table capability. In the Pivot Table field window, it is possible to select an Options button (see Figure 4.22). If this button is selected, it is possible to then select a 'Show Data as' box that allows the user to select any one of nine ways to display the data in the Pivot Table cells. One of these is the normal view, which is given in Figure 5.4. Another is 'as percent of the total' that displays the data as shown in cells A19:E13 of Figure 5.5.

It can be confirmed from the table that the marginal probability (p) that the visit was for a true emergency is equal to the joint probability that it was for a true emergency and occurred during the first shift, plus the joint probability that it was for a true emergency and occurred during the second shift, plus the joint probability that it was a true emergency and occurred during the third shift. This can be seen in Equation 5.1.

$$p(\text{True}) = p(\text{True } and \text{ First}) + p(\text{True } and \text{ Second})$$
$$+ p(\text{True } and \text{ Third}) \tag{5.1}$$
$$p(\text{True}) = .205 + .253 + .188 = .646$$

In general, it is always possible to find the marginal probability of occurrence of an event from the joint probabilities of its occurrence when viewed in a contingency table, such as that shown in Figure 5.5. The reader can confirm that the marginal probabilities for the other categories are the sum of the relevant joint probabilities.

Thus far, the discussion has concerned a joint probability that is represented by the conjunction *and*. It is also possible to discuss a joint probability that is represented by the conjunction *or*. The joint probability "or" would be stated in regard to true emergencies and time of day, as, for example, the visit was for a true emergency *or* it occurred during the first shift. The joint probability "or" is the sum of the appropriate marginal probabilities minus the appropriate joint *and* probability. For example, the probability that a visit was for a true emergency *or* that it took place during the first shift can be calculated by the formula shown in Equation 5.2.

$$p(\text{True } or \text{ First}) = p(\text{True}) + p(\text{First}) - p(\text{True } and \text{ First})$$
$$p(\text{True } or \text{ First}) = .646 + .362 - .205 = .803 \tag{5.2}$$

Figure 5.6 shows all the joint probability "or" values for arriving during one of three shifts or for coming for an emergency or for a condition that is not an emergency. The formula line shows the calculation of the joint probability $p(\text{True } or \text{ First})$ as B$13+$E11-B11. This formulation lets us drag the formula in cell B17

FIGURE 5.6. JOINT PROBABILITY "OR" FOR SHIFT AND EMERGENCY STATUS.

B17	▼	=	=B$13+$E11-B11		
	A	B	C	D	E
9	Count of Shift	Shift			
10	Emergency Status	1st	2nd	3rd	Grand Total
11	Emergency	0.205	0.253	0.188	0.646
12	Other	0.157	0.134	0.063	0.354
13	Grand Total	0.362	0.387	0.251	1.000
14					
15	Count of Shift	Shift			
16	Emergency Status	1st	2nd	3rd	Grand Total
17	Emergency	0.803	0.780	0.709	2.292
18	Other	0.559	0.607	0.542	1.708
19	Grand Total	1.362	1.387	1.251	4.000

to the other five cells and generates the joint probability "or" for each of the cells in the table. The joint probabilities "or" for each row and column have been summed in cells B19:D19 and in cells E17 and E18. In terms of probabilities, these numbers mean nothing, because all probability values must be 1 or less to have meaning. But the sum of the row probabilities or the sum of the column probabilities can be summed to the total of the joint probabilities "or" in cell E19. For a two-by-three table, such as the one shown in Figure 5.6, the sum of the joint probabilities "or" will always be 4. Four turns out to be the number of rows in the figure plus the number of columns minus 1. In fact, for any contingency table of any size, the sum of all joint probabilities "or" is always equal to the number of rows plus the number of columns minus 1.

It is possible to determine if the calculation of joint probabilities "and" are correct by determining if they sum to 1. It is equally possible to ensure that the calculation of joint probabilities "or" is correct by determining whether the probabilities sum to the number of rows plus the number of columns minus 1. For example, in a three-by-four table (three rows and four columns), the sum of all joint probabilities "or" would be $3 + 4 - 1$, or 6.

Conditional Probability

The discussion of probabilities given thus far has involved the development of probabilities with essentially no prior knowledge of events. The discussion has focused, for example, on the probability that a visit to the emergency room would be for a true emergency *and* would occur during the first shift. Now the discussion turns to another point of probability—the probability of one event occurring if it is *known* that another event has occurred. For example, suppose we know that an emergency room visit has taken place during the third shift. The task then might be to determine the probability that the visit would be a true emergency, given that it is already known that it took place during the third shift. We might also ask, What is the probability that the visit was an emergency *conditional on* its having taken place during the third shift? This is known as *conditional probability.*

The calculation of conditional probabilities can be taken directly from our discussion of marginal and joint probabilities and may be shown as given in Equation 5.3. In Equation 5.3, $p(A|B)$ is read as "the probability of A given B," which means the probability of A conditional on B having occurred, or having been known.

$$p(A|B) = p(A \text{ and } B)/p(B) \tag{5.3}$$

In regard to our example of emergency room visits, the conditional probability that a visit was for a true emergency, given that it occurred during the third shift, would be calculated as is shown in Equation 5.4.

$$\begin{aligned} p(\text{True}|\text{Third}) &= p(\text{True and Third})/p(\text{Third}) \\ p(\text{True}|\text{Third}) &= .188/.251 = .748 \end{aligned} \tag{5.4}$$

The calculation of all the conditional probabilities, given that the arrival took place either during the day or during the night, is shown in Figure 5.7. Cell B17, for example, shows the calculation of the conditional probability that the arrival was for an emergency, given that it took place during the first shift. The formula used for that calculation is shown in the formula line above the spreadsheet and can be copied into all the cells in the table. It is important to note that the conditional probabilities in Figure 5.7 are calculated for the columns. This means

FIGURE 5.7. CONDITIONAL PROBABILITIES FOR ARRIVAL DURING ANY SHIFT.

B17 ▼	= =B11/B$13			
A	B	C	D	E
9 Count of Shift	Shift			
10 Emergency Status	1st	2nd	3rd	Grand Total
11 Emergency	0.205	0.253	0.188	0.646
12 Other	0.157	0.134	0.063	0.354
13 Grand Total	0.362	0.387	0.251	1.000
14				
15 Count of Shift	Shift			
16 Emergency Status	1st	2nd	3rd	Grand Total
17 Emergency	0.567	0.654	0.748	0.646
18 Other	0.433	0.346	0.252	0.354
19 Grand Total	1.000	1.000	1.000	1.000
20				

that each conditional probability is the probability that the arrival is or is not an emergency, given that it took place during either the first, second, or third shift. Because these probabilities are calculated by column, the total of column conditional probabilities add to 1 for each column. It is also possible to calculate row conditional probabilities. The row conditional probabilities would be interpreted as the probability of coming during a particular shift, given that the visit was for an emergency or not. If conditional probabilities were calculated this way, they would sum to 1 by rows rather than by columns. In general, however, conditional probabilities are usually calculated for columns.

Conditional probabilities can also be calculated directly from data frequencies. It should be noted that the conditional probability of the visit to the emergency room being for a true emergency, given that it took place during the first shift, is just the number of visits for true emergencies taking place during the first shift, divided by all the visits taking place during the first shift. If we look at Figure 5.4, for example, we can see that there were 2,652 visits during the first shift, of which 1,504 were for true emergencies. If we divide 1,504 by 2,652, the result is .567, which is the same as what we found using the formula in Equation 5.4, or as calculated in Figure 5.7.

This introduction of the concept of conditional probability provides another opportunity to talk about the notion of independent events and independence. Earlier, independence was defined as being a situation in which the occurrence of one event had no relation to the occurrence of a second event. In particular, if a coin is flipped twice, the second flip is generally assumed to be independent of the first because the result of the first will not influence the result of the second. If the first is a head, we should not expect that a second flip will be any more likely to be a tail than a head.

The introduction of conditional probability provides another way to look at the independence of events. Two events are *independent* if all the conditional probabilities of the event are equal to the marginal probabilities of the event. This general relationship is expressed in Equation 5.5. Consider the conditional and marginal probabilities for emergency room visits, shown in Figure 5.7. The conditional probability of a true emergency, given that the visit took place during the first shift, is .567. The marginal probability of a true emergency is .646. Because these are not equal, arrival for an emergency and arrival during a particular shift are not independent of one another.

$$p(\text{A}|\text{B}) = p(\text{A}) \qquad \text{(condition for independence)} \qquad (5.5)$$

The condition of independence, as shown in Equation 5.5, holds for the earlier discussion of the flip of two coins. If a first coin, B, is flipped and its outcome is observed (head or tail), the probability of flipping a head or tail on the second toss (A) is no different than the probability of flipping a head or tail if the first flip had not been observed. Regardless of the results of flip B, the probability of flip A does not change, so $p(A|B) = p(A)$, and the events are independent. But considering visits to emergency rooms, the probability that a visit was for a true emergency, given that it took place during the first shift, is .567, but the probability that a visit is a true emergency is .646. In this case, $p(A|B) \neq p(A)$.

If we had been dealing with a table of two rows and two columns, any conditional probability that did not equal the marginal probability would have forced all conditional probabilities to be different from the marginal probabilities. The nature of a two-by-two table is such that if $p(A|B) \neq p(B)$ for any individual conditional probability in the table, it will hold for all other conditional probabilities in the table.

In a table with more than four internal cells, however, such as that in Figure 5.7, a selected conditional probability may be equal to the relevant marginal probability, and the two variables may nevertheless not be independent of one another. Consider, again, children ever born to 2,556 women. Suppose these women were divided into low and high income and the number of children ever born was categorized as 0, 1, 2, 3, and 4+, as shown in Figure 5.8. The number of women in the high- and low-income groups, with their respective numbers of children, are

FIGURE 5.8. CONDITIONAL PROBABILITIES FOR HIGH- AND LOW-INCOME WOMEN AND NUMBER OF CHILDREN.

H10		=	=H2/H$7	
	G	H	I	J
1	Children Born	High	Low	Total
2	0	102	154	256
3	1	380	302	682
4	2	317	479	796
5	3	189	342	531
6	4+	32	259	291
7		1020	1536	2556
8				
9	Children Born	High	Low	Total
10	0	0.100	0.100	0.100
11	1	0.373	0.197	0.267
12	2	0.311	0.312	0.311
13	3	0.185	0.223	0.208
14	4+	0.031	0.169	0.114
15		1.000	1.000	1.000

shown in cells H2:I6. The column conditional probabilities (the conditional probability, for example, of having 0 children, given that the woman is high income) are given in cells H10:I14. It is possible to see in that figure that the conditional probability of having 0 children, given high income, is essentially the same as the marginal probability of having no children within three decimal points. Similarly, the conditional probability of having two children, given high income, is the same as the marginal probability of having two children. But in other cells, the conditional and marginal probabilities are not equal. For example, the conditional probability of having one child, given high income, is not the same as the marginal probability for one child. Because any of the conditional probabilities in this table is not equal to the marginal probabilities, income and children born, based on these data, would not be considered to be independent.

It is important to point out, however, that the concept of independence discussed thus far is *mathematical* independence. If Equation 5.5 does not hold, then two events are not mathematically independent. By this definition, the two events, arrival for an emergency and arrival during a particular shift, are not independent. But the conditional probabilities for arrival for an emergency or for a nonemergent condition, given shift during the day, are not much different from the marginal probabilities. As Figure 5.7 shows, the conditional probability of arriving for an emergency during any particular shift is in every case no more than .1 different from the marginal probability. Viewed another way, could we think of a concept of statistical independence? The answer to this question is yes. Chapter Eight discusses statistical tests for categorical data that will allow us to determine whether the differences between the conditional and marginal probabilities shown in tables, such as those given in Figure 5.7 and Figure 5.8, can be considered independent from a statistical perspective.

Exercises for Section 5.2

1. Use the data in file Chpt 5–2.xls. This is the data file from which the discussion in Section 5.02 was developed. Do the following:
    a. Generate a contingency table such as that shown in Figure 5.4, using the Pivot Table capability of Excel.
    b. Calculate the marginal probabilities for both Shift and Emergency Status, as is shown in Figure 5.5.
    c. Calculate the joint probabilities "and" for each of the cells in the table, as is shown in Figure 5.5. Confirm that the sum of the cells is 1.
    d. Calculate the joint probabilities "or" for each of the cells in the table, as is shown in Figure 5.6. Confirm that the sum of the joint probabilities "or" is equal to rows + columns − 1.

   e. Calculate the conditional probabilities of reason for arrival, given that the patient arrives in the first, second, or third shift (replicate Figure 5.7) and confirm that reason for arrival and time of arrival are not independent.

2. Use the file created in Exercise 2 of Section 3.3 of Chapter Three (or use Chpt 5–3.xls) and do the following:
   a. Generate a contingency table with Sex as the column variable and Insurance as the row variable and calculate the marginal probabilities of each variable.
   b. Calculate joint probabilities "and" for the two variables and show them in a separate table. Confirm that the joint probabilities "and" sum to 1.
   c. Calculate joint probabilities "or" for the two variables and show them in a separate table. Confirm that the joint probabilities "or" sum to rows + columns − 1.
   d. Calculate conditional probabilities of having a particular type of insurance, given Sex, and determine if the two variables are independent.

3. Use the file in Exercise 2 (preceding) and do the following:
   a. Generate a new variable—Charges 2, where Charges 2 is 1 if Charges is greater than the average and 0 if less.
   b. Generate a contingency table with Insurance as the column variable and Charges 2 as the row variable and calculate marginal probabilities for each variable.
   c. Calculate joint probabilities "and" for the two variables and show them in a separate table. Confirm that the joint probabilities "and" sum to 1.
   d. Calculate join probabilities "or" for the two variables and show them in a separate table. Confirm that the joint probabilities "or" sum to rows + columns − 1.
   e. Calculate conditional probabilities for charges, given insurance, and show these in a separate table. Determine if the two variables are independent.

Section 5.3 Binomial Probability

As has been discussed thus far, a person comes to the emergency room for one of two reasons: either for an emergency or for a nonemergent reason. Because arrival can be for one of two reasons, this can be considered a binary event. The occurrence of binary events generally follows a known distribution, called the binomial distribution. Consider, again, a most common binary event—the flipping of a coin. The result can be either a head or a tail, and either outcome is equally likely, as either outcome has a .5 probability of occurrence. But suppose we are flipping the coin five times. Figure 5.1 showed the number of different heads that could be obtained in five flips of a coin. That table indicates that the probability of getting all heads was .03125, the probability of getting four heads was .15625, the probability of getting three heads was .3125, and the probability of getting two one or no heads were exactly the same probabilities in reverse. These probabilities for five flips of a coin follow the binomial distribution.

Figure 5.9 shows all the possible outcomes of the flip of a coin five times. Column B shows the result of the first flip, column C shows the result of the second

FIGURE 5.9. ALL POSSIBLE OUTCOMES OF THE FLIP OF A COIN FIVE TIMES.

	A	B	C	D	E	F	G	H
1		First	Second	Third	Fourth	Fifth	# Heads	Prob
2	1	H	H	H	H	H	5	0.03125
3	2	H	H	H	H	T	4	0.03125
4	3	H	H	H	T	H	4	0.03125
5	4	H	H	H	T	T	3	0.03125
6	5	H	H	T	H	H	4	0.03125
7	6	H	H	T	H	T	3	0.03125
8	7	H	H	T	T	H	3	0.03125
9	8	H	H	T	T	T	2	0.03125
10	9	H	T	H	H	H	4	0.03125
11	10	H	T	H	H	T	3	0.03125
12	11	H	T	H	T	H	3	0.03125
13	12	H	T	H	T	T	2	0.03125
14	13	H	T	T	H	H	3	0.03125
15	14	H	T	T	H	T	2	0.03125
16	15	H	T	T	T	H	2	0.03125
17	16	H	T	T	T	T	1	0.03125
18	17	T	H	H	H	H	4	0.03125
19	18	T	H	H	H	T	3	0.03125
20	19	T	H	H	T	H	3	0.03125
21	20	T	H	H	T	T	2	0.03125
22	21	T	H	T	H	H	3	0.03125
23	22	T	H	T	H	T	2	0.03125
24	23	T	H	T	T	H	2	0.03125
25	24	T	H	T	T	T	1	0.03125
26	25	T	T	H	H	H	3	0.03125
27	26	T	T	H	H	T	2	0.03125
28	27	T	T	H	T	H	2	0.03125
29	28	T	T	H	T	T	1	0.03125
30	29	T	T	T	H	H	2	0.03125
31	30	T	T	T	H	T	1	0.03125
32	31	T	T	T	T	H	1	0.03125
33	32	T	T	T	T	T	0	0.03125

flip, and so on. By examining the figure, it can be seen that there is only one way that the result can be five heads, five ways that the result can be four heads, ten ways that the result can be three heads, and so on, to one way to obtain no heads. The probability of any one of the thirty-two outcomes is given in column H. Each of these outcomes has exactly the same probability: .03125. But since there are five ways to get four heads, each of these .03125 probabilities can be added together to get the probability of getting four heads. The same can be done for three heads, and so on. The results will be exactly those shown in Figure 5.1.

But is it possible to generalize the information found in Figure 5.9 to any number of coin flips, or, for that matter, to any binary events—such as the arrival for an emergency or nonemergent condition? The answer is yes. To do so, let us first consider the probability of getting any number of heads in five flips of the coin. Let us say that we flip a coin five times and we get the outcome HHTHT, which is outcome number six in Figure 5.9. What is the probability of getting that outcome? It is the probability of a head on the first flip (.5) times the probability of a head on the second flip (.5) times the probability of a tail on the third flip (.5) times the probability of a head on the fourth flip (.5) times the probability of a tail on the fifth flip (.5). Because the probabilities of heads or tails are both .5, the probability of the outcome HHTHT is $.5 \times .5 \times .5 \times .5 \times .5$, or $.5^5$. But it is also the probability of heads raised to the third power times the probability of tails raised to the second power, or $.5^3 \times .5^2$. Think of the number of flips of a coin as being designated by n; think of the occurrence of a head—the outcome we wish to track—as the *index value* (I) and the number of heads that come up as being designated by x. Then, the probability of any single outcome (that is, of any number of heads in a specific order) in n flips of a coin is given in Equation 5.6.

$$p\begin{pmatrix} n \\ I^* \\ x \end{pmatrix} = p(I)^x(1 - p(I))^{(n-x)} \tag{5.6}$$

where $p(I)$ is the probability of the event I (for example the probability of a head in one flip of a coin) and $p\begin{pmatrix} n \\ I^* \\ x \end{pmatrix}$ is the probability of any single outcome of x events in n tries (for example the outcome HHTHT in five flips of a coin).

For example, the probability of the specific pattern of heads and tails HHTHT is $p\begin{pmatrix} 5 \\ H^* \\ 3 \end{pmatrix} = .5^3 \times 5^{(5-3)} = .03125$.

For the flip of a coin where the probability of heads and one minus the probability of heads are the same (.5), the result of Equation 5.6 is exactly the same for any single value of x (that is, for any single number of heads, such as 1 head, 2 heads, and so on). If we consider again the visit of people to an emergency room and use the empirical probabilities shown in Figure 5.4, $p(I)$ and $1 - p(I)$ are not equal. Consequently, the result of the application of Equation 5.6 will not be the same for every different number of true emergencies (x) and nonemergent conditions. Figure 5.10 shows all the possible outcomes of the visit to an emergency room of five people and their emergency or nonemergency status, *assuming that each visit is independent of all other visits*. The probability of five emergencies is given as .113. You can confirm that this is $.646^5$ or $p(I)^5 \times (1 - p(I))^{(5-5)}$. The probability

FIGURE 5.10. ALL POSSIBLE OUTCOMES OF FIVE EMERGENCY ROOM VISITS.

	A	B	C	D	E	F	G	H
1		First	Second	Third	Fourth	Fifth	# Emerg	Prob
2	1	E	E	E	E	E	5	0.113
3	2	E	E	E	E	NE	4	0.062
4	3	E	E	E	NE	E	4	0.062
5	4	E	E	E	NE	NE	3	0.034
6	5	E	E	NE	E	E	4	0.062
7	6	E	E	NE	E	NE	3	0.034
8	7	E	E	NE	NE	E	3	0.034
9	8	E	E	NE	NE	NE	2	0.019
10	9	E	NE	E	E	E	4	0.062
11	10	E	NE	E	E	NE	3	0.034
12	11	E	NE	E	NE	E	3	0.034
13	12	E	NE	E	NE	NE	2	0.019
14	13	E	NE	NE	E	E	3	0.034
15	14	E	NE	NE	E	NE	2	0.019
16	15	E	NE	NE	NE	E	2	0.019
17	16	E	NE	NE	NE	NE	1	0.010
18	17	NE	E	E	E	E	4	0.062
19	18	NE	E	E	E	NE	3	0.034
20	19	NE	E	E	NE	E	3	0.034
21	20	NE	E	E	NE	NE	2	0.019
22	21	NE	E	NE	E	E	3	0.034
23	22	NE	E	NE	E	NE	2	0.019
24	23	NE	E	NE	NE	E	2	0.019
25	24	NE	E	NE	NE	NE	1	0.010
26	25	NE	NE	E	E	E	3	0.034
27	26	NE	NE	E	E	NE	2	0.019
28	27	NE	NE	E	NE	E	2	0.019
29	28	NE	NE	E	NE	NE	1	0.010
30	29	NE	NE	NE	E	E	2	0.019
31	30	NE	NE	NE	E	NE	1	0.010
32	31	NE	NE	NE	NE	E	1	0.010
33	32	NE	NE	NE	NE	NE	0	0.006

FIGURE 5.11. PROBABILITIES OF NUMBER OF VISITS THAT ARE ACTUAL EMERGENCIES.

	T	U	V
1	Emergencies	Ways	Prob
2	5	1	0.113
3	4	5	0.308
4	3	10	0.338
5	2	10	0.185
6	1	5	0.051
7	0	1	0.006
8		32	1.000

of four emergencies out of five (for example outcome number 2 or outcome number 3) is .062. It is possible to confirm that this is $.646^4 \times .354^1$ or $p(I)^4 \times (1 - p(I))^{(5-4)}$, as expressed in Equation 5.6.

Having calculated the probabilities of occurrence of each of the thirty-two different ways in which five persons can present emergencies or nonemergent conditions in an emergency room, it is possible now to add all of the ways that each number of emergencies may be generated to produce the result shown in Figure 5.11.

Equations for the Binomial Distribution

But there is a less tedious way of getting the result in Figure 5.11 than by enumerating every possible combination of each possible set of emergency room visits (or heads and tails) and adding each of the probabilities. As both Figure 5.10 and Figure 5.11 show, the probability of getting any single number of emergencies is exactly the same for each one of the ways in which that number of emergencies can be obtained. For example, the probability of seeing three emergencies out of five arrivals at the emergency room is .034 for any of the ten ways to see three emergencies. Consequently, if there is a way to determine the number of ways that one can find three emergencies out of five visits, it would be possible simply to multiply this number times the probability of finding three emergencies in any single way (Equation 5.6). It turns out that there is a formula for finding the number of ways that one can get three emergencies out of five visits, or, more generally, x emergencies (I) out of n total observations. That formula is the general formula for the number of combinations out of any number of tries, as is shown in Equation 5.7. Equation 5.7 says that the total number of combinations, (C), for finding n emergencies (I or the Index event) out of m observations is m factorial divided by the quantity n factorial times $(m - n)$ factorial.

$$C\binom{n}{\substack{I \\ x}} = \frac{n!}{x! \times (n - x)!}$$ (5.7)

where $C\binom{n}{\substack{I \\ x}}$ is the number of different ways to get x results of I

out of n observations. (Three emergencies out of five persons coming to the emergency room, for example.)

The term *factorial* means to multiply the number to which the factorial refers by every number less than it in the number sequence. So, for example, 5! is $5 \times 4 \times 3 \times 2 \times 1$, or 120. The Excel =FACT() function will provide the value of factorials up to 170! (about 7.257E+306 or 7,257 followed by 303 zeros). Now if we wish to know the probability of seeing, for example, x emergencies in the next n persons who come to the clinic, the complete formula is as given in Equation 5.8.

$$p\binom{n}{\substack{I \\ x}} = C\binom{n}{\substack{I \\ x}} p\binom{n}{\substack{I^* \\ x}}$$ (5.8)

where $p\binom{n}{\substack{I \\ x}}$ is the total probability of n results of I out of x

observations (the binomial probability).

Figure 5.12 shows the same probabilities as Figure 5.11, except that those in Figure 5.12 were developed using the =FACT() function and the formulas in Equation 5.6, Equation 5.7, and Equation 5.8. Column D in the figure is the result of the application of Equation 5.7. Column E is the result of the application of Equation 5.6. Column F is the binomial probability, which is the result of the application of Equation 5.8. The actual setup of the formulas as implemented in Excel is shown in Figure 5.13. You will recall that the picture shown in Figure 5.13 can be generated by going to Tools/Options and checking formulas on the View tab.

The formulas for Figure 5.13 were entered only into row 2 and copied to the other rows. It is useful to look closely at Figure 5.13 to see how the $ convention was used to generate the correct cell references in each row.

Figure 5.12 was calculated using the formulas in Equation 5.6, Equation 5.7, and Equation 5.8. Excel actually provides a function that produces an easier way to determine binomial probabilities. This is the =BINOMDIST() function.

FIGURE 5.12. PROBABILITIES OF NUMBER OF VISITS USING FORMULAS.

	A	B	C	D	E	F
1	Emergencies	n!	x!*(n-x)!	Ways	p(I*) (1 way)	prob
2	5	120	120	1	0.113	0.113
3	4	120	24	5	0.062	0.308
4	3	120	12	10	0.034	0.338
5	2	120	12	10	0.019	0.185
6	1	120	24	5	0.010	0.051
7	0	120	120	1	0.006	0.006
8						1.000
9	p(I)	0.646				

FIGURE 5.13. FORMULAS USED FOR CALCULATIONS OF PROBABILITIES.

	A	B	C	D	E	F
1	Emergencies	n!	x!*(n-x)!	Ways	p(I*) (1 way)	prob
2	5	=FACT($A$2)	=FACT(A2)*FACT($A$2-A2)	=B2/C2	=$B$9^A2*(1-$B$9)^($A$2-A2)	=D2*E2
3	4	=FACT($A$2)	=FACT(A3)*FACT($A$2-A3)	=B3/C3	=$B$9^A3*(1-$B$9)^($A$2-A3)	=D3*E3
4	3	=FACT($A$2)	=FACT(A4)*FACT($A$2-A4)	=B4/C4	=$B$9^A4*(1-$B$9)^($A$2-A4)	=D4*E4
5	2	=FACT($A$2)	=FACT(A5)*FACT($A$2-A5)	=B5/C5	=$B$9^A5*(1-$B$9)^($A$2-A5)	=D5*E5
6	1	=FACT($A$2)	=FACT(A6)*FACT($A$2-A6)	=B6/C6	=$B$9^A6*(1-$B$9)^($A$2-A6)	=D6*E6
7	0	=FACT($A$2)	=FACT(A7)*FACT($A$2-A7)	=B7/C7	=$B$9^A7*(1-$B$9)^($A$2-A7)	=D7*E7
8						=SUM(F2:F7)
9	p(I)	0.646				

The =BINOMDIST() function takes four arguments. These are the number of emergency visits (5, 4, 3, 2, 1, or 0), the number of visits observed (five), the probability of an emergency (.646), and a 0 or 1 to indicate whether the value to be determined is the actual probability or the cumulative probability. Figure 5.14 shows the result of using the =BINOMDIST() function to calculate binomial probabilities. The values in column B have been calculated by the equation shown in the formula bar. The values in column C have been calculated by dragging the equation from column B to column C and changing the 0 in the final argument to a 1.

Two additional things should be pointed out. The cumulative binomial function always accumulates from the lowest number of the index value (0 emergencies) to the highest. Consequently, column C accumulates from cell C7 to cell C2. A second point to mention is that it is relatively easy to confirm that the cumulative probabilities are simply the accumulation of the probabilities at each of the number of emergencies. In other words, the cumulative value for two emergencies is the sum of the probabilities for zero emergencies, one emergency and two emergencies. This seems logical, and it is true because the number of emergencies is a discrete

FIGURE 5.14. THE =BINOMDIST( ) FUNCTION.

B2	▼	=	=BINOMDIST($A2,$A$2,$B$9,0)	
	A	B	C	D	E
1	Emergencies	Actual	Cummulative		
2	5	0.113	1.000		
3	4	0.308	0.887		
4	3	0.338	0.579		
5	2	0.185	0.241		
6	1	0.051	0.056		
7	0	0.006	0.006		
8					
9	P(E)	0.646			

numerical variable. There cannot be a half of an emergency or 3.2 emergencies. We will discuss distributions, particularly the normal distribution, where it is not possible to accumulate individual probabilities to get the cumulative probability.

A final thing should be mentioned about Figure 5.14. It is instructive to examine how the $ references have been used to be able to copy the original formula from cell B2 to cells B2:C7 to get all the correct probabilities by changing only the 0 in cell B2 to a 1 in column C.

Having spent this much time on the development of the binomial distribution, it would seem appropriate to say a few more words about why this knowledge is useful to a health worker. The binomial distribution can give the probability for the occurrence of any event that can have two outcomes. So, for example, to continue with emergency room visits, suppose a hospital emergency room administrator has data over the past year showing that exactly 20,278 true emergencies were seen in the emergency room out of 31,390 people who sought care from the emergency room. And suppose further that the emergency room administrator is pretty certain that most visits to the emergency room are independent events (they don't deal with many train wrecks or multiple car accidents). Then, the emergency room administrator can use the binomial distribution to figure out how many emergencies she might expect during an eight-hour shift (when an average of twenty-nine people will show up at the emergency room). For example, she may be interested in the probability that no more than fifteen real emergencies will appear in the emergency room. By using the =BINOMDIST(15,29,.646,1) function, she will learn that there is a probability of only about .106 that fifteen or fewer true emergencies will show up at the emergency room.

FIGURE 5.15. BINOMIAL DISTRIBUTION FOR EMERGENCIES IN AN EIGHT-HOUR SHIFT.

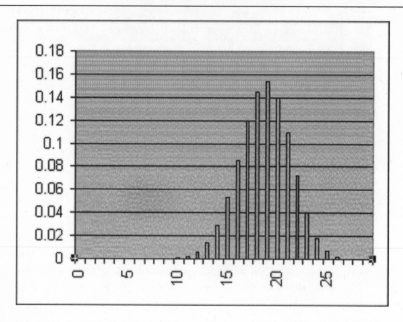

The administrator would have good reason, then, to be prepared for more than fifteen emergencies. But what would be the probability, for example, that more than twenty-five emergencies would show up during her shift? That would be found by subtracting =BINOMDIST(25,29,.646,1) from 1, the result of which is about .002. So she would be justified in assuming that only very rarely-in fewer than three eight-hour shifts each year-would she have to be prepared for more than twenty-five true emergencies. The chart in Figure 5.15 shows the entire binomial distribution for any number of emergencies (from 0 to 29) occurring during an eight-hour shift. As the figure shows, the administrator can expect between thirteen and twenty-five true emergencies during any eight-hour shift. On virtually no days will they see fewer than thirteen emergencies and rarely more than twenty-five. This same logic can be applied to any other occurrences that can take on only two values.

Answering the Question of Correctly Documented Medicare Claims

In Chapter One there is a brief discussion of the problem of incorrectly documented Medicare claims at the Pentad Home Health Agency. The agency drew a random sample of eighty records from their files, and during an audit of the records, it was determined that only 75 percent of them were correctly documented. The agency believed that any fewer than 85 percent correctly documented would lead to real reimbursement difficulties with the Medicare administration. They were concerned that they should initiate a training activity for staff to ensure that at least 85 percent would be correctly documented in the future. But they were not completely convinced that just because only 75 percent were correctly documented in the audit, fewer than 85 percent of all records were incorrectly documented. The training activity was not going to be cheap, and it would be a real waste to undertake the training if it was not really needed. What information could they call on to make a decision whether to undertake training?

Since any record can be either correctly or incorrectly documented, the outcome is binary. If we assume that the probability of one record being correctly documented is independent of whether any other is being correctly documented (not a completely obvious assumption), we can consider that the probability of appearance in our random sample of any number of correctly or incorrectly documented records will follow the binomial distribution. So if we want to know the probability that the true proportion of correctly documented records is 85 percent when we discovered 75 percent correctly documented in our sample, we could approach the question in either of two ways.

The first way would be to ask, if we have found 75 percent of our sample correctly documented, what is the probability that 85 percent of the population from which the sample came were correctly documented? Considering eighty records, 85 percent would be 68 records. So we can use the binomial distribution equations given in Equation 5.6, Equation 5.7, and Equation 5.8, or the =BINOMIAL(67,80,.75,1) function, to determine that the cumulative binomial probability of obtaining a value of sixty-seven or fewer correctly documented in any random sample of eighty records is .978. We can also determine that $1 - (=\text{BINOMIAL}(67,80,.75,1))$ is .022, which is the probability that the true proportion of correctly documented records is 85 percent or more when the sample proportion is 75 percent.

The alternative is to ask, if the true proportion of correctly documented cases in the population is 85 percent, what is the probability that only 75 percent of a sample will be correctly documented? Again, considering eighty records, 75 percent would be sixty. So we can use the binomial distribution equations or the =BINOMIAL(60,80,.85,1) function to determine that the cumulative binomial probability of obtaining sixty or fewer correctly documented records in any random sample of eighty records is .013. In either way of looking at this issue, the odds that 85 percent of the population of records could be correctly documented, given a sample proportion of 75 percent, are very small. A statistical consultant

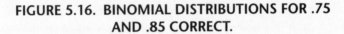

FIGURE 5.16. BINOMIAL DISTRIBUTIONS FOR .75 AND .85 CORRECT.

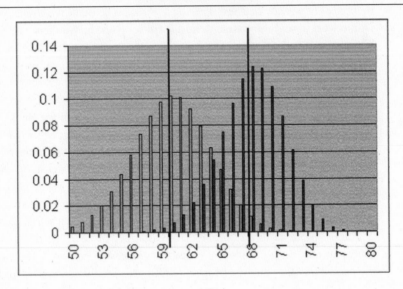

to the home health agency would almost certainly recommend initiating a training event.

Another way of considering either of these alternatives might be by picturing the actual binomial distributions for each. Figure 5.16 shows the binomial distribution for 75 percent correct out of eighty observations (the light gray distribution on the left) and the binomial distribution for 85 percent correct out of eighty observations (the black distribution on the right). These were generated using the =BINOMDIST(x,80,p,0) function, where x was all values from fifty to eighty and p was either .75 or .85. If we look first at the light gray distribution ($p = .75$), we can see that only a small proportion of that distribution (actually 2.2 percent) is to the right of the vertical black line that marks the number sixty-eight (85 percent of eighty). But if we look at the black distribution ($p = .85$), we can see that only a small proportion of that distribution (actually, 1.3 percent) is to the left of the vertical black line that marks the number sixty (75 percent of 80). This is graphic evidence that it is very unlikely that the true proportion of correctly documented records is 85 percent when the sample finds 75 percent.

One question that may remain is, why are the probabilities found from these two views not exactly the same? The answer lies in the fact that the binomial distribution is not symmetrical. The closer the actual proportion gets to 0 or to 1, the more the binomial distribution becomes skewed in the direction away from the 0 or 1 limit. This means that in most cases, the probabilities examined in the two ways given earlier will not be exactly equal. An example of a situation in which they would be equal could be given as the following. What is the probability that the true proportion of the population is .55 if a sample of 80 finds a proportion of .45? In this case, the two proportions are equidistant from the center of the probability distribution, which is .5. The proportion .55 of 80 is 44 and .45 of 80 is 36. Now if we use =BINOMDIST(36,80,.55,1), we discover that the probability of finding thirty-six or fewer out of eighty when the probability is .45 is .046. If we use $1 - $ (=BINOMDIST(43,80,.45,1)), we discover that the probability of finding forty-four or more out of eighty is .046. This happens because .45 and .55 are equidistant on opposite sides of .5, so their skewnesses are mirror images of one another.

The fact that the two different decision rules may not always produce the same probability should not be a source of great concern. In most cases, the probabilities will differ only slightly. Only infrequently would a different decision be reached from one view versus the other.

Exercises for Section 5.3

1. Use Equation 5.6 to determine the probability of any one outcome of the following:
   a. $n = 5, x = 2, p = .646$
   b. $n = 11, x = 9, p = .42$
   c. $n = 11, x = 7, p = .42$
   d. $n = 120, x = 35, p = .5$
   e. $n = 120, x = 60, p = .5$

2. Use Equation 5.7 to determine the number of separate outcomes for the following:
   a. $n = 5, x = 2$
   b. $n = 11, x = 9$
   c. $n = 11, x = 7$
   d. $n = 120, x = 35$
   e. $n = 120, x = 60$

3. Use Equation 5.8 to determine the binomial probability of the following:
   a. $n = 5, x = 2, p = .646$
   b. $n = 11, x = 9, p = .42$
   c. $n = 11, x = 7, p = .42$

d. $n = 120, x = 35, p = .5$

e. $n = 120, x = 60, p = .5$

4. Use the =BINOMDIST() function to determine the binomial probability of the following and determine if they are the same as what is given in Exercise 3.

a. $n = 5, x = 2, p = .646$

b. $n = 11, x = 9, p = .42$

c. $n = 11, x = 7, p = .42$

d. $n = 120, x = 35, p = .5$

e. $n = 120, x = 60, p = .5$

5. Use the formulas in Equation 5.6, Equation 5.7, and Equation 5.8 to replicate Figure 5.12.

a. Add the comparable values as generated by the =BINOMDIST() function as column D.

b. Add the cumulative probabilities as column E by accumulating column C from $x = 0$.

c. Add the cumulative probabilities as column F by using =BINOMDIST() with 1 as the final argument.

d. Do columns C and D and columns E and F match?

6. A local health department counsels expectant mothers coming to a prenatal clinic on cigarette smoking only if they are smokers. History has shown that about 27 percent of expectant mothers are smokers when they first come to the clinic. Assume that the clinic will see eleven new expectant mothers today.

a. Use the formulas in Equation 5.6, Equation 5.7, and Equation 5.8 to determine binomial probabilities that the health department will see no women who smoke today, one woman who smokes, two women who smoke, and so on, up to eleven women who smoke.

b. Use =BINOMDIST() to determine the same values.

c. Accumulate the values found in a (preceding) from 0 to 11.

d. Use =BINOMDIST() to determine the cumulative probabilities.

e. Make sure that the two sets of probabilities are equal to one another.

7. A dentist sees about fifteen new patients per month (the rest of her patients are repeats). She knows that on average, over the past year, about half of her patients have needed at least one filling on their first visit.

a. What is the probability that she will see ten patients or more out of fifteen who need fillings?

b. What is the probability that she will see five or fewer patients who need fillings?

  c. What is the probability that she will see between seven and ten new patients who need fillings?

 8. An emergency room head wants to know the proportion of emergency room patients who spend more than one hour before being attended to. He knows that the time of arrival at the emergency room and the time of seeing the first medical staff member are both recorded in the emergency room record. He draws a random sample of fifty records and discovers that fourteen indicate that the person spent more than one hour in waiting.

  a. What is the probability that the true proportion of persons spending more than one hour is 36 percent or more?

  b. What is the probability that the true proportion of persons spending more than one hour is 20 percent or less?

  c. What is the probability that the true proportion of persons spending more than one hour is from 24 to 32 percent?

Section 5.4 The Poisson Distribution

The Poisson distribution, like the binomial distribution, is a discrete distribution. It takes on values only for whole numbers. But whereas the binomial distribution is concerned with the probability of two outcomes over a number of trials, the Poisson distribution is concerned with the number of observations that will occur in a small amount of time or over a region of space. We have been discussing the probability of seeing a certain number of emergencies out of a number of persons who arrive at an emergency room. The binomial distribution describes these probabilities. But if we consider the actual arrival at the emergency room of anyone, emergency or not, the Poisson distribution is more likely to describe these probabilities.

  Consider again the emergency room that deals with twenty-nine people, on average, during an administrator's eight-hour shift. The administrator can figure out that this is an average of just about 0.9 persons-or just less than one person-every fifteen minutes. She also knows that it takes about fifteen minutes to go through all the administrative paperwork—checking insurance coverage, inquiring about previous visits, and so on—entailed in getting a person into the system. She knows that she will have to be prepared to deal with about one person every fifteen minutes, but she also knows that on occasion there are several people who arrive within the same fifteen-minute time interval, even when they come for different reasons. She would like to know, then, how often she will have to be prepared to deal with two people, or three or four, in any fifteen-minute time interval. She can determine this with the Poisson distribution.

FIGURE 5.17. POISSON DISTRIBUTION OF EMERGENCY ROOM ARRIVALS IN FIFTEEN-MINUTE INTERVALS.

	B2	▼	=	=POISSON(A2,$B$11,0)	
	A	B	C	D	
1	Arrivals	Probability			
2	0	0.407			
3	1	0.366			
4	2	0.165			
5	3	0.049			
6	4	0.011			
7	5	0.002			
8	6	0.000			
9		1.000			
10					
11	Average	0.9			
12					

Figure 5.17 shows the Poisson-predicted probabilities for the number of arrivals in any fifteen-minute period. The probabilities are calculated using the =POISSON() function, which takes three arguments. These are the number of arrivals (A2 in the formula line), the average number of arrivals during the period of time under consideration ($B$11 in the formula line, and generally termed λ in the context of the Poisson distribution), and a zero to indicate that the actual probability is desired.

It is important to point out that the probabilities shown in Figure 5.17 are based on three assumptions. First, the arrival of an emergency in any fifteen-minute time interval is independent of arrivals in any other fifteen-minute time interval. Second, the number of arrivals in the time interval is proportional to the size of the interval. Finally, the likelihood of more than one arrival in the time interval is very small. If the administrator accepts these assumptions, she can see from Figure 5.17 that in only a small number of fifteen-minute intervals (about two in any eight-hour shift, .063 $\times$ 32 or 2.01) will she have to deal with more than two arrivals in the same fifteen-minute interval. Moreover, she will have to deal with more than three arrivals in a fifteen-minute period in only about one fifteen-minute interval in any two eight-hour shifts (.013 $\times$ 32 or .416). On this basis, she may be well justified to be prepared to deal with up to two arrivals in a fifteen-minute time period but to let the arrival of three or more persons be treated as an unlikely event that will be handled by the mobilization of extra resources.

In the section on the binomial distribution, we spent a good deal of time showing where the binomial distribution comes from. This was for two reasons.

For one, the binomial distribution is a relatively easy distribution to understand. Second, the number of different combinations of any outcome (HHTHT, for example) is a general formula that applies to many different aspects of statistics. The Poisson distribution, however, is more difficult to derive and does not immediately apply to other aspects of statistics. So in the case of the Poisson distribution, we will just look at the formula for the distribution directly. The formula for the Poisson distribution is shown in Equation 5.9.

$$P(x) = \frac{\lambda^x e^{-y}}{x!}, \quad x = 0, 1, 2, \ldots$$

$$P(x) = 0, \qquad \text{otherwise}$$

(5.9)

Equation 5.9 says that the probability of any value x is equal to the quantity λ to the power of x times e to the power of $-\lambda$, divided by $x!$ for 0 and integer values of x, but 0 for noninteger values of x. Like the binomial distribution, the Poisson distribution is defined only for 0 and integers. The term $e^{-\lambda}$ is the value of e (approximately 2.718) raised to the negative power of the mean number of arrivals in any given interval of time.

Figure 5.18 shows the calculated values of the Poisson distribution for emergency room arrivals in fifteen-minute intervals. Column B gives the value of λ^x, where x represents zero to six arrivals. Column C is simply the value of e (2.718) raised to the power of $-\lambda$. Column D is the factorial value for each number of arrivals, zero to six. Column E uses the formula in Equation 5.9 to replicate the values in column B in Figure 5.17.

FIGURE 5.18. CALCULATED POISSON DISTRIBUTION OF EMERGENCY ROOM ARRIVALS IN FIFTEEN-MINUTE INTERVALS.

	A	B	C	D	E	F
1	Arrivals	Lambda^x	e^-Lambda	x!	Probability	
2	0	1	0.4065697	1	0.407	
3	1	0.9	0.4065697	1	0.366	
4	2	0.81	0.4065697	2	0.165	
5	3	0.729	0.4065697	6	0.049	
6	4	0.6561	0.4065697	24	0.011	
7	5	0.59049	0.4065697	120	0.002	
8	6	0.531441	0.4065697	720	0.000	
9					1.000	
10						
11	Lambda	0.9				
12						

FIGURE 5.19. CALCULATED POISSON DISTRIBUTION OF EMERGENCY ROOM ARRIVALS: EXCEL FORMULAS.

	A	B	C	D	E
1	Arrivals	Lambda^x	e^-Lambda	x!	Probability
2	0	=$B$11^A2	=EXP(-$B$11)	=FACT(A2)	=B2*C2/D2
3	1	=$B$11^A3	=EXP(-$B$11)	=FACT(A3)	=B3*C3/D3
4	2	=$B$11^A4	=EXP(-$B$11)	=FACT(A4)	=B4*C4/D4
5	3	=$B$11^A5	=EXP(-$B$11)	=FACT(A5)	=B5*C5/D5
6	4	=$B$11^A6	=EXP(-$B$11)	=FACT(A6)	=B6*C6/D6
7	5	=$B$11^A7	=EXP(-$B$11)	=FACT(A7)	=B7*C7/D7
8	6	=$B$11^A8	=EXP(-$B$11)	=FACT(A8)	=B8*C8/D8
9					=SUM(E2:E8)
10					
11	Lambda	0.9			
12					

Figure 5.19 shows the Excel formulas for the calculations in Figure 5.18. The calculations in column C use the Excel =EXP() function that raises the value of e to the power of the value in the parentheses. The calculations in column D use the =FACT() function, which provides the factorial of the number in parentheses. Both of these functions take only one argument. The formulas shown in Figure 5.19 are revealed in Excel by the selection of Tools/Options from the menu bar and the checking of the Formula box on the View tab.

Poisson distributions apply not only to the distribution of occurrences in short periods of time but also to occurrences in regions. For example, suppose a hospital supply room is responsible for maintaining a supply of, say, rubber gloves, which come in boxes of a hundred. Quality control is supposed to be very good concerning rubber gloves. However, the hospital supply room manager has found that he gets reports of an average of about two gloves in every box of a hundred that are not usable for one reason or another. Given this information, what is the probability that in any given box of gloves all will be usable? What is the probability that only one will not be usable, or that more than five will not be usable? This can also be found by using the Poisson distribution.

Figure 5.20 shows a chart of the distribution of probabilities for the number of gloves that will be unusable in a box of a hundred if the average number unusable in a box is two. The supply room manager can expect about 14 percent of the boxes to have all good gloves, an equal number, about 27 percent, to have one or two unusable gloves, and about 18 percent to have three unusable gloves. A very small percent of boxes will have as many as eight unusable gloves.

FIGURE 5.20. CHART OF POISSON DISTRIBUTION FOR GLOVES THAT ARE NOT USABLE IN A BOX OF A HUNDRED.

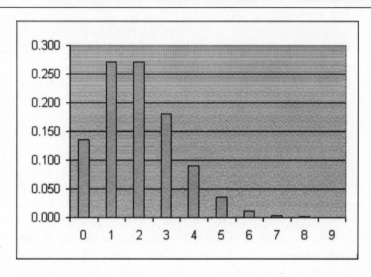

Exercises for Section 5.4

1. Replicate the poison distribution for persons arriving at the emergency room, as is shown in Figure 5.17, using
   a. The =POISSON() function
   b. The Poisson formula shown in Equation 5.9

2. Calculate the Poisson probabilities for finding unusable gloves in a box of a hundred if the average is two per box
   a. Using the =POISSON() function
   b. Using the Poisson formula shown in Equation 5.9
   c. Replicate the chart in Figure 5.20

Section 5.5 The Normal Distribution

The last topic that will be taken up in this chapter is the normal distribution. Both the binomial distribution and the Poisson distribution are distributions that describe discrete numerical variables. That is, under the appropriate circumstances, they will give us the probability of discrete events, such as the probability of a certain number of true emergencies among visitors to an emergency room or the number of people who will arrive at the emergency room in a given period of time. These are discrete events.

The normal distribution, however, provides probabilities for continuous numerical variables. Height of adult males, for example, is a continuous variable. Body temperature is another continuous variable, as is pulse rate or blood pressure. The amount of time spent in a physician's waiting room or with the physician is a continuous variable. All of these variables can be determined not by counting, which can be done with a discrete variable, but by measurement. In general, it is reasonable to say that a continuous numerical variable is the result of some measurement—with a watch, a length rule, a scale, and so forth.

The normal distribution is just one of a number of distributions that describe the properties of continuous numerical data, but in terms of elementary statistical applications, it is by far the most important and is the only continuous distribution treated in any detail in this text. The chi-square distribution and the F distribution, both continuous distributions, will be discussed, but only as these apply to hypothesis testing.

To briefly introduce the normal distribution, consider the Excel chart shown in Figure 5.21. This chart represents the normal distribution. The normal distribution is discussed in detail in Chapter Six, but several points are made about it here. First, the normal distribution has often been called a bell-shaped curve because it looks like the cross-section of a bell. Second, because the normal distribution looks like a bell, both sides of the distribution have exactly equal probabilities. For example, if the probability of being at the point -1 on the horizontal scale is

FIGURE 5.21. A NORMAL DISTRIBUTION.

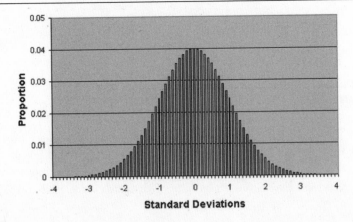

.024, then the probability of being at 1 on the horizontal scale is also .024. More-over, the probability of being between -3 and 0 is exactly the same as being between 0 and 3.

In Figure 5.21, the horizontal axis is given as Standard Deviations. The mean-ing of the term *standard deviation* is also discussed in detail in Chapter Six, but for now it is sufficient to say that in any normal distribution, 68 percent of all obser-vations will be within 1 standard deviation of the center of the distribution. Consequently, if a set of data is normally distributed-average height of adult males, for example, then it can be expected that in a large sample of adult males, 68 per-cent will have heights no less than one standard deviation below the average and no more than one standard deviation above the average. Furthermore, if the average height of adult males is normally distributed, 95 percent of all adult males will have heights between -2 and 2 standard deviations on either side of the average and 99 percent will have heights between -3 and 3 standard deviations on either side of the average.

The average height of adult males in the United States is about sixty-nine inches. Let us say that virtually all adult U.S. males are at least sixty inches tall and no more than seventy-eight inches tall. (Of course, there are some U.S. adult males, professional basketball players, for example, who are notably taller than seventy-eight inches, but that, too, is a characteristic of normal distributions. They have no upper or lower limits.) But, to continue, if the range of adult human height is sixty to seventy-eight inches and *if* height is normally distributed, then we could say that the standard deviation of height is about three inches. Consequently, we could say that 68 percent of all U.S. males are between sixty-six and seventy-two inches tall. Furthermore, we could say that 95 percent of all adult males are between sixty-three and seventy-five inches tall and 99 percent are between sixty and seventy-eight inches tall.

The use of height to discuss the normal distribution is not accidental. Height is a measure. On the measurement scale of height, a person may be at any point. He does not need to be exactly sixty-nine inches tall (although we might mea-sure him as such). The normal probability distribution is a distribution of measurement. This is in contrast to both the binomial probability distribution and the Poisson probability distribution, which are both distributions of events or counts. Because the normal distribution is a distribution of measures, it is a con-tinuous numerical probability distribution. More is said about the consequence of this fact in Chapter Six.

CHAPTER SIX

MEASURES OF CENTRAL TENDENCY AND DISPERSION: DATA DISTRIBUTIONS

There are three related, but quite different, uses of statistics. The first of these uses is descriptive. In a descriptive context, statistics are used to characterize either a total population or a sample from that population, but they go no further than characterization. The second use of statistics is inferential. In an inferential context, statistics from a sample are used to make inferences about the populations from which the samples were drawn. The third use of statistics is in hypothesis testing. Here, statistics are used to assign a probability to the likelihood that a particular statistical value could have come from some specifiable population, that two (or more) sample (or population) groups are different from one another, or that a measure taken from a sample (or from a population) is of a particular value. This chapter deals with the first of these uses of statistics: description. Subsequent chapters deal in detail with both inferential statistics and hypothesis testing.

Section 6.1 Measures of Central Tendency and Dispersion

This chapter is about data distributions. Two ways of characterizing any data distribution is by the central values around which the data cluster—measures of central tendency—and by the extent to which the data are variable—measures of dispersion.

FIGURE 6.1. TIME SPENT BY PHYSICIAN WITH PATIENTS.

	A	B	
1	Patient	Minutes with patient	
2	1	2	
3	2	8	
4	3	11	
5	4	12	
6	5	6	
7	6	10	
8	7	7	
9	8	8	
10	9	14	
11	10	8	
12	11	7	
13	12	14	

Central Tendency

One of the most important ways of characterizing either populations or samples is to provide information about what is called the central tendency of the data. There are three commonly employed measures of central tendency: the Mean, the Median, and the Mode. These three measures can be illustrated with the data shown in Figure 6.1. This figure shows the amount of time, in one-minute intervals, spent by a physician with people coming to his office practice. Patient 1 received two minutes of the physician's time, patient 2 received eight minutes, and so on.

The *mode* refers to the most commonly appearing value in a set of data. In this case, eight minutes is the most commonly appearing value and is the mode, or modal value. The physician spent eight minutes with each of three patients. Data sets can be bi- or multimodal if more than one value is represented an equal number of times. If, for example, patient 5 had received seven minutes of the physician's time, both eight minutes and seven minutes would have been modal values. In general, although the mode is usually listed as one of the three measures of central tendency, it rarely figures into any further statistical applications.

The *median* refers to the middle value in an ordered set of values, or, if there is an even number of values, it refers to the average of the two middle values. If we look at the data from Figure 6.1, as reordered in Figure 6.2, we can see that the sixth and seventh observations (out of twelve, an even number) are both eight. The average of two values of 8 are also 8, so that the median for this set of data is 8. Typically, it is more likely that the median will be used to describe a

FIGURE 6.2. ORDERED TIME SPENT BY PHYSICIAN WITH PATIENTS.

	A	B
1	Patient	Minutes with patient
2	1	2
3	5	6
4	7	7
5	11	7
6	2	8
7	8	8
8	10	8
9	6	10
10	3	11
11	4	12
12	9	14
13	12	14

set of data than the mode. It is not uncommon to see the median referenced as the measure of central tendency in such examples as median family income, median age, and median inpatient days.

The mode provides a measure of central tendency that uses only the most commonly appearing value. The median essentially provides a measure of central tendency that uses only the middle value—for an odd number of observations—or the two middle values—for an even number of observations—in an ordered array. The *mean* uses all the information in the data set to provide a measure of central tendency. The mean is a familiar concept to most readers. It is the average. Few people taking a first time statistics course are unfamiliar with how to obtain an average for a set of numbers; you just add them all up and divide by the total number.

In statistical applications, however, the average is almost always called the mean and is defined formally *for a sample*, as:

$$\bar{x} = \frac{\sum_{i=1}^{n} x_i}{n} \tag{6.1}$$

where $\bar{x}$ (pronounced x bar) designates the sample mean and $\sum$ (pronounced sigma) indicates a summation of all values x_i from $i = 1$ to $i = n$, with n being the sample size.

For the data shown in Figure 6.1, Equation 6.1 would be executed as $(2 + 8 + 11 + \cdots + 14)/12$ (the three dots mean continue adding the numbers together), and the result would be the mean, which is approximately 8.92. In this example, the median is 8 and the mean is 8.92. The mean and the median are frequently different. In certain situations, such as with personal income, the median and the mean might be substantially different, with the mean being larger than the median. This occurs because a large number of people are making a relatively small amount of money, and a very few people such as the owner of the company that makes Excel—are making a great deal of money. Such a situation usually obtains, also, in regard to hospital days or hospital costs. A large number of people stay in the hospital for short periods of time and have *relatively* smaller charges, whereas a small number of people have relatively long hospital stays and high charges. So, for both personal income and hospital days and cost per admission, the mean is higher than the median and the distribution of both are skewed to the right. If the mean of a data set is lower than the median, the data are skewed to the left.

Excel provides a function for each of the three measures of central tendency. These are =MODE(), =MEDIAN(), and =AVERAGE() (*not* =MEAN()). The =MEDIAN() and =AVERAGE() functions work just as would be expected, producing the correct value. The =MODE() function will produce the correct value if the data set has only one mode. If it has more than one mode, it will produce a result that indicates only one of the modal values—the value that appears earliest in the data set.

Most of the work we do in this book with measures of central tendency will be done with the mean. The presentation in Equation 6.1 refers specifically to the mean of a sample of observations from some larger population. In the case of the data shown in Figure 6.1 or Figure 6.2, the population would presumably be all patients who ever did or ever will come to the office of the particular physician in question. If we were to consider the mean as a measure of central tendency for the entire population of patients who ever did or ever will visit this physician, it would be designated by slightly different symbols. The mean *for a population* is defined as shown in Equation 6.2. In Equation 6.2, the sample designation $\bar{x}$ has been replaced by the population designation μ and the sample designation for all the observations in the sample, n, has been replaced by the population designation for all possible observations in the population, N.

$$\mu = \frac{\sum_{i=1}^{N} x_i}{N} \qquad (6.2)$$

where μ (the small Greek letter for m, pronounced mu) designates the population mean and N represents all patients who ever have or ever will visit the physician. The value of x_i is summed from $i = 1$ to N.

The point of using the formula in Equation 6.1 to calculate the mean of the sample is that it is what is known as an *unbiased estimator* of the true population mean defined in Equation 6.2. An unbiased estimator is a sample estimator of a population parameter for which the mean value from all possible samples will be exactly equal to the population value. Thus, since $\bar{x}$ is an unbiased estimator of μ, the mean of the values of $\bar{x}$ from all possible samples taken from the population will be exactly equal to μ. More is said of this in the next section.

Dispersion

A measure of central tendency, whether it be the mode, median, or mean, can be produced for virtually any data set. Similarly, a measure of dispersion or variation in the data can also be produced for any data set. A simple measure of dispersion, which is often mentioned in introductory statistics texts, is the range. The range is the difference between the largest and smallest values in the data set. There are also a number of modifications on the range, such as the range within which are found the lowest 25 percent of cases, the highest 25 percent of cases, the middle 50 percent of cases, and so on. The range is a measure of dispersion that is similar in concept to the median as a measure of central tendency. It uses only a limited amount of the data. Except for some descriptive purposes, the range is rarely used in statistical analysis applications and is therefore not discussed further in this book.

The measure of dispersion that, like the mean, uses all the information in the data is the *variance*, or its square root, the *standard deviation*. Both the variance and standard deviation are used extensively in statistical applications and are, in fact, the basis upon which much of statistics is constructed. The variance for a sample is defined mathematically as shown in Equation 6.3.

$$s^2 = \frac{\sum_{i=1}^{n}(x_i - \bar{x})^2}{n-1} \tag{6.3}$$

where s^2 designates the variance and Σ indicates a summation of all values of $(x_i - \bar{x})^2$ from $i = 1$ to $i = n$.

The standard deviation for a sample is calculated as shown in Equation 6.4.

$$s = \sqrt{s^2} \tag{6.4}$$

Basically, the variance is a measure of the extent to which each observation differs from the mean of all observations. For the data shown in Figure 6.1, the variance calculation is shown in Figure 6.3, an Excel spreadsheet representation

FIGURE 6.3. CALCULATION OF VARIANCE.

C17	▼	=	=VAR(B3:B14)

	A	B	C	D
1				
2	Patient	Minutes (x)	(x-xbar)^2	
3	1	2	47.84028	
4	2	8	0.840278	
5	3	11	4.340278	
6	4	12	9.506944	
7	5	6	8.506944	
8	6	10	1.173611	
9	7	7	3.673611	
10	8	8	0.840278	
11	9	14	25.84028	
12	10	8	0.840278	
13	11	7	3.673611	
14	12	14	25.84028	
15	xbar	8.9166667	132.9167	
16		variance	12.08333	
17			12.08333	
18				

of the calculation. In Figure 6.3, the patient number is shown in cells A3 to A14 and the minutes spent with the physician are shown in cells B3 to B14. Cells C3 to C14 show the calculation of the numerator portion of Equation 6.3. The mean value for the data (shown in cell B15) is subtracted from each cell: B3 to B14, and the result is then squared (the Excel formula for cell C3, for example, is (=(B3-$B$15)^2). The title in cell C2 is a convenient way to show this operation in Excel, since it is difficult to put bars above letters or to create superscripts to show the square process. The ^2 is the Excel convention for raising a value to a power. Cell C15 is the sum of the squared differences (=SUM(C3:C14)) and Cell 16 is the actual variance as calculated by the formula in Equation 6.3 (=C15/11). The number in cell C17, which is identical to cell C16, is the variance as calculated using the =VAR() function provided by Excel. This function can be seen in the formula bar above the spreadsheet, since cell C17 was the highlighted cell when the figure was copied from Excel. It is relatively easy to confirm the results shown in Figure 6.3. All that is required is to enter the data in column B into an Excel spreadsheet and follow the formula given in Equation 6.3.

IMPORTANT: An Excel function result should always agree with the result obtained using a formula that appears in this book. If these two do not agree, either the formula was not correctly done or the wrong formula was used to reproduce the result of the function. Invoking the Excel function is always a sure test of whether you understand the formula and concept.

The variance is a measure of dispersion calculated on the basis of squared differences between each observation and the mean of all observations. This produces a measure of dispersion that is not on the same scale as the measure of central tendency (the mean). The variance actually corresponds more closely to the square of the mean than to the mean itself. To get the measure of dispersion back to the same scale as the mean, the measure of dispersion that is typically used is the standard deviation, shown in Equation 6.4.

The value of the standard deviation for the data shown in Figure 6.3 is approximately 3.48. You can confirm this by using the function =STDEV(), which Excel provides to calculate the standard deviation on the data shown in Figure 6.3. You can also confirm that the =STDEV() function actually produces the square root of the variance by using the =SQRT() function to calculate the square root of the variance given in the same figure. You should find that the results of the two methods are the same.

The formulas in Equation 6.3 and Equation 6.4 are formulas that provide the variance and standard deviation for samples from a larger population. If we wished to calculate the variance and standard deviation for the entire population of patients who ever had or ever would attend the clinic in question, we would use the formula shown in Equation 6.5. The equation for the standard deviation of the population, designated δ^2, is just the square root of the value in Equation 6.5.

$$\delta^2 = \frac{\sum_{i=1}^{N}(x_i - \mu)^2}{N} \tag{6.5}$$

where δ^2 designates the variance and N indicates that the summation of $(x_i - \mu)^2$ is over all observations in the entire population.

Why Is the Sample Variance Divided by $n - 1$?

In the calculation of the most frequently used measure of central tendency—the mean, the formulas for the sample estimate of the population parameter (Equation 6.1) and the population parameter itself (Equation 6.2) are calculated essentially the same way. All the values are summed and divided by the number of separate values. For the variance, however, and similarly for the standard deviation, the population value and the sample values are not calculated in the same way. The population variance as shown in Equation 6.5 is, logically, the sum of all the squared differences between actual values and the overall mean divided by the total number of observations; but the sample variance (Equation 6.3) is divided, instead, by the total number of observations less one. On the face of it, this does not seem logical. Why should it be?

Interestingly, the answer to this question has to do, again, with unbiased estimators. As was mentioned earlier, the sample formula for the mean shown in Equation 6.1 is an unbiased estimator of the population value of the mean shown in Equation 6.2. Similarly, under a particular sampling assumption, *sampling with replacement,* the sample formula for the variance shown in Equation 6.3 will be an unbiased estimator of the population value of the variance calculated, as shown in Equation 6.5. In other words, if we took all possible samples from a population using the sampling technique of sampling with replacement, the average variance for all possible samples calculated, as given in Equation 6.3, would be exactly equal to the population variance calculated, as given in Equation 6.5. This relationship has been proved mathematically, and the proof is given, for example, in Freund and Walpole (1987). Such a proof is beyond the scope of this book. But what this book does do is use the capabilities of Excel to demonstrate that the sample variance calculated, as given in Equation 6.3, is an unbiased estimate of the population variance calculated, as given in Equation 6.5, for a very small population and a very small sample. Such a demonstration does not guarantee that it will work for any population or for any sample, but it at least demonstrates that it is reasonable.

Let us imagine a very small population that consists of only four observations. These four observations take on the following four values: 2, 4, 5, and 7. If this is the entire population, it is relatively easy to confirm that the mean, μ, for this population is 4.50, using the formula in Equation 6.2, and the variance δ^2 is 3.25, using the formula in Equation 6.5. To examine the effect of taking all possible samples, we can limit ourselves to all the possible samples of a given size. Whatever the outcome for a sample of any size, the outcome for all samples of other sizes will be the same.

First, what is sampling with replacement? Suppose we want a sample of size 2, and we randomly select one observation from our very small population, which turns out to be 5. Now we will draw a second observation from the population to complete the sample of two. In sampling with replacement, we return the observation 5 to the population so that it has an equal chance, along with all other observations, of being drawn in the second selection. If we were sampling

FIGURE 6.4. ALL SAMPLES OF 2 FROM A POPULATION OF 4.

	A	B	C	D	E	F	G	H
1		Population	Sample	First	Second	Mean	Variance	
2		2	1	2	2	2	0	
3		4	2	2	4	3	2	
4		5	3	2	5	3.5	4.5	
5		7	4	2	7	4.5	12.5	
6			5	4	2	3	2	
7			6	4	4	4	0	
8	Mean	4.50	7	4	5	4.5	0.5	
9	Variance	3.25	8	4	7	5.5	4.5	
10			9	5	2	3.5	4.5	
11			10	5	4	4.5	0.5	
12			11	5	5	5	0	
13			12	5	7	6	2	
14			13	7	2	4.5	12.5	
15			14	7	4	5.5	4.5	
16			15	7	5	6	2	
17			16	7	7	7	0	
18								
19					Overall average	4.5	3.25	
20								

without replacement and drew the observation with the value of 5 on the first draw, that observation would not be available for the second draw, which would be limited to the observations with values of 2, 4, and 7.

If we are taking samples with replacement, there are N^n different samples of size n that can be taken from a population of size N. (If we are taking samples without replacement, there are $N!/(n!(N-n)!)$ different samples of size n that can be taken from a population of size N, a substantially smaller number. This is discussed in more detail later, but you should recognize this as being part of the binomial distribution formula.) In the case of our population of four observations, there are 4^2, or sixteen, different samples of size 2 that can be taken from the population with replacement. These samples are shown in Figure 6.4.

Cells B2:B5 in Figure 6.4 are the values taken on by each of the four members of the population. The value in B8 is the mean of the population calculated with the Excel function =AVERAGE(B2:B5). The value in cell B9 is the variance of the population calculated with the Excel function =VARP(B2:B5), which calculates the population variance as given in Equation 6.5. The cells C2:C17 just number the sixteen different samples of size 2 that can be taken from the population of 4 with replacement. Cells D2:D17 show the first observation in each sample, and

E2:E17 show the second. Cells F2:F17 represent the means of each sample calculated, using =AVERAGE() for each of the corresponding two cells in D and E. For example, cell F2 is calculated as =AVERAGE(D2:E2). Cell F19 is calculated as =AVERAGE(F2:F17). It can be seen that it matches the value in B8. Similarly, cells G2:G17 are calculated by the Excel function =VAR(), with the appropriate references in columns D and E. Note that the =VAR() function divides by $n - 1$ rather than by n. The number in cell G19 is calculated as =AVERAGE(G2:G17) and is the average of all the sample variances. It is exactly equivalent to cell B9. If, instead of using =VAR() to calculate the sample variances in G2:G17, =VARP() had been used, the average of all sample variances (cell G19) would have been not 3.25 but, rather, 1.625—a value much smaller than the true population variance.

This is a demonstration of the appropriateness of using the formulation in Equation 6.3 as the sample variance if we want a measure that will be an unbiased estimate of the population variance as calculated in Equation 6.5. But two things should be remembered. First, although it is a demonstration (and it works every time), it is not a proof. Also, this relationship between Equation 6.3 and Equation 6.5 holds only for samples taken with replacement. In most cases, samples are not taken with replacement. If you draw a sample of people for interviews, you would not want to interview the same person twice if it happened by chance that he or she got into the sample twice. When sampling without replacement, the formulation in Equation 6.3 is not an unbiased estimate of the population variance. But, in general, the size of a sample relative to the size of a population makes it highly unlikely that any single population item will be selected more than once, so that sampling with replacement might be assumed. Interestingly, when sampling without replacement, the average of all sample variances calculated by Equation 6.3 turns out to be numerically equal to the variance of the population calculated by replacing N in Equation 6.5 with $N - 1$.

One other point should be made in regard to unbiased estimates of dispersion. The typical measure of dispersion used is the standard deviation or the square root of the variance. The average value of the standard deviation of all possible samples from any population will not be equal to the standard deviation of the total population, calculated by any means. This is because, in general, $\sqrt{\Sigma x_i} \neq \Sigma \sqrt{x_i}$.

Why Is the Measure of Dispersion So Complicated?

Why is it necessary to use something as complicated as the sum of the squared difference between each observation and the mean as the measure of dispersion (or the square root of that value, which is even more complicated)? Could there not be a simpler measure of dispersion that did not involve the complicating problem of squaring and taking square roots? For example, could we not use simply the difference between each value and the mean or the absolute value of the difference between each value and the mean?

One such possibility might be the sum of the differences between each value and the mean of all values, which could be shown as:

$$\sum_{i=1}^{n} (x - \bar{x}) \tag{6.6}$$

Unfortunately, this strategy does not work well. Since the mean is the numerical midpoint of the distribution, the sum of all the negative numbers will always equal the sum of all the positive numbers derived from the operation given in Equation 6.6, so the result of this operation is always zero for every data set. Because of this, Equation 6.6 cannot serve as a useful measure of dispersion.

But what if a measure of dispersion was the *absolute value* of the difference between each observation and the mean of all observations? Such a possibility would be expressed as Equation 6.7:

$$\sum_{i=1}^{n} |x - \bar{x}| \tag{6.7}$$

Unfortunately, this criterion also does not work well for a measure of dispersion if our measure of central tendency is the mean. In Equation 6.6, subtracting the mean from every value and summing the results always produces zero. Summing the difference between each observation and any constant other than the mean will produce a result greater or less than zero. In this sense, Equation 6.6 is *centered* on the mean. One assumption we are making is that any measure of dispersion we ultimately choose should be centered on the mean.

To understand the notion of *centered* in the context of Equation 6.7, consider the table shown in Figure 6.5. This table shows a column (A16 to A22) of seven data points that take on the values 1 through 7, respectively. It is easy to confirm that the mean of these seven items is 4. Cells B15 to H15 contain seven possible constants that may be substituted for the mean in Equation 6.7, including the true mean of 4. The formula line in Figure 6.5 shows that the cell B16 is the absolute difference between A16 and B15. Cell B17 is the absolute difference between A17 and B15. The remaining values are calculated in the same way. The sums of the absolute differences in each column are given in cells B23 through H23. The value 12 in cell E23, which corresponds to the mean, is the smallest of the sum of absolute differences. In this sense, the result of Equation 6.7 is centered on the mean *in this data set*. If any number other than the mean is used as the constant subtractor, the result of the sum of absolute differences will be greater than the value

FIGURE 6.5. SUM OF ABSOLUTE DIFFERENCES.

	B16			=	=ABS($A16-B$15)			
	A	B	C	D	E	F	G	H
14		Constant						
15	Data	1	2	3	4	5	6	7
16	1	0	1	2	3	4	5	6
17	2	1	0	1	2	3	4	5
18	3	2	1	0	1	2	3	4
19	4	3	2	1	0	1	2	3
20	5	4	3	2	1	0	1	2
21	6	5	4	3	2	1	0	1
22	7	6	5	4	3	2	1	0
23		21	16	13	12	13	16	21

FIGURE 6.6. SUM OF ABSOLUTE DIFFERENCES, EXAMPLE 2.

	B30			=	=ABS($A30-B$15)			
	A	B	C	D	E	F	G	H
28		Constant						
29	Data	1	2	3	4	5	6	7
30	1	0	1	2	3	4	5	6
31	2	1	0	1	2	3	4	5
32	2	1	0	1	2	3	4	5
33	2	1	0	1	2	3	4	5
34	7	6	5	4	3	2	1	0
35	7	6	5	4	3	2	1	0
36	7	6	5	4	3	2	1	0
37		21	16	17	18	19	20	21

when the mean is employed. In general, a working assumption is that whatever measure of dispersion is chosen, it should be centered on the mean in the same sense that it produces a minimum sum of differences at, and only at, the mean.

But Equation 6.7 does not always produce the minimum value at the mean. In fact, it turns out that Equation 6.7 always produces a minimum value at the median. To see an illustration of this, consider the data shown in Figure 6.6. This table again shows seven observations (cells A30 to A36), but in this case, it is not difficult to confirm that the mean of the data elements is 4, whereas the median is 2. Again, the values in the cells B30 to H36 are the absolute differences between each data point and the constant values listed in B29 to H29. Now it can be seen that the minimum value of the absolute differences (16 in column C) is not centered on the mean of 4 but, rather, on the median of 2. This is the primary reason that the absolute differences between each value and the mean are not

FIGURE 6.7. SUM OF SQUARED DIFFERENCES.

	B44	▼	=	=($A44-B$15)^2				
	A	B	C	D	E	F	G	H
42		Constant						
43	Data	1	2	3	4	5	6	7
44	1	0	1	4	9	16	25	36
45	2	1	0	1	4	9	16	25
46	2	1	0	1	4	9	16	25
47	2	1	0	1	4	9	16	25
48	7	36	25	16	9	4	1	0
49	7	36	25	16	9	4	1	0
50	7	36	25	16	9	4	1	0
51		111	76	55	48	55	76	111

generally used as a measure of dispersion when the mean is the measure of central tendency. (It can also be shown that for data sets that have even numbers of cases, the absolute difference is centered in the sense discussed here on both values that define the median and all possible numerical values between them.)

Now what of the sum of squared differences (Equation 6.3) as a measure of dispersion? Does it provide a measure that is centered on the mean? Consider Figure 6.7. This figure shows the sum of squared differences for the data originally displayed in Figure 6.6. Now, the minimum value of the sum of differences (squared) is at the mean of 4, so the sum of squared differences is centered at the mean. The reader might wish to confirm that for the data in Figure 6.5, the sum of squared differences is a minimum at the mean. It will turn out that for any data set, the sum of squared differences has the desirable property that it is centered at the mean in the sense that the sum of squared differences between the data elements and any constant will be a minimum when the true mean is the constant.

Exercises for Section 6.1

1. Use the Hospital charges worksheet in the file Chpt 4–1.xls.
   a. Calculate the mean and median for Age, LOS, and Charges by using the Excel functions =AVERAGE() and =MEDIAN().
   b. Based on these, in what direction are these distributions skewed, if at all.
   c. Calculate the variance and standard deviation of Age, LOS, and Charges by using the formulas in Equation 6.3 and Equation 6.4.
   d. Calculate the variance and standard deviation of Age, LOS, and Charges by using the =VAR() and =STDEV() functions. Make sure that the results in c match those in d.

2. Use the SWC worksheet in the file Chpt 4–1.xls.
   a. Calculate the mean and median for U5MR, IMR, and LEB by using the Excel functions =AVERAGE() and =MEDIAN().
   b. Based on these, in what direction are these distributions skewed, if at all.
   c. Calculate the variance and standard deviation of U5MR, IMR, and LEB by using the formulas in Equation 6.3 and Equation 6.4.
   d. Calculate the variance and standard deviation of U5MR, IMR, and LEB by using the =VAR() and =STDEV() functions. Make sure that the results in c match those in d.

3. A complete population consists of the values 1, 2, 5, 6, and 9.
   a. Demonstrate that the mean of the means of all samples of size 2, taken with replacement from the population, will equal the true population mean.
   b. Demonstrate that the mean of the variances of all samples of size 2, taken with replacement from the population, will equal the true population variance. (The sample variance in Excel is =VAR() and the population variance is =VARP().)
   c. Demonstrate that the mean of the variances of all samples of size 2, taken without replacement from the population, will equal a value for the true population calculated using the *sample* variance formula.

4. Use the population given in Exercise 3.
   a. Demonstrate that the mean of the means of all samples of size 3, taken with replacement from the population, will equal the true population mean.
   b. Demonstrate that the mean of the variances of all samples of size 3, taken with replacement from the population, will equal the true population variance. (The sample variance in Excel is =VAR() and the population variance is =VARP().)
   c. Demonstrate that the mean of the variances of all samples of size 3, taken without replacement from the population, will equal a value for the true population calculated using the *sample* variance formula.

5. Fourteen women delivering at a hospital on a single day had made the following number of prenatal visits prior to their delivery:

3	4	6	4	15
4	6	12	5	5
4	4	9	3	

   a. Using the model given in Figure 6.5, Figure 6.6, and Figure 6.7, show that $\sum_{i=1}^{n}|x_i - \bar{x}|$ is centered at the median in the sense discussed previously.
   b. Using the same model, show that $\sum_{i=1}^{n}(x_i - \bar{x})^2$ is centered at the mean.

Section 6.2 The Distribution of Frequencies

The measures of central tendency and dispersion presented in Section 6.1 represent one way to characterize a set of data. A second way to characterize a data set is by the way in which it is distributed over its range of values, commonly known as a frequency distribution. The frequency distribution was discussed in some detail in Chapter Four. In that discussion, the frequencies generated with the =FREQUENCY() function were based on bin ranges developed by dividing the range from highest to lowest data values by some arbitrary number, such as six, to create six frequency intervals. This section discusses the frequency distribution further, basing the bin ranges on standard deviations of the data.

Frequency Distributions and Standard Deviations

A frequency distribution can be based on arbitrary bin ranges (for example, six equal-size ranges, from the smallest to the largest value in the data set). But they can also incorporate information about the mean and standard deviation of the data to help in the understanding of those data. The example considered here will use the Human Development Index (HDI) for the countries of the world, as given by the United Nations Development Program (UNDP) for 1999 (http://www.undp.org/hdro/statistics/downloadtables.html). The HDI is developed from measures of life expectancy, literacy, and GNP per capita for each country. The entire data set used in developing the HDI and the HDI for each country for which UNDP gives an HDI value for 1999 is contained in the Excel file Chpt 6–1.xls.

The HDI index is given in column J in the Excel file Chpt 6–1.xls. To create a frequency distribution incorporating information about the mean and standard deviation, it is first necessary to calculate those values for the HDI index. This can be done using the =AVERAGE() and =STDEVP() functions. (Since this data set represents virtually all countries of the world for which the requisite data are available, it is being treated as a population rather than as a sample.) The actual mean of the HDI index is .684 and the standard deviation is .181.

The use of the mean and standard deviation in creating a frequency distribution is shown in Figure 6.8. In Figure 6.8, column B contains the countries of the world ranked by HDI index number. There are actually 162 countries ranked in column B, but only the first thirteen are shown in the figure. Column C contains the HDI score for the top thirteen countries. The maximum score (for Norway) is .939. The minimum score (which is not shown and is for Sierra Leone) is .258. The mean of the HDI score across countries is shown in D2 as .684 and the standard deviation is shown in D3 as .181. Beginning in E6 is the sequence of

FIGURE 6.8. FREQUENCY DISTRIBUTION WITH MEAN AND STANDARD DEVIATION, HDI DATA.

	F6	▼		=	=$E$2+E6*$E$3		
	A	B	C	D	E	F	G
1	HDI Rank, 1999		HDI99				
2	1	Norway	0.939	Mean	0.684		
3	2	Australia	0.936	StDev	0.181		
4	3	Canada	0.936				
5	4	Sweden	0.936		StDevs	Bin Values	Frequency
6	5	Belgium	0.935		-3	0.140	0
7	6	United States	0.934		-2	0.321	5
8	7	Iceland	0.932		-1	0.502	32
9	8	Netherlands	0.931		0	0.684	25
10	9	Japan	0.928		1	0.865	70
11	10	Finland	0.925		2	1.046	30
12	11	Switzerland	0.924		3	1.227	0
13	12	Luxembourg	0.924				162
14	13	France	0.924				

numbers, $-3, -2, \ldots 3$. This sequence represents a distance from the mean in numbers of standard deviations ranging from -3 to 3. These distances are actually calculated in F6:F12. The equation that is used to calculate the distances is shown for F6 in the formula line as =$E$2+E6*$E$3. This Excel formula notation means that when the formula is copied from F6 to F7 through F12, the formula will refer to the relevant consecutive cells from E7 to E12 but will always refer to E2 (the mean) and E3 (the standard deviation).

The frequency distribution is shown in G6:G12; it was calculated using the =FREQUENCY(B2:B163,F6:F12) function. You will recall that it is always necessary to use Ctrl/Shift/Enter to get the =FREQUENCY() function to work correctly because it is one of the functions that computes a value for more than one cell at a time. Two things might be noted about the frequency distribution. First, the sum of the frequency distribution given in F15 as 162 (=SUM(F6:F14)) confirms that all of the countries are included in the frequency distribution. Second, the HDI value for every country is contained in the range from three standard deviations below the mean to two standard deviations above the mean. (Remember that the bin value refers to the top of a particular range so that -2 contains all countries with HDI scores between .140 and .321.)

A look at the histogram created by this frequency distribution of the HDI data is also of interest. The histogram for these data is shown in Figure 6.9. Several

FIGURE 6.9. GRAPH OF HDI VALUES.

	E	F	G	H	I	J	K	L	M	N
					'-3 to -2					
1										
2	Mean	0.684								
3	StDev	0.181								
4										
5	StDevs	Bin Values	Frequency	Percent						
6	-3	0.140	0	0.00						
7	-2	0.321	5	0.03	-3 to -2					
8	-1	0.502	32	0.20	-2 to -1					
9	0	0.684	25	0.15	-1 to mean					
10	1	0.865	70	0.43	mean to 1					
11	2	1.046	30	0.19	1 to 2					
12	3	1.227	0	0.00	2 to 3					
13			162							
14										
15										
16										

things might be mentioned in regard to this figure. First, the histogram includes data only for the range from -3 to 3 standard deviations. Typically, most of the observations in almost any data set will be in the three standard deviation range. A second point of interest is that column I contains bin labels that were not used in the calculations in any way but were used to label the horizontal dimension of the graph. This was discussed in Chapter Four under construction of graphs. It should be remembered that the bin values actually used in the =FREQUENCY() formula represent the top of the bin range, so, for example, the -2 in Cell E8, which is associated with the value .321 in Cell F8, actually refers to the range from -3 to -2 standard deviations. Column H represents the percentage of countries in each bin range.

The histogram itself shows a distribution of the frequencies that is not atypical for many distributions; that is, the observations tend to cluster near the mean and be fewer farther from the mean. Ninety-five of the 162 countries (58 percent) have HDI scores within one standard deviation of the mean. When one counts the number of countries within two standard deviations of the mean, there are 157 of the 162 (97 percent). This type of distribution of individual cases around the mean is typical of many distributions found in the real world. In many cases, data are distributed approximately in what is known as a normal distribution. The normal distribution was introduced in Chapter Five. There, it was indicated that the normal distribution is symmetrical with an equal number of observations above and below the mean. A second characteristic of the normal distribution is that approximately 68 percent of the observations are within one standard deviation of the mean and 95 percent of the observations are within two standard deviations. The distribution in Figure 6.9 is not actually symmetrical (seventy countries are in the range of one standard deviation above the mean, whereas only twenty-five are within the range of one standard deviation below). Still, the percentages of 58 percent at one standard deviation and 97 percent at two are not far from the normal distribution percentages of 68 percent and 95 percent.

The Normal Distribution

The normal distribution was introduced in Chapter Five and discussed briefly in the last section. This section provides additional detail on the normal distribution and the importance of the mean and standard deviation in the normal distribution.

A normal distribution is one that is symmetrical and which has approximately 68 percent of its observations within one standard deviation of the mean and 95 percent within two. In addition, a normal distribution has about 99 percent of its observations within three standard deviations of the mean. Excel provides a number of options for constructing and visualizing a normal distribution. Figure 6.10 shows a normal distribution generated by Excel. The distribution in Figure 6.10 shows the classic normal distribution form. As can be seen, the distribution is symmetrical and takes on what has been called the "bell-shaped" curve because it looks somewhat like the side view of a bell.

FIGURE 6.10. NORMAL DISTRIBUTION.

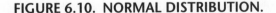

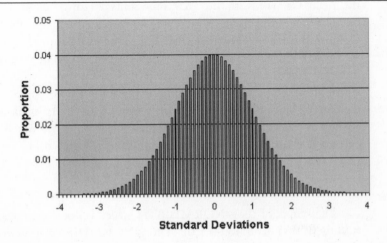

FIGURE 6.11. CALCULATIONS FOR NORMAL DISTRIBUTION.

	C2	▼	=	=1/SQRT(2*PI()*1)*EXP((-1/2)*((A2-0)/1)^2)	
	A	B	C	D	E	F
1	StDev	Normal Dist	Normal Dist2			
2	-4	0.0001338	0.0001338			
3	-3.9	0.0001987	0.0001987			
4	-3.8	0.0002919	0.0002919			
5	-3.7	0.0004248	0.0004248			
6	-3.6	0.0006119	0.0006119			
7	-3.5	0.0008727	0.0008727			
8	-3.4	0.0012322	0.0012322			
9	-3.3	0.0017226	0.0017226			
10	-3.2	0.0023841	0.0023841			
11	-3.1	0.0032668	0.0032668			
12	-3	0.0044318	0.0044318			
13	-2.9	0.0059525	0.0059525			
14	-2.8	0.0079155	0.0079155			
15	-2.7	0.0104209	0.0104209			
16	-2.6	0.013583	0.0135830			
17	-2.5	0.0175283	0.0175283			
18	-2.4	0.0223945	0.0223945			

The way in which the normal distribution in Figure 6.10 was constructed in Excel is informative about the kinds of information that can be obtained from Excel. Figure 6.11 shows a portion of the Excel spreadsheet that was used to produce the normal distribution shown in Figure 6.10. Column A, labeled StDev, represents the distance from the mean in standard deviation units. Cell A2 is shown as −4, which means that the cell represents four standard deviation units below the mean. Cell A3, with the −3.9, represents 3.9 units below the mean, and so on. The values in column A increase to 4 in cell A82 (not visible in the figure). Column B is labeled Normal Dist. The value in B2 is produced by the Excel =NORMDIST() function and represents the proportion of the normal distribution that falls at the point represented by −4. The proportion of the normal distribution falling at any single point is given in Equation 6.8. The values in Column C, labeled Normal Dist2, represent the normal distribution values calculated by the formula shown in Equation 6.8. The way in which the formula is expressed in Excel is shown in the formula line in Figure 6.11.

$$f(x) = \frac{1}{\sqrt{2\pi\sigma}}e^{-(1/2)[(x-\mu)/\sigma]^2} \qquad (6.8)$$

The syntax of the =NORMDIST(), which is not shown in Figure 6.11, is =NORMDIST(Cell Ref,0,1,0). The =NORMDIST() function takes four arguments: (1) the cell reference (Cell Ref) for which the point proportion of the normal distribution is desired (-4, -3.9, etc.), (2) the mean of the distribution (which, in this case, is given as 0), (3) the standard deviation of the distribution (here given as 1), and (4) a value of 0, indicating that the distribution desired is the normal probability density function and NOT the cumulative normal distribution (more about that distribution later).

Looking at Figure 6.10, it should be recognized that there is a very small proportion of the observations in a normally distributed data set that lies outside the range -3 to $+3$ standard deviations. In fact, a normal distribution has about 99 percent of its observations in the -3 to $+3$ range on either side of the mean. However, some proportion of a normal distribution (albeit a very small proportion) is out beyond four standard deviations, five standard deviations, and even twenty standard deviations. The probability of being out at those extremes is finite, but very, very small. Although it is not obvious from Figure 6.10, about 68 percent of the observations lie in the range from -1 to $+1$ standard deviations and about 95 percent lie in the range from -2 to $+2$ standard deviations.

It is basically correct to say that 68 percent of all observations in a normal distribution are within one standard deviation on either side of the mean value, that 95 percent are within two standard deviations, and so on. But an interesting characteristic of normal distributions is that they are based on scales that are continuous rather than discrete. For example, if one were measuring the height of U.S. adult men, the recorded measurement would be limited by the measuring device to record the height in measurement intervals, probably no smaller than quarters of an inch at the most precise. But if there were a more sophisticated measuring technique, it might be possible to discover that someone who was measured as being five feet, ten and a half inches tall might actually be five feet, ten and 7/16th inches tall. With a still more sophisticated measurement tool, it might be discovered that that person was actually five feet, and ten and 455/1000th inches tall. Still more sophisticated . . . but you get the point.

A consequence of this theoretical ability to measure things on what might be considered a true scale of infinite possibilities means that the probability that any given observation will be at any one specific spot in the normal distribution (for example, exactly one standard deviation above the mean) is actually zero. If a finite number of objects is distributed over an infinite number of sites (points in the scale), the probability that any one object will fall on any specific site will be the number of observations divided by infinity, which will always come out to zero. The consequence of this is that the actual proportion of observations between two points in a normal distribution (say, two standard deviations below to two standard deviations above the mean) cannot be calculated from the formula in Equation 6.8. Instead, the actual proportion of observations within any interval in the normal distribution must be taken from the cumulative normal distribution. This distribution is discussed in detail in the following subsection.

Cumulative Normal Distributions and Excel

The cumulative normal distribution sums all the probabilities of the normal distribution up to a given specific value. For example, suppose the mean weight of newborns is 3,600 grams (about eight pounds) and the standard deviation is 850 grams. If the weight of newborns is normally distributed, the cumulative normal distribution, then, using Excel, could tell us that we would expect that just under 10 percent of all newborns should be under 2,500 grams, the cut-off for low birth weight. This could be calculated with the =NORMDIST() function as =NORMDIST(2500,3600,850,1), where 2,500 equals the low birth weight level, 3,600 is the mean weight in grams, 850 is the standard deviation, and 1 indicates that the cumulative distribution is desired. It is also possible to predict that, for example, only about 5 percent of all newborns will weigh more than 5,000 grams (about eleven pounds) by subtracting =NORMDIST(5000,3600,850,1) from 1.

The value of the cumulative normal distribution is that it allows the determination of the exact probability of any observation when a normal distribution is assumed. Figure 6.12 shows a graph of the cumulative normal distribution based on standard deviations from the mean. The figure shows that the cumulative normal distribution starts at zero in the range to the left of three standard deviations below the mean. It increases (because it accumulates all previous percentages) to a maximum approaching one (100 percent) in the range to the right of three standard deviations above the mean.

FIGURE 6.12. CUMULATIVE NORMAL DISTRIBUTION.

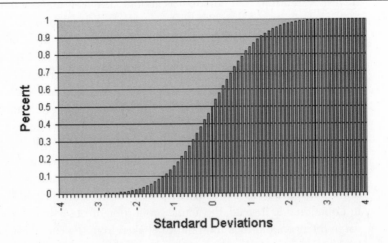

The actual value of any point on the cumulative normal distribution can be found by using the =NORMDIST() function, with the first argument being the value of the point of interest, the second being the mean of the distribution, the third being the standard deviation, and the fourth being the value 1, to denote that the cumulative normal distribution is being requested. The values of the cumulative normal distribution represent the area under a normal curve to the left of any number. The actual value is the integral of the area under the curve from $-\infty$ to the number in question, but it can be approximated using one of several methods. The formula in Equation 6.9 is the way the area under the cumulative normal distribution is calculated by Excel, and it duplicates the result of the Excel =NORMDIST(x,mean, stdev,1) function. This formula is an approximation, rather than an exact solution, but is far more readily obtained than any exact solution.

$$p(x) = 1 - Z(x)(b_1 t - b_2 t^2 - b_3 t^3 - b_4 t^4 - b_5 t^5) \qquad (6.9)$$

where

$$Z(x) = \frac{1}{\sqrt{2\pi e^{-x^2/2}}} \qquad t = \frac{1}{1 + px}$$

$$p = .23164\ 19$$

$$b_1 = .31938\ 1530 \qquad b_2 = -.35656\ 3782$$

$$b_3 = 1.78147\ 7937 \qquad b_4 = -1.82125\ 5978$$

$$b_5 = 1.33027\ 4429$$

Equation 6.9 works for values of x greater than 0. If the value of x is less than 0, it is necessary to subtract $p(x)$ from 1 in order to get the probability from $-\infty$ to the value of x less than 0. For example, if you wished to obtain the cumulative proportion at -1, as shown in Figure 6.12 (approximately 15 percent, by the graph), it would be necessary to find the cumulative proportion at the value of 1, as shown in Figure 6.12, and subtract that value from 1 to get the cumulative proportion at -1.

There is no particular reason why you, as a user of this book, will need to know the formulas in Equation 6.8 or those in Equation 6.9. But we are always interested in how things happen. If Excel provides a value for the cumulative normal distribution, we like to know, if possible, where Excel got the value. Thus the equations are given. You may use them as you wish.

Figure 6.13 shows the values generated by a cumulative normal distribution based on the assumption that U.S. newborns average 3,800 grams and that the distribution of the weight of newborns has a standard deviation of 850 grams. Column A shows .5 standard deviation units from the mean of 3,600. Column B

FIGURE 6.13. CUMULATIVE NORMAL PROBABILITIES FOR THE WEIGHT OF NEWBORNS.

	C3		=	=NORMDIST(B3,$E$3,$E$4,1)	
	A	B	C	D	E	F
1		Weight of Newborns				
2		Weight	Probability			
3	-3.5	625	0.000233	Mean	3600	
4	-3	1200	0.002375	StDev	850	
5	-2.5	1600	0.009313			
6	-2	2000	0.029894			
7	-1.5	2400	0.07901			
8	-1	2800	0.173307			
9	-0.5	3200	0.318967			
10	0	3600	0.5			
11	0.5	4000	0.681033			
12	1	4400	0.826693			
13	1.5	4800	0.92099			
14	2	5200	0.970106			
15	2.5	5600	0.990687			
16	3	6000	0.997625			
17	3.5	6400	0.999506			
18						

shows the weight in grams that corresponds to each standard deviation unit from the mean, assuming a mean of 3,600 grams and a standard deviation of 850 grams. Column C is the probability that was obtained, as the formula line indicates, with the =NORMDIST() function. The first argument is the weight given in column B, the second is fixed as the mean given in cell E3, the third is the standard deviation given in cell E4, and the final argument is the 1 denoting cumulative distribution.

To understand the logic and use of the cumulative normal distribution, suppose there is an interest in knowing what proportion of newborns will weigh less than 2,000 grams (two standard deviations below the mean). To determine this, given the assumption that the average is 3,600 grams and the standard deviation is 850 grams, it is only necessary to look at the probability given in cell C6 in Figure 6.13. According to that cell, only about 3 percent of newborns would weigh as little as 2,000 grams. What if the interest was in knowing what proportion of newborns would weigh more than some amount at birth—say, 4,800 grams? Still, assuming a mean of 3,600 and a standard deviation of 850, it is possible to see that the probability associated with 4,800 grams (cell C13) is .92.

But this is the proportion of births that will weigh 4,800 or less. To get the proportion that will weigh 4,800 or more, it is necessary to subtract the proportion at 4,800 from 1; so, the actual proportion that will weigh more than 4,800 grams at birth is 1 − .92, or .08.

Finding the probability of any occurrence that can be described by a normal distribution with a known mean and standard deviation can be accomplished with the use of the =NORMDIST() function. Suppose the weight of thirteen-year-old girls is normally distributed with a mean of a hundred pounds and a standard deviation of fifteen pounds. What is the likelihood of finding a thirteen-year-old girl who weighs less than seventy pounds? The answer can be found in Excel with =NORMDIST(70,100,15,1), which returns the result of about .02. Suppose the temperature of healthy adults is normally distributed with a mean of 98.6 degrees Fahrenheit and a standard deviation of .5 degrees. What is the probability of observing a healthy adult with a temperature of 101 degrees Fahrenheit or more? The answer can be found using Excel as =NORMDIST(101,98.6,.5,1), which produces .9999 to four decimals. But now, we do not want to know the probability of finding a healthy adult with a temperature *below* 101 but, rather, the probability of finding a health adult with a temperature of 101 or above. That would be found as 1 − .9999, or .0001 at four decimal places. Because the probability of finding a healthy adult with a temperature of 101 is so small, we would typically conclude that such a person could not be healthy.

Exercises for Section 6.2

1. Use Hospital charges worksheet in the file Chpt 4–1.xls.
   a. Based on the mean and standard deviation for LOS, generate a frequency distribution in terms of one-standard deviation units around the mean.
   b. Develop the Excel chart to show the frequency distribution generated in a.

2. Use the SWC worksheet in the file Chpt 4–1.xls.
   a. Based on the mean and standard deviation for IMR, generate a frequency distribution in terms of one-standard deviation units around the mean.
   b. Develop the Excel chart to show the frequency distribution generated in a.

3. Use the data set Chpt 6–1.xls and do the following:
   a. Calculate the mean and standard deviation of the HDI index.
   b. Generate a frequency distribution for the HDI index in terms of one-standard deviation units from the mean.
   c. Develop an Excel chart to show the frequency distribution generated in b.
   d. Compare the result to the graph shown in Figure 6.9.

4. Use the mean and standard deviation for LOS as used in Exercise 1.
   a. Develop the probability distribution in terms of one-standard deviation units that would be expected if LOS were normally distributed. Include at least three standard deviations on each side of the mean.
   b. Develop an Excel chart to show the frequency distribution generated in a.

5. Assume that the height of U.S. males is normally distributed with a mean of seventy inches and with a standard deviation of three inches.
   a. Generate the normal distribution probabilities for the height of adult males in one-inch units, including at least three standard deviations on each side of the mean.
   b. Develop an Excel chart to show the frequency distribution generated in a.

6. Assume that adult diastolic blood pressure is normally distributed with a mean of 75 mmhg and a standard deviation of 5 mmhg.
   a. Generate the normal distribution probabilities for the diastolic blood pressure in one-mmhg units, including at least three standard deviations on each side of the mean.
   b. Develop an Excel chart to show the frequency distribution generated in a.

7. Assume the mean and the standard deviation of the height of adult males as given in Exercise 5. Use the =NORMDIST() function to determine the following:
   a. The proportion of men who are less than sixty-five inches tall
   b. The proportion of men who are less than sixty-nine inches tall
   c. The proportion of men who are greater than seventy-one inches tall
   d. The proportion of men who are greater than sixty-eight inches tall
   e. The proportion of men between sixty-seven and seventy inches tall

8. Assume the mean and standard deviation of diastolic blood pressure as given in Exercise 6. Use the =NORMDIST() function to determine the following:
   a. The proportion of people who have diastolic blood pressure less than 76 mmhg
   b. The proportion of people who have diastolic blood pressure less than 72 mmhg
   c. The proportion of people who have diastolic blood pressure greater than 73 mmhg
   d. The proportion of people who have diastolic blood pressure greater than 79 mmhg
   e. The proportion of people who have diastolic blood pressure between 72 and 78 mmhg

9. Assume that waiting time in an emergency room is normally distributed with a mean of thirty-eight minutes and a standard deviation of ten minutes. Use the =NORMDIST() function and determine the following:
   a. The proportion of people who wait less than thirty minutes
   b. The proportion of people who wait less than twenty minutes
   c. The proportion of people who wait more than forty minutes
   d. The proportion of people who wait more than fifty minutes
   e. The proportion of people who wait between twenty-five and forty-five minutes

Section 6.3 The Sampling Distribution of the Mean

The previous subsection discussed the variance and the standard deviation as measures of dispersion that apply both to populations and to samples taken from populations. The discussion was concerned with the dispersion of the individual entities that make up the population or sample. So, for example, when waiting time for patients was discussed, it was the dispersion of the waiting times for individual patients that was the subject of the variance or standard deviation calculation. In this section we take up a somewhat different concept—the sampling distribution of the mean.

The Standard Error with a Known Variance

Consider a population made up of all discharges from a hospital for the past year. The hospital has two hundred beds and an average stay of 5.2 days. The total number of hospital discharges over the year is approximately twelve thousand. The standard deviation calculated for all stays is 4.12 days (the formula used is that in Equation 6.5 because this is the population of all discharges for the year). These twelve thousand discharges are distributed, as shown in Figure 6.14. As the figure shows, the length of stay for the twelve thousand discharges is skewed to the right, as would be expected, since the length of stay can never be less than zero days, and the standard deviation is large, relative to the mean length of stay. (Approximately 47.5 percent of a normally distributed variable should be within two standard deviations below the mean-half of the 95 percent two standard deviations on both sides of the mean, but two standard deviations below the mean would go down to -3.) So, although the standard deviation can be readily calculated for these hospital discharges, it must be remembered that the meaning of standard deviation is not what it would be if the length of stay was actually normally distributed.

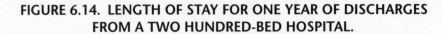

**FIGURE 6.14. LENGTH OF STAY FOR ONE YEAR OF DISCHARGES
FROM A TWO HUNDRED-BED HOSPITAL.**

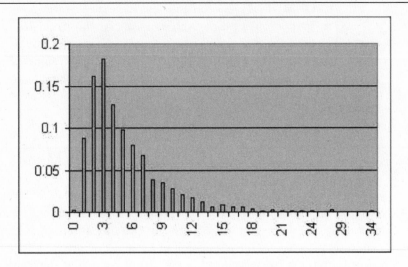

We know the actual mean length of stay of the population of discharges. It is 5.2 days. But suppose we did not know the mean length of stay, and the only way we could get an estimate of it was to draw successive samples from all discharges. To keep the discussion relatively simple, we will say that it is only possible to draw samples of size 100. So we will be drawing successive samples of 100 discharges in order to estimate the true mean. Suppose we draw a first sample of a hundred discharges and the mean for the sample is 5.76 days. This is an estimate of the true population mean, but, clearly, it is not the true mean. But we do not know this, because all we have at this point is the one sample estimate. So we draw a second sample of 100 to estimate the true mean. This time we get a value of 5.17 as an estimate of the mean of the total population. We continue to draw samples of size 100 from the discharges until we have 250 separate samples.

Since we now have 250 samples means, we decide that the value we will accept for the true mean of the population will be the mean value of the 250 samples. When we calculate the mean of the 250 sample means, we discover that it is 5.22. So 5.22 becomes the estimate to represent the true mean of the population. But that is not the end of the story. Clearly, the mean values from our 250 samples have a distribution of their own. What can we say about that distribution? To look at that distribution, we are going to graph it in standard deviation units from the mean. But we are not going to use population, or even sample standard deviation units. We are going to use the standard deviation units of the *sample means.*

FIGURE 6.15. DISTRIBUTION OF 250 SAMPLE MEANS.

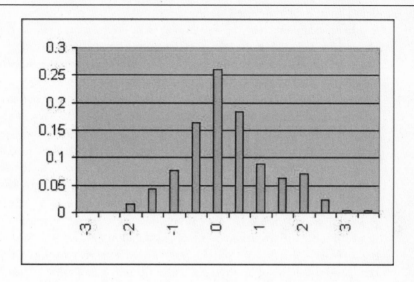

The standard deviation of the sample means is .402. The largest sample mean in the set of 250 was 6.45 and the smallest was 4.29. Given the standard deviation of .402, we would expect that about 95 percent of the sample means would be between 4.42 and 6.02, which is two standard deviations on either side of the mean of the samples, *if the 250 means are normally distributed.* The distribution of the 250 sample means is shown in Figure 6.15.

Figure 6.15 shows a very different picture when compared with Figure 6.14. Although the actual discharges as shown in Figure 6.14 are heavily skewed to the right, the means of 250 samples selected from that original data, shown in Figure 6.15, are almost normal in their distribution. It is not totally obvious from Figure 6.15, but there are about 70 percent of all sample means within one standard error of the mean of all samples (the normal distribution has 68 percent). There are also about 97 percent of the mean values within two standard deviations of the mean of all samples (the normal distribution has 95 percent). So the distribution shown in Figure 6.15 is seen to be a fairly close approximation of a normal distribution.

This finding that the means of 250 samples approximates a normal distribution reveals an interesting characteristic of sampling—or, rather, the means of samples. When the sample size is relatively large (30 or more in the sample is usually considered relatively large) the distribution of sample *means* tends to be normal, regardless of the nature of the distribution of the actual values. This characteristic of the distribution of sample means will be very useful when the notion of confidence limits is examined in Chapter Seven.

In an examination of the distribution of sample means, a relatively new notion was introduced. This is the standard deviation of the sample means. Up until this time, the discussion of standard deviations has focused on the individual observations. When the standard deviation of actual lengths of stay was calculated for the hospital data, it was 4.12 days. But when the standard deviation of the 250 sample means was calculated, it turned out to be only .402 days. A question that might now be asked is whether there is any defined relationship between the standard deviation of the individual observations and the standard deviation of the sample means. This leads to the introduction of the concept of the *standard error*. The standard error is the standard deviation of the sample means for samples of a given size. If the true population variance is available, the standard error is given as shown in Equation 6.10. This shows that there is a very specific relationship between the standard deviation of the population and the standard error of the means of samples drawn from the population. This relationship is precisely that the standard error of the means is the standard deviation of the individual observations divided by the square root of the sample size.

$$S.E._{\bar{x}} = \frac{\delta}{\sqrt{n}} \qquad (6.10)$$

The formula in Equation 6.10 provides an interesting comparison. If we go back for a moment to the variance rather than the standard deviation, we can recall from Figure 6.4 that the mean of the variance of all possible samples of size 2 from a population of four will be exactly equal to the variance of the four actual observations. Similarly, the standard deviation of all four observations divided by the square root of the sample size of 2 will be exactly the same as the standard deviation of the means from all possible samples of size 2 taken from the population of four. This is demonstrated in Figure 6.16. This figure is the same as that in Figure 6.4, except that it now shows the population standard deviation divided by the square root of the sample size (cell B10) and the standard deviation of the *means* of all samples of size 2 (cell F20). These two values are exactly the same. (It should be noted that the standard deviation of the means of all samples is calculated using the population standard deviation function =STDEVP(). This is appropriate, since this set of means is the population of all mean values.)

Now let us return to our 250 samples of size 100. The standard error of the mean for samples of size 100 using Equation 6.10 is 4.12 divided by the square root of 100, or .412. This is close to the standard deviation of the means that was calculated from the 250 samples we selected (.402), but it's not identical. Why the

FIGURE 6.16. COMPARISON OF THE POPULATION VARIANCE DIVIDED BY TWO AND THE VARIANCE OF THE MEAN OF ALL SAMPLES OF SIZE 2.

	A	B	C	D	E	F	G
F20			=	=STDEVP(F2:F17)			
1		Population	Sample	First	Second	Mean	Variance
2		2	1	2	2	2	0
3		4	2	2	4	3	2
4		5	3	2	5	3.5	4.5
5		7	4	2	7	4.5	12.5
6			5	4	2	3	2
7			6	4	4	4	0
8	Mean	4.50	7	4	5	4.5	0.5
9	Variance	3.25	8	4	7	5.5	4.5
10	StDev/sqrt(2)	1.27475	9	5	2	3.5	4.5
11			10	5	4	4.5	0.5
12			11	5	5	5	0
13			12	5	7	6	2
14			13	7	2	4.5	12.5
15			14	7	4	5.5	4.5
16			15	7	5	6	2
17			16	7	7	7	0
18							
19					Overall average	4.5	3.25
20				Standard Deviation of Means		1.27475	
21							

difference? It is simply because we do not have all the possible samples of size 100 that could be selected from the twelve thousand discharges (with sampling with replacement, there would be $12,000^{100}$ such samples—a very large number indeed). However, if we did have the means of all those samples, they would be equal to the standard error as calculated in Equation 6.10, or exactly .412.

The Standard Error with an Estimated Variance

Equation 6.10 is fine if the population variance is known. But, in general, the population variance is not known. Typically, unlike the example previously discussed, we would have only one sample—with one sample mean and one sample standard deviation. How, then, would we be able to determine the standard error (the standard deviation of the sampling distribution of the means of all samples)? The best estimate of the standard deviation of the population when we have only one sample is the standard deviation of the sample values. So the standard error is typically estimated as given in Equation 6.11. More about the importance of the standard deviation of individual samples in calculating the standard error of the mean is provided in Chapter Seven.

$$S.E._{\bar{x}} = \frac{s}{\sqrt{n}} \qquad (6.11)$$

The Standard Error When Sample Size Is Large, Relative to Population Size

Virtually all populations that we may have any interest in are finite; that is, they have a countable number of elements. All the hospital admissions for a year is a finite population. The infant mortality rate for all the countries of the world represents the infant mortality rate of a finite population. All the health departments in a state represent a finite population. But in some cases, a sample is large relative to a finite population and sometimes it is not. A sample of twenty health departments from all those in a state is a large sample relative to the population if there are only sixty-five health departments in the entire state. A sample of two hundred hospital discharges from all discharges for a year is not large relative to the population if the hospital has fifteen thousand discharges per year. However, in the former case, it is appropriate to reduce the standard error calculated by Equation 6.11 by multiplying times a value that is commonly called the *finite population correction*, or *fpc*.

The *fpc* is given by the formula in Equation 6.12. As the equation shows, the *fpc* is the square root of the population size minus the sample size divided by the population size minus 1. With a population of fifteen thousand discharges and a sample of two hundred, it is easy to confirm that the value of the *fpc* would be about .99, and probably not worth bothering with. However, for a sample of twenty health departments from a population of sixty-five, the *fpc* would be about .84 and probably small enough to make a useful difference in the standard error.

$$fpc = \sqrt{\frac{(N - n)}{(N - 1)}} \qquad (6.12)$$

If the finite population is to be used in the calculation of a standard error, the entire formula would be as shown in Equation 6.13.

$$S.E._{\bar{x}} = \frac{s}{\sqrt{n}} \sqrt{\frac{(N - n)}{(N - 1)}} \qquad (6.13)$$

Drawing Multiple Samples of Any Size

The random number generation add-in that is part of the Tools/Data Analysis package in Excel provides a way to draw multiple random samples from a

FIGURE 6.17. PROBABILITIES OF PRENATAL VISITS.

	A	B	
1	Prenatal Visits	Proportion of Women	
2	1	0.0588	
3	2	0.1104	
4	3	0.1710	
5	4	0.1981	
6	5	0.1702	
7	6	0.1175	
8	7	0.0795	
9	8	0.0418	
10	9	0.0237	
11	10	0.0121	
12	11	0.0068	
13	12	0.0045	
14	13	0.0030	
15	14	0.0019	
16	15	0.0007	
17			

population. Although this would never be done in a real research project, it is useful as a learning devise, particularly in regard to understanding the way in which the means of a large number of samples are distributed.

To see how Excel can be used to draw a large number of separate samples from a defined population, suppose we have a population of women who have come for prenatal visits. We will assume that this is a very large population. The distribution of the visits and the probability of making a specific number of visits are shown in Figure 6.17. As the figure shows, there is about a 6 percent chance of making one visit, an 11 percent chance of making two visits, a 17 percent chance of making three, and so forth. No woman made more than fifteen prenatal visits.

We will draw a large number of samples of size 30 from this population. The drawing of the samples will use the Data Analysis Add-In. The Data Analysis Add-In is found under Tools. Selecting Tools and Data Analysis, the Data Analysis window, shown in Figure 6.18, will come up. In the Data Analysis Window we select Random Number Generation.

FIGURE 6.18. DATA ANALYSIS WINDOW.

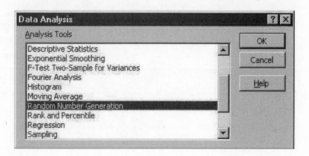

FIGURE 6.19. RANDOM NUMBER WINDOW.

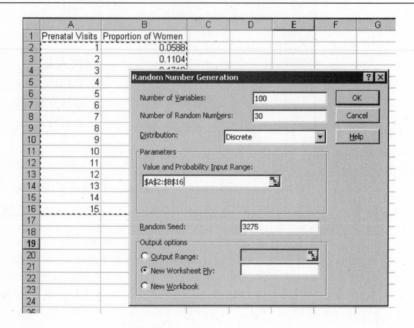

Selecting Random Number Generation will produce the window shown in Figure 6.19. The random number generation window (shown along with the part of the spreadsheet that contains prenatal visits and the proportion of women making those visits) contains several items. The first category of information that needs to be supplied is the number of samples desired, called by Excel, Number of Variables. We are going to generate a hundred separate random samples, so we put a hundred into the number of variables window. Each sample we generate will include thirty observations, so we put thirty into the number of random numbers window. Figure 6.19 shows a dotted line from A2 to B16, the range that is put into the value and probability input range. Column A represents the discrete visits (from 1 to 15) and column B represents the probability of any woman making each number of visits during her pregnancy. In the random seed box we put 3,275, which was generated using the =RAND() function, dropping the decimal point and taking only the first four digits. The last piece of information required by the random number generation window is where the output will go. We will put it on a new sheet.

When we press OK, Excel will generate a hundred samples of prenatal visits of size 30, based on the probabilities given in column B. The result of the generation of these hundred samples is as shown in Figure 6.20. This figure shows only a portion of the spreadsheet in which the random numbers have been generated. Each column in the spreadsheet shown in Figure 6.20 represents a separate sample. The numbers in each column represent the number of visits made by the women selected to be part of each sample of thirty. The first woman selected as part of the first sample (A1) made three visits to the clinic. The second woman selected for the first sample made four visits to the clinic, and so on. Because there are thirty observations in each sample, the numbers in each column actually run to row 30. Because there are a hundred samples, the numbers in the columns run to column CV.

FIGURE 6.20. RANDOM SAMPLES OF VISITS.

	A	B	C	D	E	F	G
1	3	4	2	2	2	6	3
2	4	3	4	5	5	9	1
3	3	3	3	7	7	2	5
4	2	4	4	2	4	4	4
5	4	4	7	4	4	4	7
6	3	4	1	5	3	3	2
7	5	5	6	2	5	5	5
8	4	4	4	7	3	5	3
9	4	3	9	4	6	6	4
10	2	2	4	4	7	11	7
11	7	6	11	3	2	5	6
12	3	13	3	3	6	9	10
13	4	11	4	7	3	6	5
14	5	5	10	5	1	4	4
15	4	3	2	2	6	6	3
16	8	4	4	2	2	4	1

FIGURE 6.21. EXAMPLE OF CALCULATIONS OF MEANS, STANDARD DEVIATIONS AND STANDARD ERRORS FOR A HUNDRED SAMPLES.

	B34	▼	=	=B33/SQRT(30)			
	A	B	C	D	E	F	G
25		5	4	5	4	4	5
26		6	3	3	3	3	5
27		6	8	3	3	7	4
28		3	4	1	3	4	3
29		9	3	6	12	5	9
30		3	6	6	6	8	1
31							
32	Mean	4.533333	4.933333	5.033333	4.2	4.433333	5.1
33	St Dev	1.995397	2.504249	2.697168	2.21904	1.851064	2.577756	2.53
34	St Error	0.364308	0.457211	0.492433	0.405139	0.337956	0.470632	0.4
35							

Given these hundred samples of size 30, we can calculate the mean, standard deviation, and standard error of each sample, as shown in Figure 6.21. In this figure, a first column has been added to the spreadsheet to provide a place to put the labels for mean, standard deviation, and standard error. This figure shows the last six numbers selected in the first six samples and in row 32—the mean of the number of visits for the thirty women in each sample. Row 33 shows the standard deviation as estimated by this sample, and row 34 shows the standard error. The calculation for the standard error for column B—the first sample—is shown in the formula bar.

Let us now look at the distribution of means from a large number of samples. Figure 6.22 shows the distribution of sample means from 250 samples of size 100 taken from the population of women who have come for prenatal visits. The x axis represents standard deviation units from the mean. The designation -2 shows those samples with mean values from -3 to -2 standard deviations from the mean. The designation -1 shows those samples with mean values from -2 to -1, standard deviations from the mean, and so on. It is clear from this figure that sample means from relatively large samples approximate a normal distribution, even though the original data may not.

This section discusses the use of Excel to generate a large number of samples with given attributes. It is important to remember, however, that, in general, one never draws more than one sample. The discussion here is presented solely for the purpose of helping the reader understand the use of the discrete sampling option in the Random Sample add-in. This example is referred to again in Chapter Seven, which discusses the calculation of confidence limits.

FIGURE 6.22. DISTRIBUTION OF MEANS FROM 250 SAMPLES OF SIZE 100.

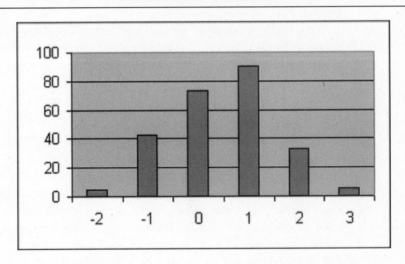

Exercises for Section 6.3

1. Determine the standard error of the mean for each of the following:
   a. A random sample of a hundred persons whose blood pressure has been measured when the known standard deviation is 2.5 mmhg
   b. A random sample of thirty-eight men when the known standard deviation for height is three inches
   c. A random sample of sixty-five persons who are waiting in an ER when the known standard deviation for waiting time is ten minutes
   d. The LEB for sixteen countries randomly selected from the SWC sheet of the file Chpt 4–1.xls when the countries on the sheet represent the entire population of countries (Consider using the finite population correction.)
   e. The IMR for twenty states randomly selected from the fifty states given on the U.S. IMR worksheet of the file Chpt 4–1.xls (Consider using the finite population correction.)

2. Determine an *estimate* of the standard error of the mean for the following:
   a. Waiting time in an emergency room for a random sample of thirty-six people selected from the emergency room wait worksheet of the file Chpt 6–2.xls, assuming that the records shown represent the population of emergency room visits for a month

   b. U5MR for a random sample of twenty countries selected from the SWC worksheet of the file Chpt 4–1.xls (Consider using the finite population correction.)

   c. BP for a random sample of forty-two persons selected from the BP worksheet of the file Chpt 6–2.xls, assuming that the records shown represent the population of persons who have had blood pressure checked at a single clinic in the past month

   d. Number of prenatal visits for a sample of sixty women selected at random from the population of women shown in Figure 6.17

3. Use the emergency room wait worksheet of the file Chpt 6–2.xls and do the following:

   a. With the discrete sampling option, select a hundred samples of size 30 from the population of waits. (It is necessary to assign a probability of 1/832 to each of the 832 waits before drawing the samples. This probability should appear in column C.) Be sure to generate a random seed using =RAND().

   b. Calculate the mean, standard deviation, and standard error of each of the hundred samples.

   c. Generate a frequency distribution of the means of the hundred samples, based on one-standard deviation units around the mean of all sample means.

   d. Display the resulting frequency distribution in a column graph and give some interpretation as to whether the distribution looks approximately normal or not.

   e. Save this file for later use.

4. Use the prenatal visits for the women shown in Figure 6.17 (Visits worksheet of Chpt 6–3.xls) and do the following:

   a. With the discrete sampling option, select 250 samples of size 100 from the population of women. Be sure to generate a random seed using =RAND().

   b. Calculate the mean, standard deviation, and standard error for each of the 250 samples.

   c. Generate a frequency distribution of the means of the 250 samples, based on one standard deviation unit around the mean of all sample means.

   d. Display the resulting frequency distribution in a column graph and give some interpretation as to whether the distribution looks approximately normal or not.

   e. Save this file for later use.

Section 6.4 Mean and Standard Deviation of a Discrete Numerical Variable

The introduction of the prenatal visits shown in Figure 6.17 gives an opportunity to briefly discuss the mean and standard deviation of a discrete numerical variable. Although most of this chapter is devoted to continuous numerical variables that can take on any values in the number scale, discrete numerical variables can only take on whole number values. With a variable that only takes on whole number values, it is possible to introduce a different definition of the mean and standard deviation. This definition is given in Equation 6.14.

$$\mu = \sum_{k=1}^{T} x_k p(x_k) \tag{6.14}$$

and

$$\delta = \sqrt{\sum_{k=1}^{T} (x_k - \mu)^2 p(x_k)}$$

where k designates each separate value of x, T represents the total of all different values of x, and p represents the probability associated with each value of x.

What the two formulas in Equation 6.14 say is that the population mean of a discrete numerical variable is given as the sum of all values that the variable takes on, multiplied by the probability of any one of those values. The population standard deviation is the square root of the sum of the difference between each value that the variable takes on and the population mean multiplied by the probability of any one of the values.

A demonstration of the calculation of both the mean and standard deviation of a discrete numerical variable is shown in Figure 6.23. Columns A and B represent the number of visits made by women and the proportion of women making each number of visits as originally shown in Figure 6.17. These columns have been renamed to indicate that they represent the variable x (column A) and the probability of the value of x, $p(x)$ (column B). Column C represents the multiplication of each value of x by the probability of x. The sum of column C is given in C18. This is the population mean. Column D represents the square of the difference between each value of x and the mean of x (in cell C18), multiplied by the probability of x. The sum of values in column D is given in cell D18. This is the population variance. The standard deviation—the square root of the variance—is given in cell D19.

FIGURE 6.23. CALCULATION OF THE MEAN AND STANDARD DEVIATION OF A DISCRETE NUMERICAL VARIABLE.

	D2	▼	= =(A2-$C$18)^2*B2	
	A	B	C	D
1	Visits (x)	Proportion (p(x))	x*p(x)	(x-mu)^2*p(x)
2	1	0.0588	0.0588	0.7499
3	2	0.1104	0.2208	0.7298
4	3	0.1710	0.513	0.4221
5	4	0.1981	0.7924	0.0646
6	5	0.1702	0.851	0.0313
7	6	0.1175	0.705	0.2399
8	7	0.0795	0.5565	0.4690
9	8	0.0418	0.3344	0.4915
10	9	0.0237	0.2133	0.4649
11	10	0.0121	0.121	0.3566
12	11	0.0068	0.0748	0.2810
13	12	0.0045	0.054	0.2483
14	13	0.0030	0.039	0.2131
15	14	0.0019	0.0266	0.1689
16	15	0.0007	0.0105	0.0761
17				
18			4.5711	5.0071
19				2.2377
20				

It should be recognized that the results obtained by the formulas in Equation 6.14 produce exactly the same results as the formulas in Equation 6.1 and Equation 6.5. The difference lies in the fact that the latter formulas treat each observation individually, whereas the former deals with the values of the variable and the proportion of times the values appear in the data set. To understand this point, suppose we just moved the decimal points in Figure 6.23 four digits to the right (the same as multiplying each probability by 10,000). This would produce the numbers 588, 1,104, 1,710, and so on, in column B. If we now translated this into actual numbers of the variable x, that would mean 588 women with one visit to the prenatal clinic, 1,104 women with two visits, 1710 women with three visits, and so one. There would be seven women with fifteen prenatal visits. In total, there would be ten thousand women, each with a specific number of prenatal visits. We could now calculate the mean and standard deviation for these women by using the formulas given in Equation 6.1 and Equation 6.5 and get exactly the same values as those given in cells C18 and D18 in Figure 6.23.

Exercises for Section 6.4

1. Using the data shown in Figure 6.17 (Visits worksheet in Chpt 6–3.xls), replicate the figure to calculate the mean and standard deviation for prenatal visits.

2. Chapter Five discussed the probabilities of having zero through seven children (Figure 5.2) in a population of 2,556 women. Use those data (or the Births worksheet in Chpt 6–3.xls) and calculate the mean and standard deviation of this population of 2,556 women by using the appropriate formulas from this section.

3. A health agency does an audit of six hundred of its records and discovers the distribution of recording errors as shown on the Errors worksheet in Chpt 6–3.xls. Use these data to calculate the mean and standard deviation of the errors in records, using the appropriate formulas in this section.

4. A hospital knows that .646 of the persons coming to the emergency room come for true emergencies. Using the formulas in this section and the binomial distribution, calculate the mean and standard deviation for any ten arrivals at the emergency room.

Section 6.5 The Distribution of a Proportion

In Chapter Five, the binomial distribution was discussed. The binomial distribution is the distribution that describes the way in which a sequence of events, all independent of one another and each having two possible outcomes, will be distributed. One example that introduced the binomial distribution was the probability of arrival at an emergency clinic of any given number of emergencies out of forty-three arrivals. When the number of observations is relatively large (say, thirty or more) and when the probability associated with either outcome of the observations is in the range .2 to .8, the binomial distribution can be relatively effectively approximated by the normal distribution.

You will recall from Chapter One the home health agency that wanted to estimate the proportion of correctly filled Medicare forms for all eight hundred clients from a sample of eighty forms taken at random. If fewer than 85 percent of the sample forms were filled out correctly, this would signal the need for relatively costly training to ensure that the forms were filled out correctly. The sample of eighty forms showed that only sixty (or 75 percent) were filled out correctly. The immediate result of this would probably be to alert the agency to the need to initiate this costly remedial training. But before they proceed, they might be interested in the probability that the true population proportion could be

FIGURE 6.24. PORTION OF CORRECT AND INCORRECT FORMS.

	A2	▼		=	=STDEVP(A5:A84)/SQRT(A3)	
	A	B	C	D	E	F
1	0.75					
2	0.048412	0.048412				
3	80					
4	Correct					
5	1					
6	1					
7	1					
8	1					
9	0					
10	1					
11	1					
12	0					
13	1					

85 percent. To determine this probability, they can treat the distribution of the proportion as if it is normal with a mean at .75 and a standard error as given in Equation 6.15.

$$S.E._{p} = \sqrt{p \times (1 - p)/n} \qquad (6.15)$$

The value of Equation 6.15 would be exactly the same if =STDEVP()/SQRT(n) were applied to a series of ones and zeros in which 75 percent were ones (or zeros). This idea is demonstrated in Figure 6.24. The figure shows a determination of whether the Medicare forms were filled out correctly or not for the first nine forms (A5 to A13). There are actually eighty forms represented in column A (A3 is provided by =COUNT(A5:A84)). The .75 in A1 represents the average for all eighty forms, which is the same as the proportion. The standard error of the distribution is given in A2 as calculated using =STDEVP() divided by the square root of 80. Notice that in calculating this standard error, it is assumed that the sample actually represents the entire population, thus the =STDEVP(). If this were not done, the standard error calculated using Equation 6.15 would not equal the result using the actual observations. The standard error calculated using Equation 6.15 is shown in B2.

Now the probability that the true population proportion of correct forms could be .85, given that the sample yielded a proportion of .75, can be calculated using the =NORMDIST() function. Recall that in Chapter Five this probability was calculated using the actual binomial distribution as either 2.2 percent or 1.3 percent, depending on whether the distribution around .75 or around .85 was considered. Figure 6.25 shows the result of the use of the =NORMDIST()

FIGURE 6.25. CALCULATION OF PROBABILITY OF 85 PERCENT CORRECT.

C4		= =1-NORMDIST(0.85,A1,B2,1)		
	A	B	C	D	E
1	0.75				
2	0.048412	0.048412			
3	80				
4	Correct		0.019433		
5	1				
6	1				
7	1				

FIGURE 6.26. PROBABILITY OF 70 PERCENT OR LESS.

C5		= =NORMDIST(0.7,A1,B2,1)		
	A	B	C	D	E
1	0.75				
2	0.048412	0.048412			
3	80				
4	Correct		0.019433		
5	1		0.15085		
6	1				
7	1				

function to determine this same probability. It turns out to be quite similar: 1.9 percent. The difference from the other two values is due to the fact that the binomial distribution is not exactly symmetrical.

Suppose, now, that the home health agency was concerned that if the true population value was 70 percent or less correct, a training event would not be sufficient, but that the entire process of keeping the home health records would have to be wholly reorganized. How might they determine the probability that the true proportion was 70 percent or less, given a sample value of 75 percent? Again, they would use the =NORMDIST function as shown in Figure 6.26. As this figure shows, the probability that the true population value could be as low as 70 percent or less, given a sample value of 75 percent, is .15. On the basis of this result, it is unlikely that the home health agency will decide to restructure their entire process of record keeping.

In determining the probability of being at .85 or higher, the =NORMDIST() function was subtracted from 1 (.019433 in Figure 6.25). In determining the probability of being at .7 or lower, the =NORMDIST() function was not subtracted from 1. How was that decision made? In general, it is important to realize what the magnitude of a desired probability is likely to be. If we realize that the distribution around .75 is essentially normal, we know that the farther from .75 we go, the smaller will be the likelihood of finding the true mean value there. If we are interested in the probability of being away from .75 on either side, either higher or lower, we must expect that the probability will be less than .5. If we did not subtract the =NORMDIST() function from 1 in Figure 6.25, the probability would have been about .98. Clearly that is not less than .5 and therefore must be incorrect. Conversely, when we look at the calculation as being below .7, we see that it is away from .75 on the other side. Again, the result must be less than .5, and so =NORMDIST() alone is the appropriate function. If we had been interested in knowing the probability that the true mean of the population would have been .85 *or less*, given a sample value of .75, we would have used the =NORMDIST() function alone, which would have yielded about 98 percent. Because we are now interested in a range that actually includes the sample proportion, we can see that the probability must be more than .5—which it is.

But if you are interested in a foolproof way of knowing whether to subtract the =NORMDIST() function from 1 or not, here is a general rule. If you wish to know the probability that the true population value is above proportion $p1$, given a sample proportion p_s, you subtract the =NORMDIST() function from 1, regardless of whether the hypothesized true population value is above or below the sample value. If you wish to know the probability that the true population value is below proportion $p2$, given a sample proportion p_s, you do not subtract the =NORMDIST() function from 1. This is demonstrated in Figure 6.27. As the figure shows, when the inequality sign points to the right, one subtracts =NORMDIST() from 1. When the inequality sign points to the left, one does not subtract the =NORMDIST() function from 1.

It was said earlier that the normal distribution when used with a proportion is an approximation of the binomial distribution, which actually applies to a proportion, because a proportion is inevitably a dichotomous outcome. We have seen, in comparing the discussion of the correct forms in Chapter Five with the

FIGURE 6.27. USE OF THE =NORMDIST() FUNCTION.

	A	B	C
1			
2	Sample	Population	Formula
3	0.75	>.85	=1-NORMDIST()
4		<.85	=NORMDIST()
5		>.7	=1-NORMDIST()
6		<.7	=NORMDIST()
7			

discussion here, that the binomial distribution and normal distribution produce similar values but not exactly equal values. Why then would we use the normal distribution to find the binomial probabilities?

The reason resides primarily in the difficulty of finding the result. Until the advent of computer programs like Excel, figuring the actual binomial distribution for a probability was much more difficult than obtaining the normal distribution probabilities. Even now, with the use of Excel, it is not possible to obtain binomial distribution probabilities for more than 1,029 observations, because the factorial calculations that are involved in the binomial distribution formula result in numbers too large for Excel to handle. In consequence, it is often impossible to use exact binomial probabilities to determine the likelihood of binomial events.

Exercises for Section 6.5

1. Use the formula in Equation 6.15 to determine the following standard errors:
   a. $p = .3, n = 80$
   b. $p = .5, n = 80$
   c. $p = .3, n = 250$
   d. $p = .5, n = 250$

2. A dental group practice of eighteen dentists upgraded their computer system and in the process suspects that they lost information on recalls for many of their patients. They drew a simple random sample of two hundred patient records and discovered that twenty-two of those had follow-up calls that were not included in the new computer system. Use the =NORMDIST() function to determine the following:
   a. The probability that the true proportion of missed follow-up calls is less than 10 percent among all records
   b. The probability that the true proportion of missed follow-up calls is greater than 20 percent among all records

3. A state health department is concerned about full immunization among children in their state. They draw a sample of 150 children born between one and two years ago from state birth records and follow up on the children to determine if they are fully immunized. They discover that ninety of the children are fully immunized. Use the =NORMDIST() function to determine the following:
   a. The probability that the true proportion of fully immunized children is 90 percent or more
   b. The probability that the true proportion of fully immunized children is less than 50 percent

Section 6.6 The *t* Distribution

The normal distribution has been the subject of several sections in this chapter. The normal distribution is a distribution that is based on the notion of an infinite number of observations. Thus far, whenever normal distribution has been discussed in this book, it has been stated that a distribution tends to be normal—or that the data are approximately normally distributed. This, in part, has been because the normal distribution assumes an infinite number of observations. An important distribution for statistics is a distribution that approximates the normal distribution but does not assume infinite observations. This distribution is called the *t* distribution.

What Is a *t* Distribution?

Whereas the normal distribution assumes an infinite number of observations, the *t* distribution assumes a finite number of observations. Because the normal distribution assumes an infinite number of observations, there is a single normal distribution. Because the *t* distribution depends on the number of observations in question, there is a whole family of *t* distributions, each corresponding to a separate number of observations—or more precisely, to a separate *degrees of freedom.*

Degrees of Freedom

The concept of degrees of freedom will arise a number of times in our discussion of statistics, because it is central to the probability of an outcome. Before discussing the *t* distribution in more detail, it is desirable to clarify what the concept of degrees of freedom means. Suppose we have a set of four numbers that we know will add to 10. We are going to select those four numbers any way we choose, but at the end they have to add to 10. If we think about the first number, it could be anywhere on the number scale, from $-\infty$ to ∞, but let us say that the first number we choose is 4. We can now select the second number, and it, too, is limited only by $-\infty$ to ∞. But let us say that the second number is -5. Now the third number can be selected, again with no limitations—but imagine that we select 8 as the number. What happens now? The scenario so far is shown in Figure 6.28. We have selected the numbers 4, -5, and 8 as the first three numbers and we now wish to select the fourth number. But the total must be 10. For this to be true, we have no choice for the fourth number. It must be 3. Because we wished to choose four numbers that all added to 10, we had three degrees of freedom. We could choose any numbers we wished for the first three numbers (thus the degrees of freedom),

FIGURE 6.28. DEGREES OF FREEDOM.

	A	B	
1	Number	Value	
2	1	4	
3	2	-5	
4	3	8	
5	4	?	
6	Sum	10	
7			

FIGURE 6.29. TWO *t* DISTRIBUTIONS.

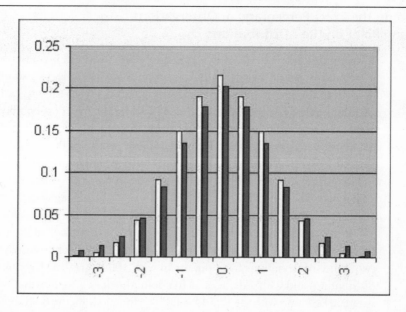

but we were constrained to pick the only number that would make the four numbers add to 10 as the fourth number. Here we have seen that the degrees of freedom are the number of values under consideration less 1. In a very large number of statistical applications, the degrees of freedom will be the number of observations less 1, or as it is often given, $n - 1$.

Let us go back now to the *t* statistic. The *t* distribution, which approximates the normal distribution, depends on the degrees of freedom. A *t* distribution with 100 degrees of freedom (a sample of size 101) will be more nearly normal in shape than a distribution with 4 degrees of freedom (a sample of size 5). Figure 6.29

shows two different t distributions. The white distribution is the t distribution for degrees of freedom equal to 100. The dark gray distribution is the distribution for degrees of freedom equal to 4. The horizontal axis shows standard deviations from the mean.

The distribution for 100 degrees of freedom is nearly normal. The proportion of cases within one standard deviation on either side of the mean is .68, and the proportion within two standard deviations is .95. The distribution for degrees of freedom equal to 4 appears approximately normal (and it is), but as can be seen from the figure, there are fewer observations in the middle of the distribution and more at the extremes. With the distribution for 4 degrees of freedom, only about 63 percent of the distribution is within one standard deviation of the mean and about 88 percent is within 2.

Finding the Exact Percentage of Observations at any Point on the t Distribution

At many times in the course of a statistical analysis, it will be important to know what proportion of a t distribution is beyond, for example, two standard deviations from the mean, or three standard deviations from the mean. One of the capabilities that Excel provides is that of finding the exact probability associated with any portion of a t distribution, given the degrees of freedom. In the past, before the widespread availability of computer programs that would do statistics, and particularly before Excel, the only way to determine this probability was from a table of probabilities of the t distribution. Most statistics books, even today, have such tables. The use of the tables is generally described along with the tables themselves at some point in the body of the book.

But Excel eliminates the need for such tables. If we look at the two distributions given in Figure 6.29, what is the exact probability of being outside the range of two standard deviations from the mean with 100 degrees of freedom (the white distribution) and with 4 degrees of freedom (the dark gray distribution)? The answer can be found with the Excel =TDIST() function. Figure 6.30 shows the exact probability of being outside one, two, and three standard deviations of the mean for 100 degrees of freedom and for 4 degrees of freedom. The formula bar shows the =TDIST() function, which takes three arguments. The first is the number of standard deviations from the mean (column A). The second argument is the number of degrees of freedom (given in B2 and C2). The third argument is the number of tails to consider in the distribution. The number of tails can be 1 if the exact probability of being *either* above or below a particular standard deviation number is desired (that is, in only one tail of the distribution). The number of tails will be

FIGURE 6.30. EXACT PROBABILITIES OF *t* DISTRIBUTIONS.

	B4 ▼	= =TDIST($A4,B$2,2)	
	A	**B**	**C**
1		DF	
2	Standard Deviations	100	4
3	Two tails		
4	1	0.319724	0.373901
5	2	0.048212	0.116117
6	3	0.003408	0.039942
7	One tail		
8	1	0.159862	0.18695
9	2	0.024106	0.058058
10	3	0.001704	0.019971
11			

2 if the exact probability of being *both* above OR below a certain number of standard deviations is desired (that is, in both tails of the distribution). Rows 4, 5, and 6 show the two-tail probabilities, whereas rows 8, 9, and 10 show the one-tail probabilities. As Figure 6.30 demonstrates, for example, only about 5 percent of the distribution with 100 degrees of freedom is beyond two standard deviations (two tail), whereas nearly 12 percent of the distribution is beyond two standard deviations (two tail) with 4 degrees of freedom.

Excel also provides another useful function related to the *t* distribution. This is the =TINV() function. The function =TINV() will return the exact value of *t* (that is, the number of standard deviations from the mean) for any probability. So, for example, if one wishes to know the number of standard deviations, it is necessary to go out from the mean in order to include 95 percent of all observations in a *t* distribution with 100 degrees of freedom; that number can be found with =TINV(0.05,100). The result of the =TINV() function written, as in the last sentence, will be 1.98. This means that it is necessary to go out 1.98 standard deviations on either side of the mean to find the interval within which 95 percent of the observations will fall.

One important point about the =TINV() function is that it always returns the two-tail distance from the mean in standard deviation for any probability. For example, if one wanted the one-tail probability distance for a probability of .05 and degrees of freedom equal to 100, it would be necessary to use the function =TINV(.1,100).

Exercises for Section 6.6

1. What is the number of degrees of freedom in each of the following?
   a. A sample of ten observations
   b. A sample of a hundred observations
   c. A sample of 250 observations
   d. A sample of a thousand observations

2. What is the two-tail probability in each of the following?
   a. $n = 10$, *S.E.* from the mean = 2
   b. $n = 10$, *S.E.* from the mean = 3
   c. $n = 100$, *S.E.* from the mean = 2
   d. $n = 100$, *S.E.* from the mean = 3
   e. $n = 250$, *S.E.* from the mean = 2
   f. $n = 250$, *S.E.* from the mean = 3

3. What is the one-tail probability in each of the following?
   a. $n = 10$, *S.E.* from the mean = 2
   b. $n = 10$, *S.E.* from the mean = 3
   c. $n = 100$, *S.E.* from the mean = 2
   d. $n = 100$, *S.E.* from the mean = 3
   e. $n = 250$, *S.E.* from the mean = 2
   f. $n = 250$, *S.E.* from the mean = 3

4. How many standard errors from the mean are the following assuming two-tail results?
   a. $p = .05, n = 10$
   b. $p = .12, n = 10$
   c. $p = .05, n = 100$
   d. $p = .12, n = 100$

5. How many standard errors from the mean are the following assuming one-tail results?
   a. $p = .05, n = 10$
   b. $p = .12, n = 10$
   c. $p = .05, n = 100$
   d. $p = .12, n = 100$

Reference

Freund, J. E., and Walpole, R. E. *Mathematical Statistics.* (4th ed.) Englewood Cliffs, N.J.: Prentice Hall, 1987.

CHAPTER SEVEN

CONFIDENCE LIMITS AND HYPOTHESIS TESTING

It has been noted that one of the most important functions of statistics, and the one to which the remainder of this book is devoted, is the determination of whether two variables could be considered to be independent of one another. This is a determination that is made on a sample of observations but is understood to apply to an entire population. The central task of determining independence is the establishment of confidence limits and the testing of hypotheses about the data.

Section 7.1 What Is a Confidence Interval?

A confidence interval is the range within which we expect a true population value—for example, a mean—to lie. Confidence intervals are established from samples and are used to predict a population value when it is not possible, either because of cost or for some other reason, to measure the true value directly. For example, suppose a hospital financial officer wishes to know the average cost of services provided to inpatients in the hospital. But the only record that the hospital maintains for most hospital stays is information about the insurance reimbursable amount and total charges, both of which are based primarily on length of stay and diagnosis. The only way to get the actual cost of services for any inpatient stay is to examine the specific hospital record, determine which services were provided, and assign a cost to each of these services, based on time and motion studies that had been carried out by the hospital. Perhaps an average-sized hospital might have ten to fifteen thousand discharges in a given year. If the financial officer were to try to examine each of these to determine the average cost of services provided to inpatients, the magnitude of the task would be prohibitive.

Conversely, the financial officer might reasonably expect that such an assessment could be made for a sample of hospital discharges, say a hundred discharges. If the financial officer selected a random sample of a hundred hospital discharges from all discharges for the past year, it should be possible to estimate, on the basis of this sample, the true mean cost of services for inpatients. In doing this, the financial officer would calculate a mean value for the sample and infer that this is the mean for all discharges. But as we saw in Chapter Six, the mean value for one sample would not necessarily be the same as the mean value of a second sample. We learned there that, in fact, if we selected many samples, the means from these many samples would tend to be normally distributed around the mean of all samples (and also around the true mean of all discharges).

So now, the financial officer might be interested not only in the point estimate of costs per discharge but also in the range within which the true population mean of costs for all discharges might lie if he were able to measure the cost of all discharges. To examine this question, we need to return to the data from the twelve thousand hospital discharges examined in Chapter Six. But this time, instead of looking at length of stay, we are going to look at hospital costs.

The hospital financial officer cannot—because of the time involved—get the true cost of discharges for the year, but, for the sake of discussion in this book, let us assume that we have accomplished this and that it is $5,905.75. The distribution of costs in standard deviation units is shown in Figure 7.1. Column A shows standard deviation units above and below the actual mean of $5,905.75. Column B shows the actual dollar amount at the top of each standard deviation range. Column C shows the proportion of discharges in the range up to the dollar amount shown in column B. For example, the value $5,905.75 in column B represents those discharges that cost between $1,125.29 and $5,905.75. All other cells in B are interpreted similarly.

It appears, then, from Figure 7.1, that just over 65 percent of all hospital discharges have costs in the range of one standard deviation below the mean (those in cell C4). Twenty three percent of all discharges have costs in the range of one standard deviation above the mean (those in cell C5). Only .8 percent of discharges have costs below one standard deviation below the mean (cell C3). The remainder of the discharges have costs ranging from one standard deviation above the

FIGURE 7.1. DISTRIBUTION OF COSTS FOR TWELVE THOUSAND DISCHARGES.

	A	B	C
1	Stand Dev	Cost	Proportion
2	-2	$ (3,655.16)	0.0000
3	-1	$ 1,125.29	0.0080
4	0	$ 5,905.75	0.6530
5	1	$ 10,686.20	0.2335
6	2	$ 15,466.66	0.0575
7	3	$ 20,247.11	0.0275
8	4	$ 25,027.56	0.0110
9	5	$ 29,808.02	0.0045
10	6	$ 34,588.47	0.0020
11	7	$ 39,368.93	0.0015
12	8	$ 44,149.38	0.0010
13	9	$ 48,929.84	0.0005
14			

mean to nine standard deviations above the mean. Clearly, actual costs are not normally distributed, but we can have some confidence from Chapter Six that if we take samples of a large enough size, the means of those samples will be approximately normally distributed. And it is the mean that we wish to estimate rather than any individual discharge cost.

So, for example, suppose the financial officer chose a random sample of a hundred discharges from among all the hospital discharges for the year in question and determined after an examination of the records that the mean for the one hundred discharges was exactly $6,586.30. The officer might then infer that the true average cost of hospital stays was $6,586.30. But he or she realizes that this is only an estimate about the population mean based on a sample. So having had a course in statistics in graduate school, the financial officer decides to determine a confidence interval for this mean value in such a way that he has a high probability of predicting the range in which the true mean cost per patient is likely to be found. The financial officer remembers that sample mean values are distributed approximately as a t distribution, with degrees of freedom equal to the sample size minus 1. So he decides that two standard errors on either side of the mean will give him the approximate range in which he will have a 95 percent likelihood of finding the true mean of the population. (In fact, 1.98 standard deviations on either side of the mean will give him the exact 95 percent likelihood of finding the true mean, but 2 is close enough in most applications.)

Calculating Confidence Limits

The financial officer calculates the standard error of the mean by using the formula in Equation 6.11 in Chapter Six and determines that the standard error is $526.27. Based on this, he determines that there is a 95 percent likelihood that the true mean cost per hospital stay lies between $5,533.75 and $7,638.84. The way in which he carried out the calculations is given in Equation 7.1. As the equation indicates, the limits are the sample mean plus or minus the appropriate value of t times the standard error of the mean. The exact 95 percent value of t is 1.98 for a sample of a hundred observations, but 2 is close enough. The exact percent of the means expected to fall within two standard errors of the mean with a sample of size 100 is 95.2 percent.

$$CL = \bar{x} \pm t \times S.E._{\bar{x}} \qquad (7.1)$$

where CL designates the confidence limits and t represents the number of standard errors on either side of the mean required to encompass a desired proportion of the t distribution (generally 95 percent).

Finding the exact t values for any level of confidence can be done by using the =TINV() function in Excel. To find the exact t value for a 95 percent confidence limit and a sample of 100, for example, the function would be =TINV(.05,99), where .05 is 1 minus the confidence level desired (this is usually called alpha) and 99 is the degrees of freedom for a sample of size 100. If you wanted to find the t value for a 99 percent confidence limit with a sample of 30, the function would be =TINV(.01,29) and would produce a t value of 2.76. The range 2.76 standard deviations on both sides of a mean from a sample of 30 would produce the 99 percent confidence limits.

It should be recognized that the =TINV() function always returns the two-tail value for t. If you wanted to know the t value for a one-tail test—for example, the 95 percent probability *below* which the mean value for the population would lie for a sample of—say, 100, it would be necessary to double the value of alpha. The appropriate statement in Excel would be =TINV(.1,99), which would produce a t value of 1.66.

Having made the point in the paragraph immediately preceding, it is useful to say a few words about a one-tail test. When both upper and lower confidence limits are found (such as are pictured in Figure 7.2), the 5 percent of all possible sample means that are outside the 95 percent limits could be either above the upper limit or below the lower limit. Frequently, the interest is in establishing 95 percent (or other percentage value) limits relative only to a single direction from the mean. For example, suppose the hospital financial officer is interested only in determining what the highest value of true hospital charges could be, based on

FIGURE 7.2. CONFIDENCE LIMITS FROM TEN SAMPLES.

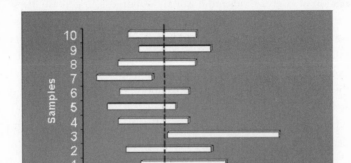

the sample mean of $6,586.30 and a standard error of $526.27. What is the upper limit *below which* he is 95 percent confident that the true average hospital cost will lie?

The financial officer is uninterested in the lower limit of the distribution. The consequence of this lack of interest in the lower limit of the distribution means that the 5 percent of possible mean values outside the limits (1 − .95) must all be at the top end of the distribution. With the limits at both ends, 2.5 percent of 1 − .95 is at each end of the continuum. If it is desired to have 5 percent at the top end of the continuum only, it is not necessary to go out as far from the sample mean in terms of standard errors. For a sample of size 100, the upper limit (the only limit of interest) would be $6,586.30 + $526.27 · 1.66, or $7,459.91. In other words, the financial officer can be 95 percent certain that the true average hospital cost lies *below* $7,459.91.

What Does the 95 Percent Confidence Limit Mean?

Having found the 95 percent confidence limits for the cost of cases discharged from the hospital, what has the financial officer actually found? He has not found limits within which the true mean has a 95 percent likelihood of falling. The true mean is either in his 95 percent range or it is not. If it is, the probability that the mean is in the range (which it is, given that the true mean is $5905.75) is 1. If it is not, the probability that the true mean is in the range is 0. So what does the 95 percent confidence limit actually mean? To understand, we must look at Figure 7.2. Figure 7.2 shows the confidence intervals calculated for the mean of cost per discharge for ten samples of a hundred discharges drawn from the population of twelve thousand hospital discharges. (In general, these data would never be available because only one sample would be selected; but since this is a book, we can do whatever we want.) The left end of each bar representing a confidence interval is at the lower limit of the interval, and the right end of the bar is at the upper limit of the interval. The bar itself represents the range within which the true mean has a 95 percent likelihood of being found. The dashed vertical line at $5,905 represents the true mean of the population.

Confidence limits for ten sample means are shown in Figure 7.2. The confidence limits for samples 1, 2, 4, 5, 6, 8, 9, and 10 actually contain the true sample mean. The confidence limits for samples 3 and 7 do not. If we were to draw many samples of a given size (here, $n = 100$) and calculate the 95 percent confidence limits for each (approximately two standard errors on either side of the sample mean), 95 percent of the confidence intervals would contain the true mean. This is what is meant when 95 percent confidence limits are constructed. If a large number of samples were taken and the confidence limits were calculated, ninety-five of a hundred of them would be expected to contain the true mean. But whether any one of the confidence limits does or does not contain the true mean is either 1 or 0.

Exercises for Section 7.1

1. Use =TINV() and Equation 7.1 to calculate the exact 95 percent upper and lower confidence limits for the following:
   a. $n = 40$, mean $= 32$, S.E. $= 1.23$
   b. $n = 40$, mean $= 32$, S.E. $= 3.23$
   c. $n = 140$, mean $= 32$, S.E. $= 1.23$
   d. $n = 140$, mean $= 32$, S.E. $= 3.23$

2. Use $t = 2$ and Equation 7.1 to calculate approximate 95 percent upper and lower confidence limits for the following:
   a. $n = 40$, mean $= 32$, S.E. $= 1.23$
   b. $n = 40$, mean $= 32$, S.E. $= 3.23$
   c. $n = 140$, mean $= 32$, S.E. $= 1.23$
   d. $n = 140$, mean $= 32$, S.E. $= 3.23$

3. How well do the values in Exercise 2 approximate those in Exercise 1?
4. Use =TINV() and Equation 7.1 to calculate the exact 99 percent upper and lower confidence limits for the following:
   a. $n = 40$, mean $= 32$, S.E. $= 1.23$
   b. $n = 40$, mean $= 32$, S.E. $= 3.23$

    c. $n = 140$, mean $= 32$, S.E. $= 1.23$
    d. $n = 140$, mean $= 32$, S.E. $= 3.23$

5. Use =TINV() and Equation 7.1 to calculate the exact 95 percent upper confidence limit *only* (95 percent of observations below the upper limit) for the following:
    a. $n = 40$, mean $= 32$, S.E. $= 1.23$
    b. $n = 40$, mean $= 32$, S.E. $= 3.23$
    c. $n = 140$, mean $= 32$, S.E. $= 1.23$
    d. $n = 140$, mean $= 32$, S.E. $= 3.23$

6. Use the Infants worksheet in the file Chpt 2–2.xls. Assume that this is a random sample of weights of one-year-olds from a much larger defined population and calculate the exact 95 percent upper and lower confidence limits for the weight of one-year-olds in the population.

7. Use the Hospital charge worksheet in the file Chpt 4–1.xls. Assume that the data represent a random sample from a larger population.
    a. Calculate the exact 95 percent upper and lower confidence limits for the population mean of LOS.
    b. Calculate the exact 95 percent upper and lower confidence limits for the population mean of charges.
    c. Calculate the exact 95 percent upper limit only for the population mean of charges—that is, the value below which 95 percent of all sample means will be expected to fall.
    d. Calculate the exact 95 percent upper and lower confidence limits for the population proportion, which is female.

8. Use the emergency room wait worksheet in the file Chpt 6–2.xls and =RAND() to draw a random sample of sixty records from the 832 on the sheet. Calculate the exact 95 percent upper and lower confidence limits for the population mean.

Section 7.2 Calculating Confidence Limits for Multiple Samples

Section 7.1 discussed the drawing of numerous samples of a given size. This was also discussed in the third subsection of Section 6.3 in Chapter Six. In that subsection, we generated a hundred samples of size 30 from a file that contained the probability of having a specified number of prenatal visits, from 0 to 15 for

FIGURE 7.3. CALCULATION OF MEANS AND LIMITS.

B39	▼	=	=AND(B37>$B$35,B38<$B$35)				
	A	B	C	D	E	F	G	H
25		5	4	5	4	4	5	
26		6	3	3	3	3	5	
27		6	8	3	3	7	4	
28		3	4	1	3	4	3	
29		9	3	6	12	5	9	
30		3	6	6	6	8	1	
31								
32	Mean	4.533333	4.933333	5.033333	4.2	4.433333	5.1	
33	St Dev	1.995397	2.504249	2.697168	2.21904	1.851064	2.577756	2.534!
34	St Error	0.364308	0.457211	0.492433	0.405139	0.337956	0.470632	0.46:
35	mu	4.5711						
36	t	2.045231						
37	Upper limt	5.278427	5.868436	6.040473	5.028604	5.124532	6.062551	5.646
38	Lower limit	3.788239	3.998231	4.026194	3.371396	3.742134	4.137449	3.753:
39	Contain mu?	TRUE	TRUE	TRUE	TRUE	TRUE	TRUE	TRU
40		91						
41								

a population of women. Selected numbers from the first seven of the hundred samples were shown in Figure 6.20, and the calculation of the mean, standard deviation, and standard error for the first six samples were shown in Figure 6.21. We will use these one hundred samples to calculate the upper and lower 95 percent confidence limits for each sample and determine what proportion of the limits contain the actual mean value for the population.

The calculation of the upper and lower confidence limits is shown for the first six samples of the hundred in Figure 7.3. The number of prenatal visits for the last six women in the first six samples is shown in cells 25 through 30 in columns B through G. A new column has been inserted at A to allow labels to be put in rows 32 to 39. The mean value of the first sample (cell B32) is 4.533, the mean of the second is 4.933, and so on. The standard deviation of the first sample (cell B33) is 1.995 and the standard error of the mean (cell B34, the standard deviation divided by the square root of 30) is .364.

Mu (μ, cell B35) is the true mean of the population, calculated in Figure 6.23. Cell B36 contains the exact 95 percent value for t calculated by Excel, using =TINV(.05,29). Row 37 is the upper limit and row 38 is the lower limit for the 95 percent confidence interval. The values in these two rows are calculated as given in Equation 7.1. Row 39—labeled "Contains mu?"—is a logical statement that tests whether the true mean of the population (cell B35) is between the upper and lower limits. The logical statement is as that shown in the formula line in Figure 7.3, and uses the =AND() function. The =AND() function takes two arguments, as the formula line indicates. The =AND() function returns a value of TRUE if both statements in the arguments are true, and it returns a value of FALSE, otherwise. So if the true mean as given in B35 is either above or below any one of the sample limits, the =AND() function will return FALSE. The 91 in cell B40 is produced by the =COUNTIF() function that was used to count the number of TRUE entries in row 39. It turns out that for this series of a hundred samples, 91 samples had upper and lower 95 percent limits that contained the true mean. In general, we would have expected ninety-five of a hundred samples to have upper and lower limits that contained the true mean. But these are probabilities, and for a series of a hundred samples, it is not likely that the actual true value of ninety-five of a hundred will be generated.

This section discusses the use of Excel to determine upper and lower confidence limits for a large number of samples with given attributes as a means to demonstrate the meaning of the notion of confidence limits. It is important to remember, however, that, in general, one never draws more than one sample. The discussion here is presented solely for the purpose of helping you understand what confidence limits actually mean.

Exercises for Section 7.2

1. Use the file generated by selecting a hundred samples of thirty waiting times (see Exercise 3 of Section 6.3).
   a. Calculate the exact 95 percent upper and lower confidence limits for each sample.
   b. Use the =AND() statement, as given in Figure 7.3, to determine whether the confidence limits for each sample contain the true population mean.
   c. Use =COUNTIF() to determine whether the proportion of samples of the hundred actually contain the true mean of the population within the 95 percent limits.
   d. Can you account for the result you got in c?

2. Use the file generated by selecting 250 samples of a hundred from the prenatal visits for women (see Exercise 4 of Section 6.3).
   a. Calculate exact 95 percent upper and lower confidence limits for each sample.
   b. Use the =AND() statement, as given in Figure 7.3, to determine whether the confidence limits for each sample contain the true population mean.

   c. Use =COUNTIF() to determine whether the proportion of samples of the
      250 actually contain the true mean of the population within the 95 percent
      limits.
   d. Can you account for the result you got in c?

Section 7.3 What Is Hypothesis Testing?

In a statistical context, hypothesis testing is the process of determining from a sample whether something could be true of a population. In particular, the something
is usually a mean value or a proportion for the population. For example, suppose
a county public health nurse is concerned about whether children in her county
are growing at the normal rate for all children in the United States. She decides
to collect some data and test the hypothesis that children in her area of responsibility are normal in height relative to all children. Rather than assess all children
of all ages, she decides to assess a specific age and sex group and use that to
provide an indicator of all children in her county. She decides to assess the height
of six-year-old boys as her yardstick for assessing all children.

   The public health nurse knows that height for age scales indicate that the
national average height for six-year-old boys is approximately normally distributed, with a mean of forty-eight inches and a standard deviation of ten inches.
That is essentially the same as saying that 95 percent of all six-year-old boys are
between twenty-eight and sixty-eight inches. The public health nurse knows that
she has the resources to select a random sample of a hundred six-year-old
boys from the schools in her county and measure the height of each of the boys.
She will compare the results of this sample with what is known for the overall
population of six-year-old boys to determine if the children in her county are
growing at the expected rate.

   To do this, the public health nurse will be looking at the results of the sample
to see if those results could have come from a population of six-year-old boys in
which the true average height was forty-eight inches. Implicitly, the nurse might
say, "I will take a sample of six-year-old boys to see if I can support the view
that the average height of the entire population in the county is forty-eight inches."
From the standpoint of hypothesis testing, however, the nurse would be saying that
her initial hypothesis is that six-year-old boys in her county are forty-eight inches
tall. This hypothesis might be stated formally as:

   H0: The average height of six-year-old boys (h) is equal to forty-eight inches. Or,
   H0: h = 48.

This is sometimes called the null hypothesis—thus, the designation H0. And H0 is often pronounced not *H zero* but, rather, *H naught*. In general, though, in this text, H0 is referred to as the initial hypothesis.

Every initial hypothesis has an accompanying alternative hypothesis, usually designated H1, against which it is being tested. In general, the most frequently posited alternative is simply:

H1: The average height of six-year-old boys (h) is not equal to forty-eight inches. Or,
H1: h $\neq$ 48.

Every hypothesis test is a test of whether H0, the initial hypothesis, is consistent with the data that come from a sample. If the data that come from the sample are of such a nature that H0 is consistent with the data, then H0 is accepted. If the data that come from the sample are of such a nature that H0 is not consistent with the data, then H0 is rejected and the alternative hypothesis, H1, is accepted by default. A statistical test is never a direct test of H1 but is always a test of H0.

But how can we tell if the data are or are not consistent with the initial hypothesis—H0? In the first subsection of Section 7.1, we calculated confidence limits for sample values. In regard to hypothesis testing, if the H0 value that we have posited—that is, the value we expect the population mean or proportion to be—is contained within specified confidence limits about the sample mean, we will accept H0. If the H0 value we have posited is not within the confidence limits determined for the sample mean, we will reject H0. As has already been said, the rejection of H0, our initial hypothesis, automatically means the acceptance of H1, our alternative hypothesis.

Suppose, then, the nurse has taken a sample of a hundred six-year-old boys from the population of six-year-old boys in the schools in her county. When she did so, she discovered that the mean height of the boys in her sample was forty-nine inches, with a standard deviation of ten inches. She wishes to set the confidence limits at approximately 95 percent, so that with a sample of a hundred, her confidence limits will be a lower limit of forty-seven inches (49-[2*10/sqrt(100)]) and an upper limit of fifty-one inches (49+[2*10/sqrt(100)]). Since her originally hypothesized value of forty-eight inches is contained within the 95 percent confidence limits of her sample average height of forty-nine inches, the public health nurse will not reject the initial hypothesis. Thus, she will conclude that the average height for six-year-old boys in her county is the same as the national average (forty-eight inches).

But let us consider another example. Suppose the sample that the public health nurse took had a mean value of forty-five inches, still with a standard deviation of ten inches. On the basis of these data, she would calculate 95 percent confidence limits for her sample mean as forty-three inches and forty-seven inches. Now, the value of the initial hypothesis, forty-eight inches, is no longer contained in the confidence interval the nurse has calculated. As a consequence, from the standpoint of hypothesis testing, she would reject the initial hypothesis of forty-eight inches and accept the alternative hypothesis, which is that the average height of six-year-old boys in her county was not forty-eight inches. In fact, because her sample result was less than the initially hypothesized mean, she would probably decide that the average height for six-year-old boys in her county was less than the national average.

Exercises for Section 7.3

1. Suppose the twenty people who have made clinic visits, as represented on the Visits sheet of Chpt 3–1.xls, are considered to be a random sample of all the people who have ever come or will ever come to the clinic in question.
   a. Test the hypothesis at the 95 percent level of confidence that the average Visit Time for the population is thirty-seven minutes (H0: VT = 37), against the alternative hypothesis that the Visit Time is not thirty-seven minutes (H1: VT ≠ 37), and state your conclusion.
   b. Test the same hypothesis at the 99 percent level of confidence and state your conclusion.
   c. Test the hypothesis at the 95 percent level of confidence that average Charges for the population is $75 (H0: C = $75), against the alternative hypothesis that Charges is not $75 (H1: C ≠ $75), and state your conclusion.
   d. Test the same hypothesis at the 99 percent level of confidence and state your conclusion.

2. Suppose the one hundred hospital discharges on the Hospital charges worksheet in Chpt 4–1.xls represent a random sample of all Medicare-eligible persons discharged from a specific hospital.
   a. Test the hypothesis at the 95 percent level of confidence that average Charges for the population is $6,000 (H0: C = $6,000), against the alternative hypothesis that average Charges is not $6,000 (H1: C ≠ $6,000), and state your conclusion.
   b. Test the same hypothesis at the 99 percent level of confidence and state your conclusion.

    c. Test the hypothesis at the 95 percent level of confidence that average LOS for the population is 7.5 days (H0: LOS = 7.5), against the alternative hypothesis that LOS is not 7.5 (H1: LOS ≠ 7.5), and state your conclusion.

    d. Test the same hypothesis at the 99 percent level of confidence and state your conclusion.

3. Use the emergency room wait spreadsheet in file Chpt 6–2.xls.

    a. Draw a simple random sample of sixty records, using any method you choose.

    b. Test the hypothesis at the 95 percent level of confidence that the average wait time is 38.4 minutes (H0: W = 38.4), against the alternative that the average wait time is not 38.4 minutes (H1: W ≠ 38.4), and state your conclusion.

    c. Test the same hypothesis at the 99 percent level of confidence and state your conclusion.

Section 7.4 Type I and Type II Errors

In arriving at the decisions previously discussed, the public health nurse runs the risk of making two types of errors. When she concluded on the basis of the sample mean of forty-five inches that the average height for six-year-old boys in her county *was not* forty-eight inches, she ran the risk of making the type I error. The type I error is the error of concluding that the initial hypothesis is false when it is, in fact, true. When she concluded on the basis of the sample mean of forty-nine inches that the average height of six-year-old boys in her county *was* forty-eight inches, she ran the risk of making the type II error. The type II error is the error of concluding that the initial hypothesis is true when it is, in fact, false. Let us look further at both the type I and the type II error.

To begin with, consider the possibility that the true mean height of six-year-old boys in the public health nurse's county is really forty-eight inches and that the standard deviation is ten inches. If the nurse were to draw an infinite number of samples of size 100 from this population of six-year-old boys, the resulting distribution of the mean values of those samples might be as shown in Figure 7.4.

In looking at Figure 7.4, it is possible to see that it depicts a normal distribution with the midpoint (and the mean) at forty-eight inches. There is a vertical dotted line at forty-six inches and one at fifty inches. These two lines represent the cutoff point for two standard errors on either side of the mean, or the 95 percent confidence limits. The figure represents the fact that if the nurse drew an infinite number of samples of size 100 from the population of six-year-old boys in her

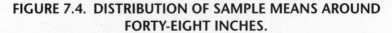

FIGURE 7.4. DISTRIBUTION OF SAMPLE MEANS AROUND FORTY-EIGHT INCHES.

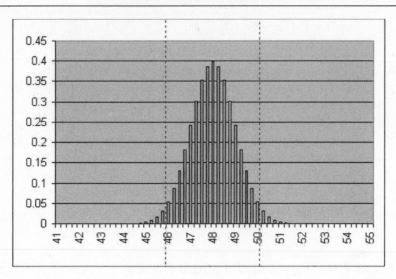

county—assuming that the true mean is forty-eight inches—the mean of 95 percent of those samples would be between forty-six and fifty inches. The mean of 5 percent of the samples would be either above or below the dotted cutoff lines, or outside the 95 percent limits. Thus, when the nurse draws her one sample to assess the hypothesis that the true mean of the height of six-year-old boys in her county is forty-eight inches, she has five chances in a hundred of drawing a sample that will have a mean value greater than fifty inches or less than forty-six inches. And it should be noted that this would happen even when the true mean is forty-eight inches. Any result outside the upper limit of fifty inches or the lower limit of forty-six inches will result in her rejecting the initial hypothesis and consequently making the type I error of concluding that the true mean height of six-year-old boys in her county is not forty-eight inches. The probability of making the type I error is called *alpha*, and in this case, it is set by the public health nurse at 5 percent by her decision to use the 95 percent confidence limits.

Consider again the two possible samples that the nurse might have drawn—one with a mean of forty-nine inches and the other with a mean of forty-five inches. In the first case, she would conclude that the true mean was forty-eight inches and would be making no error (still assuming that the true mean is forty-eight inches). In the second, she would conclude that the true mean is not forty-eight inches and would have made the type I error.

FIGURE 7.5. DISTRIBUTION OF SAMPLE MEANS FOR FORTY-EIGHT POUNDS AND FORTY-NINE POUNDS.

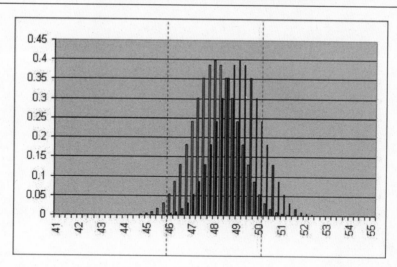

Now consider the alternative possibility—the type II error. Figure 7.5 shows the distribution of the sample means for all possible samples of size 100 from a population in which the true mean is forty-eight inches, already shown in Figure 7.4. Figure 7.5 also shows the distribution of the means for all possible samples of size 100 from a population in which the true mean is actually forty-nine inches. Figure 7.5 shows, too, the vertical dashed lines that represent the 95 percent confidence limits for a true mean of forty-eight inches.

Now suppose the true mean of the population of six-year-old boys in the county in which the public health nurse is working is actually forty-nine inches. Admittedly, this is not greatly different from forty-eight inches. But it is different. But could the nurse detect this difference on the basis of her sample of a hundred boys? Based on her 95 percent criteria, she would reject the initial hypothesis of forty-eight inches when the true mean was forty-nine inches, with only about a 20 percent likelihood (the portion of the distribution around forty-nine inches that is to the right of the right vertical dashed line). She would have about an 80 percent likelihood (the portion of the distribution being around forty-nine inches to the left of the right vertical dashed line) of accepting the initial hypothesis of forty-eight inches when, in fact, the true mean is not forty-eight inches but forty-nine inches. In this case, she has an 80 percent chance of making the type II error of accepting the initial hypothesis when it is not true. The probability of making the type II error is known as *beta*, and in this case, it is about .8.

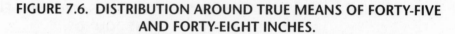

FIGURE 7.6. DISTRIBUTION AROUND TRUE MEANS OF FORTY-FIVE AND FORTY-EIGHT INCHES.

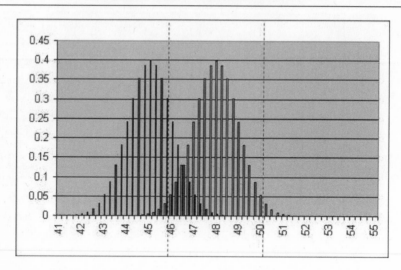

But what of the sample in which she got a mean of forty-five inches? She could not make the type II error because she rejected the initial hypothesis of forty-eight inches. But if the true mean of the population were in fact forty-five inches, is there any possibility of type II error relative to the initial hypothesis? The answer is yes. To see this, consider the distribution of the sample means from a population in which the true sample mean is forty-five inches. This distribution is shown, along with the distribution around forty-eight inches, in Figure 7.6. Again, the two dashed vertical lines representing the 95 percent confidence limits for a true mean of forty-eight inches are also shown in Figure 7.6.

Now, an examination of Figure 7.6 shows that perhaps 30 percent of the distribution of the sample means around a true mean of forty-five inches, will be to the right of the left vertical dashed line. This is the region in which the initial hypothesis is accepted. In this case, then, even when the true mean is forty-five inches, there is approximately a 30 percent likelihood—beta—of making the type II error, of accepting the initial hypothesis of forty-eight inches—when it is false.

The Mutual Dependence of Alpha and Beta

In Figure 7.6, the confidence limits around the true mean of forty-eight inches are set at 95 percent, thus making alpha equal .05. In setting alpha equal to .05, and assuming a population standard deviation of 10 and a sample size of 100, the lower confidence limit is at forty-six inches. This means that beta for a true population mean of forty-five inches—the portion of the distribution around forty-five inches that is right of forty-six inches—is about 30 percent, or .30. It is possible to reduce beta for a true mean value of forty-five inches by increasing alpha for a mean of forty-eight inches. For example, instead of decreeing that alpha should be .05, suppose we were willing to have alpha be equal to .32, which is equivalent to saying that we are willing to take a .32 percent risk of making a type I error, rejecting H0 when it is true. That would mean that we would put the upper and lower confidence limits only one standard error from the mean. The result is shown in Figure 7.7. In Figure 7.7, the vertical dashed lines are now at forty-seven and forty-nine inches. Any sample result to the left of the lower dashed line or the right of the upper dashed line will now lead to the rejection of the initial hypothesis that the mean value is 48 percent. But look also at what has happened to beta for a true mean of forty-five inches, relative to the initial hypothesis of forty-eight inches. The portion of the distribution around forty-five inches that is to the right of the lower vertical dashed line probably represents only about 10 percent of the total distribution around forty-five. Thus, by increasing alpha, we have decreased beta. This is a general result. Increasing alpha will always lead to the decrease in beta, all other things being equal.

FIGURE 7.7. SIXTY-EIGHT PERCENT CONFIDENCE LIMITS FOR A DISTRIBUTION AROUND FORTY-EIGHT INCHES.

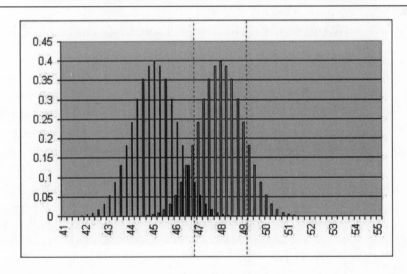

The Reality of Many Betas

In Section 7.3, the initial hypothesis was introduced as h = forty-eight inches and the alternative hypothesis was introduced as h ≠ 48. If the initial hypothesis is rejected, it means that the height of six-year-old boys in the county in which the public health nurse is working could be anything other than forty-eight inches. It could be thirty-nine inches, it could be forty-nine inches, it could be fifty inches, or it could be fifty-five inches. What does this mean in terms of beta or type II error?

A general notion of what many alternative realities regarding the true height of six-year-old boys may mean is shown in Figure 7.8. This figure shows the distribution around a true mean of forty-eight inches, a true mean of fifty inches, and a true mean of fifty-two inches. The figure also shows the 95 percent confidence limits for a true value of forty-eight inches as the vertical dashed lines at forty-six and fifty inches. If the initial hypothesis is that the true mean is forty-eight inches and the alternative is that the true mean is not forty-eight inches, the true mean might be fifty inches or it might be fifty-two inches (or any other value).

If the true mean is fifty inches, then the value of beta for the initial hypothesis of forty-eight inches is exactly 50 percent. That is, half the distribution of sample means around a true mean of 50 are left of the upper dashed line and in the region in which H0 will be falsely accepted. If the true mean is fifty-two inches, then the value of beta for the initial hypothesis of forty-eight inches is probably in the region of 3 percent. Only about 3 percent of the distribution of sample means around a true mean of fifty-two inches is below the vertical dashed line at

FIGURE 7.8. DISTRIBUTIONS AROUND THREE TRUE MEANS.

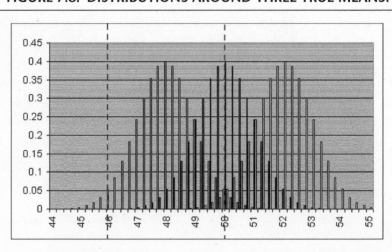

fifty inches. The point of this discussion is that there is an infinite set of beta values, each associated with one of the infinite number of possible values that an alternative hypothesis of h ≠ 48 inches could possibly take on.

It is increasingly common to wish to specify both alpha and beta in current statistical applications. Frequently, one might encounter a statement in a report of a statistical analysis, such as "alpha = beta = .05." As we have seen, there is an infinite set of beta values, each associated with a different real alternative possibility for the value being assessed as the initial hypothesis. If the initial hypothesis says that the Medicare case total charges across all hospitals in a state comes to $5,300, then the alternative hypothesis that the average is not $5,300 would have a beta value for every other possible average case charge imaginable. In order to set a beta value equal to any specific probability, it is necessary to state the alternative hypothesis as a specific value rather than as simply not H0.

Consider again the public health nurse interested in the height of six-year-old boys. She might be interested in this because she wants to assure herself and the appropriate county authorities that growth among children in her county is normal, relative to the rest of the United States. If six-year-old boys in her county were smaller in stature than six-year-old boys in general, it might signal the need for efforts to ensure adequate nutrition, such as school lunch programs. If six-year-old boys are taller in stature than six-year-old boys in general, this might not be a cause for concern, but it might lead to a question of why this may have occurred. It is likely that her main concern, however, would be that the six-year-old boys in her county should not be found to be smaller in stature than six-year-old boys in general. If this were to be found, some action on the part of the county authorities might be warranted.

Determining Beta

Suppose the nurse wished to make sure that she could test the initial hypothesis that the height of six-year-old boys in her county was forty-eight inches, against an alternative hypothesis that would allow her to set the type II error (beta) at some predetermined level. If that were the case, she would have to determine ahead of time how different an alternative height might be before it would be important enough to lead to a decision to institute an intervention. The nurse knows that the average height of U.S. six-year-old boys is forty-eight inches and that the standard deviation is approximately ten inches. So she would not be concerned if six-year-old boys in her county averaged somewhat less than forty-eight inches—say, as little as forty-six inches. But she has decided that if she finds six-year-old boys in her county average as little as 44.6 inches, some intervention is indicated.

So the public health nurse restates her initial and alternative hypotheses as follows:

H0: The average height of six-year-old boys (h) is equal to forty-eight inches. Or, H0: h = 48.

And

H1: The average height of six-year-old boys (h) is equal to 44.6 inches. Or, H1: h = 44.6.

Now two things have happened. First, the public health nurse has determined that she will accept H0 for any value of height greater than some lower limit around forty-eight inches, because she has specified an alternative value *below* forty-eight inches, thus creating what is known as a *one-tail test*. A one-tail test is one in which the initial hypothesis can be rejected only in one end of the normal distribution, in this case, the lower end. Second, she has provided a specific value for the alternative hypothesis so that she can assess the value of beta, the likelihood of making type II error.

To consider the one-tail test first, in the statement of the original alternative hypothesis, H1: h ≠ 48, h could be greater or lesser than forty-eight. Thus the region in which H0 would be rejected would be at either end of the distribution around forty-eight inches. So it is necessary to have half the region of rejection (2.5 percent of the distribution around forty-eight inches) at the upper tail of the curve, and half (again 2.5 percent) at the lower tail of the curve. Since the alternative hypothesis H1: h = 44.6 now specifies that the alternative is less than forty-eight, any value at the upper end of the distribution around forty-eight will be irrelevant to rejecting H0. Thus it is reasonable and accepted by most statisticians to determine that all of the 5 percent region of rejection will be in the lower half of the distribution around forty-eight inches. In a normal distribution, about 1.7 standard errors on either side of the mean will cut off about 5 percent of the distribution *on either side* (the exact number of standard errors required can be found by =TINV(.1,d.f.)). So the lower limit for rejecting H0 (the only limit of interest relative to the present alternative hypothesis) will be approximately 46.3 inches (48-[1.7*10/sqrt(100)]), rather than the previous forty-six inches.

Consider the second point; specifying the actual value of beta. By specifying the alternative hypothesis as H1: h = 44.6, it is possible to say that the upper 5 percent region in which we will accept H0 when in fact H1 is true, will be about 1.7 standard errors above the value of 44.6, or about 46.3. So now it is possible to say that alpha = beta = .05 for the test:

H0: h = 48.
H1: h = 44.6.

FIGURE 7.9. DISTRIBUTIONS AROUND 48 AND 44.6 INCHES.

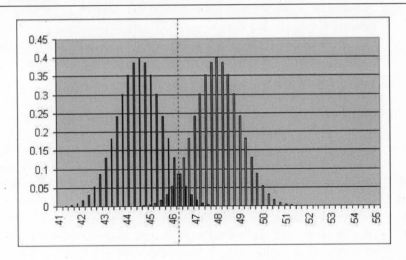

This is shown in Figure 7.9. Figure 7.9 shows the sampling distribution of the means around a true population mean of forty-eight inches (the distribution to the right) and the sampling distribution around a true mean of 44.6 inches (the distribution to the left). The vertical dashed line representing the lower 95 percent limit for the distribution around forty-eight inches is now at about 46.3 inches, or 1.7 inches below the mean of forty-eight. The vertical dashed line is also about 1.7 inches above the alternative mean of 44.6 inches. The two distributions now overlap in such a way that the probability of making type I error, of rejecting H0 when it is true, is equal to the probability of making type II error, of accepting H0 when it is false (or alternatively of rejecting H1 when it is true). Both the type I and the type II error is approximately 5 percent. It must be remembered, however, that the ability to specify alpha depends on the exact specification of a value for the alternative hypothesis.

Controlling Beta

The ability to specify alpha = beta = .05 as shown in Figure 7.9 depends on the specification of the alternative hypothesis. In this case, it was posited as being exactly that alternative that would create the results desired given that the standard deviation of the height of six-year-old boys is approximately ten inches and a sample of a hundred is being selected. But suppose the public health nurse had decided that if the six-year-old boys in her county averaged forty-six inches in height rather than forty-eight, some intervention to assure adequate nutrition of school children was warranted. How could the nurse test the hypothesis, H0: h = 48 against the alternative hypothesis, H1: h = 46 and ensure that alpha = beta = .05?

The solution to this problem lies in the fact that the standard error of the mean is inversely related to the sample size. To see this, imagine that instead of selecting a sample of 100 six-year-old boys on which to test the initial hypothesis, the nurse had selected a sample of 290 six-year-old boys. (This county is a large metropolitan area, so a sample of 290 six-year-old boys is not unreasonable). With a sample of 290 six-year-old boys, the standard error of the sampling distribution now becomes about .6 and 1.7 standard errors below the mean of forty-eight (the point below which H0 will be rejected) now lies at forty-seven inches. Similarly, the region for the distribution around forty-six inches, above which H0 will be accepted, also lies at forty-seven inches. Figure 7.10 shows this result. By comparing Figure 7.10 with Figure 7.9, it is possible to see that the second set of distributions is now much more narrowly dispersed about the two means. Also, the vertical dashed line at forty-seven inches now cuts off about 5 percent of the lower end of the upper distribution and about 5 percent of the upper end of the lower distribution. Again, alpha = beta = .05 (approximately). Thus, if the alternative hypothesis is given as a specific number value, and one knows the probable standard deviation of the data, it is possible to determine the size of the sample that will be required to ensure that alpha = beta = .05 (or any other confidence limit that may be deemed acceptable).

FIGURE 7.10. TWO DISTRIBUTIONS FOR A SAMPLE OF 290.

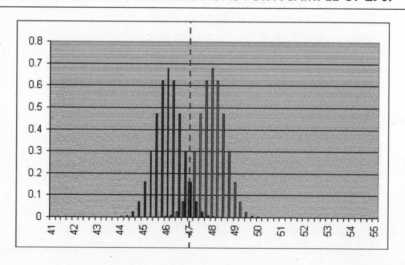

Calculating the Value of Beta for Any Alternative Hypothesis

The researcher sets the value of alpha. If the researcher wishes to make sure that type I error will be no greater than .05, then the researcher can use 95 percent confidence limits, whether upper and lower or either upper or lower individually, to determine the sample values that will lead to the rejection of H0. So, with the case of the public health worker discussed here, she can decide that she will reject H0 if the value found in her sample is more than approximately two standard errors (or approximately 1.7 standard errors if it's a one-tail test) away from the mean. When she got a sample value of forty-five inches, she determined that the value of H0 of forty-eight inches was not contained in the 95 percent confidence limits for forty-five inches, so she rejected H0. The likelihood that she was in error is 5 percent.

However, beta is determined not by the level of confidence, but, as seen earlier, it is an artifact of the sample size, of the standard deviation of the data, and of the setting of a specific alternative hypothesis. So how can the researcher know what the value of beta is for an assessment such as that carried out by the public health worker? First and foremost, it is necessary to specify an alternative hypothesis before any determination of beta can be made. As we have seen, there are an infinite number of values of beta, one for each of the infinite number of values other than that specified by H0. So the first step is to select an alternative hypothesis that is meaningful in practice.

Suppose the alternative hypothesis was, as discussed in the fourth subsection of Section 7.4, that the height of six-year-old boys in the county in question was forty-six inches and the public health nurse wished to know what the value of beta—that is, the probability of accepting H0 when in fact H1 was true—would be if she were limited to a sample of a hundred and continuing to assume a standard deviation in height of six-year-old boys as ten inches. Since she has decided that the alternative is less than forty-eight inches, she has automatically moved from a two-tail test to a one-tail test. She is only interested in knowing if the alternative is *less than* forty-eight inches. So her region of rejection of H0 would be only the lower end of the distribution around a true mean of forty-eight inches. She calculates the lower limit for forty-eight inches and finds that it is 46.34 inches (48-10/sqrt(10)*1.67). Now she can subtract the value of H1 (forty-six inches) from the lower limit for H0 to get .34. When she divides this by the standard error (10/sqrt(10)), she gets a value of .34 again, because the standard error is 1. But this now represents the value of t that the lower limit for H0 is above the mean for H1. She can now use this value in the =TDIST() function to determine the exact probability of beta. The =TDIST() function in this case is written =TDIST(.34,99,1), where the .34 refers to the number of t units, 99 refers to the degrees of freedom, and 1 refers to a one-tail probability.

The formula for finding the exact value of beta may be expressed as shown in Equation 7.2. Basically, the value of beta is found by subtracting the value of H1 from the relevant limit (upper or lower) for H0, dividing the result by the standard error to convert it to t units, and then using that t value to find the proportion of the distribution around H1 that lies within the limits of acceptance for H0, using the =TDIST() function. It should be noted, however, that this equation, as given, only works when H1 is less than the lower limit of H0—if H1 actually specifies a lower value than H0, or when H1 is greater than the upper limit of H0—if H1 specifies a higher value than H0. If H1 is closer to H0 than the limit of H0, however, it is always true that beta will be greater than 50 percent.

$$t_\beta = |H0(L) - H1|/S.E. \tag{7.2}$$

and

$$\beta = TDIST(t_\beta, df, 1)$$

where H0(L) is the upper *or* lower limit for H0, H1 is the value
of H1 and *S.E.* is the standard error that applies to H0
(assumed to apply to H1 as well).

Small Alpha or Small Beta and the Cost of Research and Intervention

In the best of all possible worlds, researchers (including the public health nurse) would not have to choose between a small alpha (traditionally set at .05 or .01) and a small beta (generally hoped by the researcher to be equal to alpha). But, as the previous sections indicate, the size of beta will depend both on the extent to which a specific alternative hypothesis differs from the initial hypothesis and on sample size. If the difference between the initial hypothesis and the alternative is small, relative to the standard deviation of the data, it will require a large sample to ensure that the value of both alpha and beta are relatively small.

Consider again the public health nurse assessing the height of six-year-old boys. But this time, assume that the public health nurse is not deciding whether there should be a school supplemental nutrition program but is instead trying to assess the effectiveness of a supplemental nutrition program for kindergarten children that has been in place in the county for some time. Six-year-old boys would generally be expected to be in the first grade, so they would have had the benefit of the program during the previous year. The nurse believes that if the nutrition program is effective, one result will be an increase in stature of the six-year-old boys. So she wishes to draw a sample to see if six-year-old boys in the county could be assessed as being taller on average than all six-year-old boys in the nation.

But the nurse is not optimistic enough to think that the supplemental nutrition program will make a great difference in the height of six-year-old boys. She believes that on the average, the six-year-old boys in her county may be one inch taller than all U.S. boys. Couched in terms of hypothesis testing, her initial hypothesis would not typically be that six-year-old boys in her county averaged forty-nine inches but, rather, that they are no different from six-year-old boys in general. Thus her hypotheses would be:

H0: h = 48.
H1: h = 49.

It has already been shown in Figure 7.5 that for a sample of a hundred six-year-old boys, the region of nonrejection for H0 extends from forty-six to fifty inches (for a two-tail test at alpha = .05). Furthermore, only about 20 percent of the distribution around a true mean of forty-nine inches lies above the region of rejection for H0. Thus, even if the true average height of six-year-old boys in her county is forty-nine inches—confirming her belief that the supplemental nutrition program has made a difference, she is not likely to be able to demonstrate that with a sample of a hundred if she maintains alpha at .05. So, in order to have a reasonable likelihood of rejecting her initial hypothesis (h = 48)—if in fact it is false, she must draw a larger sample.

How large would the sample have to be to provide her with alpha = beta = .05 for an initial hypothesis of forty-eight inches and an alternative of forty-nine? First, it should be remembered that the nurse has specified the alternative hypothesis as being h = forty-nine inches, so that she is only interested in a statistical test of whether the average for six-year-old boys in her county is greater than forty-eight. Thus, for an alpha = .05, she need go only about 1.7 standard errors above forty-eight inches to set the limit. Now, if the standard deviation of the height of six-year-old boys remains ten inches, she must draw a sample large enough so that the standard error of the distribution, multiplied by 1.7, will be equal to .5 inches. The logic of this is shown in Figure 7.11.

Figure 7.11 shows the distribution around forty-eight inches and the distribution around forty-nine inches for a sample large enough for the upper 95 percent (one-tail) limit for forty-eight inches to be 48.5 inches. Five percent of the distribution of mean values from samples in which the true mean of the population is forty-eight inches will fall above 48.5 inches. Similarly, 5 percent of the mean values from samples in which the true mean of the population is forty-nine inches will fall below 48.5 inches. In this case, alpha = beta = .05. In order to achieve this, with a standard deviation of height in the population of six-year-old boys at ten inches, the nurse would have to select and measure a sample of about 1,150 six-year-old boys.

FIGURE 7.11. UPPER LIMIT FOR ALPHA = BETA = .05.

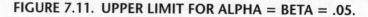

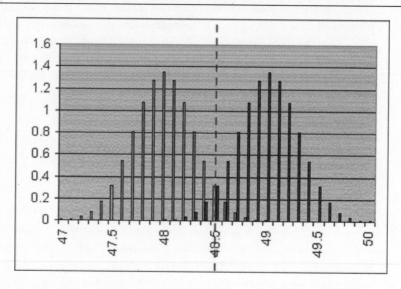

It is certainly feasible for the public health nurse to measure 1,150 six-year-old boys. But it is a much bigger job than measuring a hundred six-year-old boys. Moreover, the county health officer may not be willing to grant her the time and resources away from her other duties to carry out a survey this large. Suppose the county health officer, agreeing with the nurse that it may be useful to assess the effectiveness of the supplemental nutrition program for kindergartners, agrees that the nurse can have the time and resources to select and measure a sample of five hundred six-year-old boys. What then can be said of her perception that the program might have increased the height of six-year-old boys by one inch on the average?

If the nurse follows the prevailing tenants of statistical testing, which is to try to insure against making the type I error (rejecting the null hypothesis when it is true), she will set the upper 95 percent limit at about 48.75 inches, and the result will be as seen in Figure 7.12. Figure 7.12 shows the dashed vertical line at about 48.75 inches, so that 5 percent of the region of rejection of H0 will be above that value. But because the nurse has only a sample of five hundred, about 40 percent of the distribution around the mean of 49 percent is below the dashed line. So while the nurse has only a 5 percent chance of rejecting H0 when it is true (type I error) she has about a 40 percent chance of accepting H0 when it is false, and, in fact, H1 is true (a type II error).

Both science and conventional logic is on the side of allowing a 40 percent type II error, in the event that the nurse can select only a sample of five six-year-old

FIGURE 7.12. POSITIONING ALPHA AT .05.

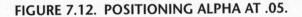

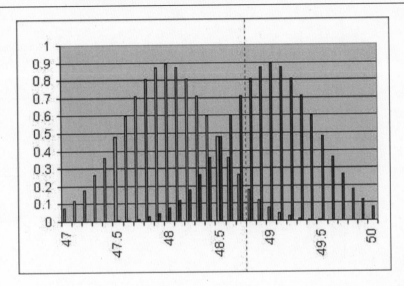

boys. It is generally deemed less unattractive to say nothing happened—unless we are absolutely sure that something did happen—than to say that something happened when we are not absolutely sure that it did. Thus, both science and conventional logic place greatest emphasis on avoiding the type I error.

But let us leave the realm of science for a moment and enter the realm of evaluation. The supplemental nutrition program has been in place for several years and has in fact become a fixture in the county. County supervisors have allocated funds for the program (to supplement grant funds received from the federal government) for the next ten years. In essence, the supplemental nutrition program is already paid for. Only if it were shown that the program did not make any difference would the county supervisors be inclined to take the politically unattractive steps necessary to disband it. The program essentially costs less money at this stage than no program.

Under these circumstances, the public health nurse would be most concerned about not making the type II error, the error of accepting H0 when it is false, or in terms of the program, the error of assuming that it had no effect when it actually did. If this were the case, the nurse—given that she is constrained to a sample of five hundred—might consciously set alpha large enough so that the probability of the type II error—beta—would be .05, even if this means that alpha must be larger than .05. If the nurse set beta for H0: h = 48 and H1: h = 49 to .05, the result would be as that shown in Figure 7.13. As Figure 7.13 shows, the area of

FIGURE 7.13. LOW BETA VALUE.

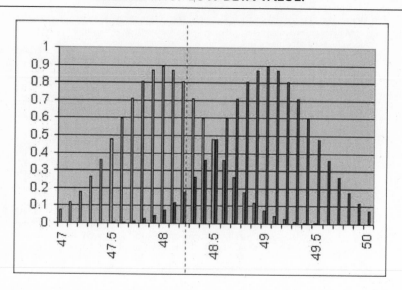

acceptance of H0 has now been moved down to about 48.25 inches. Any sample value larger than that will be assumed to have come from a population in which the true mean value is forty-nine inches, and the supplemental nutrition program will be deemed to have had an effect by its having increased the height of six-year-old boys. In this case, it is alpha that is large, being about .4, whereas beta is about .05.

Although the logic discussed here might be reasonable, it is, in fact, rarely the case that a researcher would be willing to accept a value of alpha as high as .4. Occasionally, alpha might be set as high as .1, or even .15. But higher levels of alpha, even to reduce beta in situations such as those previously described, would be very unlikely.

Exercises for Section 7.4

1. What is a type I error?
2. What is a type II error?
3. What is the meaning of alpha (α) and of beta (β).
4. Consider the hypothesis about adult men: H0: Diastolic BP = 86 and H1: Diastolic BP $\neq$ 86, to be tested at the 95 percent level of confidence.
   a. Is alpha known in principle? If yes, can its value be stated from the information given? If yes, what is alpha?

b. Is beta known in principle? If yes, can its value be stated from the information given? If yes, what is beta?

5. Consider the hypothesis: H0: average age at first birth for mothers in the United States is 23.7 years, and H1: average age for mothers in the United States is twenty-one years, to be tested at the 99 percent level of confidence.
   a. Is alpha known in principle? If yes, can its value be stated from the information given? If yes, what is alpha?
   b. Is beta known in principle? If yes, can its value be stated from the information given? If yes, what is beta?

6. Consider the hypothesis: H0: average cost per stay in a large hospital is $6,200, and H1: average cost per stay is $5,600, to be tested at the 95 percent level of confidence. A sample of 120 records has been selected and assessed for cost. The standard deviation of the costs is $3,100.
   a. Is alpha known in principle? If yes, can its value be stated from the information given? If yes, what is alpha?
   b. Is beta known in principle? If yes, can its value be stated from the information given? If yes, what is beta?

7. Consider the hypothesis: H0: the average number of prenatal visits among women to county health department prenatal clinics in a state is seven, and H1: the average number of prenatal visits is 5.5, to be tested at the 95 percent confidence level. A sample of records of seventy-five women with completed pregnancies has been randomly selected from among all those women coming to the health department clinics, and a standard deviation of 2.5 visits was found.
   a. Is alpha known in principle? If yes, can its value be stated from the information given? If yes, what is alpha?
   b. Is beta known in principle? If yes, can its value be stated from the information given? If yes, what is beta?

8. Consider the hypothesis: H0: the proportion of nonemergency visits at an emergency room facility is .35, and H1: the proportion of nonemergency visits is .45, to be tested at the 95 percent confidence level. The sample that will be used to test this will be a random sample of eighty records from all emergency room records for the past three years.
   a. Is alpha known in principle? If yes, can its value be stated from the information given? If yes, what is alpha?
   b. Is beta known in principle? If yes, can its value be stated from the information given? If yes, what is beta?

Section 7.5 Selecting Sample Sizes

In dealing with confidence limits and type I and type II error, the issue of sample size has come up several times. In particular, it was noted that in order for the public health nurse to be able to distinguish between H0 = 48 and H1 = 49, she would have to have a sample of 1,150 six-year-old boys. How was that number derived? If you recall the formula in Equation 7.1, 95 percent confidence limits are set by multiplying the t value for 95 percent (approximately 2) by the standard error of the mean. This value is then added or subtracted from the mean to get the upper or lower limits of the confidence interval. What can be effectively varied in this formulation is the size of the standard error. As the sample size increases, the standard error will decrease, because it is the standard deviation divided by the square root of the sample size. Let us see what this means in regard to the confidence limits for a sample of six-year-old boys.

We have said that the standard deviation of the height of six-year-old boys is ten inches. Given that standard deviation, we can calculate the standard error for any given sample size. Knowing the standard error, we can calculate the size of the interval on either side of the sample mean value that will include the true population mean in 95 percent of all the samples. This is essentially the confidence interval; but for simplification of what will be said later, half of the confidence interval will be called the measurement error and it will be designated (ME). (ME) is defined as shown in Equation 7.3. As you can see, Equation 7.3 is just Equation 7.1 with the mean removed. It represents half of the total 95 percent confidence interval. In no case should (ME) be confused with the standard error.

$$(ME) = t \times S.E._{\bar{x}} \tag{7.3}$$

Figure 7.14 shows the effect of sample size on the standard error, the measurement error (ME), and the upper 95 percent limit for a mean of forty-eight

FIGURE 7.14. EFFECT OF SAMPLE SIZE ON STANDARD ERROR AND MEASUREMENT ERROR.

	C2		= =$A$2/SQRT(B2)		
	A	B	C	D	E
1	StDev	Sample	StError	ME	Upper 48
2	10	100	1.000	2.000	50.000
3		500	0.447	0.894	48.894
4		1150	0.295	0.590	48.590

inches, assuming a two-tail test (that is, t in either Equation 7.1 or Equation 7.3 is 2; if a one-tail test were assumed, t would have to be approximately 1.7). For a sample of size 100, the standard error is 1 and (ME) is 2. For a sample of 500, the standard error is .447 and (ME) is .894. For 1,150, the standard error is .295 and (ME) is .590. Although it is not necessarily immediately obvious from Figure 7.14, the size of both the standard error and (ME) decrease as the square root of the increase in sample size. For example, 1,150 is 11.5 times larger than 100. The standard error for a sample of 1,150, .295, is 3.39 times smaller than the standard error for a sample of 100, or 1. The square root of 11.5 is 3.39. This is a general result. The size of the standard error, and hence the size of ME, decreases as the square root of the increase in sample size. So if sample size doubles, for example, (ME) decreases by 1.44. If sample size increases by a factor of 9, (ME) decreases by a factor of 3.

So if you know the standard deviation, you can set the standard error, and thus the confidence interval, virtually anywhere you like, as long as you have the resources required for the sample size needed. The actual formula for determining the sample size, given knowledge of the standard deviation and a good idea of how large (ME) should be, is given in Equation 7.4. This equation says that the sample size n is equal to the square of the value of t times the square of the standard deviation divided by the square of whatever the error of measurement; (ME) is expected to be.

$$n = \frac{t^2 s^2}{(ME)^2} \qquad\qquad (7.4)$$

Equation 7.4 would seem to have an intellectually soothing quality. If you know how much measurement error you can tolerate (for example, in the case of the public health nurse who wished to distinguish between an average height of forty-nine inches and an average height of forty-eight inches, measurement error required .5 inches), then you can set the sample size necessary for that error. Apart from the problem that the sample size set may be quite large and therefore quite expensive, there is another problem. This is the problem of knowledge of the variance (s^2) in Equation 7.4. In general, it is necessary to collect some data and calculate the variance before the variance is known. So, in order to determine how large a sample is required, it is already necessary to have some sample data. This is in the nature of a statistical catch-22.

There is one realm, however, in which the standard deviation can be known before any data are collected. The variance of a proportion can be calculated directly from the proportion as the square root of the proportion times 1 minus the proportion. So, for example, if you have some general knowledge of the size of a proportion to be estimated, it is possible to determine the sample size necessary to be within some specified measurement error by Equation 7.5.

$$n = \frac{t^2 p(1 - p)}{(ME)^2} \tag{7.5}$$

Exercises for Section 7.5

1. Calculate the approximate sample size required for each of the following at 95 percent confidence:
   a. Standard deviation = 10, (ME) = .5, two tail.
   b. Standard deviation = 10, (ME) = .5, one tail.
   c. Standard deviation = 10, (ME) = 1.5, two tail.
   d. Standard deviation = 10, (ME) = 1.5, one tail.
   e. Standard deviation = 35, (ME) = 5, two tail.
   f. Standard deviation = 35, (ME) = 5, one tail.
   g. Standard deviation = $3,200, (ME) = 400, two tail.
   h. Standard deviation = $3,200, (ME) = 400, one tail.

2. A hospital administrator wants to measure average cost per stay in his institution. He is willing to be within $200 of the true value with a probability of 95 percent. An initial investigation of a random sample of ten records determined that the standard deviation of cost was $3,987. How large a sample will need to be taken to meet the administrator's needs?

3. After learning of the size of sample needed in Exercise 2, the administrator decided that he would be willing to be within $500. How big a sample does he need to reach this level of error?

4. A state public health worker wants to determine the average number of visits to prenatal clinics expectant mothers are making to health department clinics in the state. She believes that the standard deviation of visits is three visits. On the basis of her belief, how large a sample must she have to test H0: visits = 7 against the alternative H1: visits = 6 with alpha = beta = .05?

5. The proportion of true emergencies coming to an emergency room is believed to be 60 percent. How large a sample of visits would the emergency room administrator have to take to confirm this 60 percent with a measurement error (ME) of .05?

CHAPTER EIGHT

STATISTICAL TESTS FOR CATEGORICAL DATA

As indicated elsewhere in this book, a major part of statistical analysis is to assess the independence of two or more variables. The t test assesses the independence of two variables, one measured on a numerical scale and the other measured on a categorical scale that takes only two values. ANOVA assesses the independence of two or more variables, one measured on a numerical scale and the others measured on categorical scales that may take on any number of values, although typically the number of values would be limited to fewer than five or six. Regression assesses the independence of two or more variables, all of which can be measured on a numerical scale. The chi-square statistic (χ^2) is a statistical analysis that can be used to establish the independence of two or more variables, each of which is measured on a categorical scale.

Section 8.1 Independence of Two Variables

Chapter Five introduced the subject of independence of two variables. In that chapter it was noted that independence could be thought of as mathematical independence or alternatively as statistical independence. This chapter takes up these two topics again, with a more detailed discussion of statistical independence, as a way of introducing the chi-square.

Mathematical Independence

The initial concept of mathematical independence has been discussed previously, in Chapter Five. But to reconsider that discussion here, suppose a hundred persons visited the emergency room in the community hospital over the past twenty-four-hour period. Thirty of those people came for true emergencies and seventy came for some condition that would not be considered a true emergency. Also, sixty of the people came during the day (say, from 6 A.M. to 6 P.M.), whereas the other forty came at night. The marginal values of this joint distribution are shown in Figure 8.1. Now if we had no other information about the people who came to the emergency room, how would we expect the people to be distributed in the four internal cells of the table—cells B2:C3? Or, from another perspective, what is the most likely distribution of people in those four cells? After a little thought, most people would conclude that the most likely distribution of people in the four cells—B2:C3-would be as shown in Figure 8.2. It is possible that some people might not even know immediately why they arrived at the frequency distribution shown in B2:C3. If questioned, however, they would probably come up with reasoning that involved the idea that, for example, total emergencies are 30 percent of all visits, so emergencies during the day should be 30 percent of all visits that occur during the day. Similarly, emergencies during the night should be 30 percent of all visits that occur during the night. Once either of those decisions is made, the rest of the cells are fixed by the marginal values.

FIGURE 8.1. MARGINAL FREQUENCIES.

	A	B	C	D
1		Day	Night	Total
2	Emergency			30
3	Other			70
4	Total	60	40	100
5				

FIGURE 8.2. MARGINAL FREQUENCIES WITH MOST PROBABLE INTERNAL FREQUENCIES.

	A	B	C	D
1		Day	Night	Total
2	Emergency	18	12	30
3	Other	42	28	70
4	Total	60	40	100
5				

When a person decides that the number of emergencies during the day should be eighteen, because eighteen is 30 percent of sixty, all other cells are fixed. If eighteen is assigned to the Day/Emergency cell, twelve must be assigned to the Night/Emergency cell, because the sum of the two cells must equal thirty. Similarly, if eighteen is assigned to the Day/Emergency cell, then forty-two must be assigned to the Day/Other cell, because the sum of the two cells must be sixty. The twenty-eight in Night/Other is fixed in the same way. Because a decision can be made about the number of observations in only one cell of the table, given the marginal totals, a two-by-two table has only one degree of freedom. In general, any $r \times c$ (rows $\times$ columns) table will have $(r - 1) \times (c - 1)$ degrees of freedom. In the table in Figure 8.2, there are two rows and two columns, thus $(r - 1) \times (c - 1)$ equals 1.

The distribution of observations shown in Figure 8.2 is one that is characterized by *mathematical independence*. Mathematical independence is defined as a situation in which the marginal probabilities in a table, such as that shown in Figure 8.2, are equal to the conditional probabilities. As we have seen in Chapter Five, marginal probabilities are just the probabilities associated with the frequency distribution of a single variable. The table in Figure 8.2 has two marginal probabilities, one for the distribution of coming during the day or night, and one for the distribution of coming for an emergency or for another reason. Again, as seen in Chapter Five, Conditional probabilities are the probability—for example, of coming for an emergency *on the condition* that the person came during the day—or during the night.

Figure 8.3 shows the marginal probabilities of coming for an emergency or coming for another reason as .3(30/100) and .7(70/100). Figure 8.3 also shows the conditional probabilities of coming for an emergency on the condition that (or given that) one came during the day—or during the night. For example, the conditional probability of coming for an emergency, given that one came during the day, is .3(18/60), whereas the conditional probability of coming for another reason during the day is .7(42/60). If we designate the marginal probability of coming for an emergency as $p(E)$ and the conditional probability of coming for

FIGURE 8.3. MARGINAL AND CONDITIONAL PROBABILITIES.

	A	B	C	D
6		Day	Night	Total
7	Emergency	0.3	0.3	0.3
8	Other	0.7	0.7	0.7
9	Total	60	40	100
10				

an emergency, given that one came during the day, as $p(E|D)$, then mathematical independence is defined as $p(E) = p(E|D)$. Since the table shown in Figure 8.2 and Figure 8.3 has only one degree of freedom, finding that any one of the conditional probabilities in the table equals any one of the marginal probabilities is equivalent to finding all conditional probabilities equivalent to all corresponding marginal probabilities.

It should be clear that this has examined conditional and marginal probabilities in only one direction—by columns. We could equally well have looked at the marginal probability of coming during the day $p(D)$ or during the night $p(N)$. For the table in Figure 8.2, we would have found that, for example, the probability of coming during the day $p(D)$ is exactly equal to the probability of coming during the day, given that one came for an emergency $p(D|E)$. In most cases, though, it is conventional to examine conditional probabilities by columns rather than by rows.

As indicated here, the definition of mathematical independence for two categorical variables is that the marginal and corresponding conditional probabilities are equal. For a two-by-two table, it is necessary only to examine one conditional probability to make this determination. In a larger table, however, it may be necessary to examine more than one conditional probability to ensure mathematical independence. In general, it will be necessary to look at as many conditional probabilities as there are degrees of freedom in the table before declaring mathematical independence.

Statistical Independence of Two Variables

Before proceeding to discuss statistical independence of two variables, it is important to be sure that what was discussed in the first subsection of Section 8.1 is fully understood. Mathematical independence means that there is no relationship between the time of day (or night) that people arrive at the emergency clinic and whether they come for an emergency or not. Considered another way, knowing if a person arrived during the day or during the night does not improve any prediction of whether they came for an emergency or not.

But consider now that the data examined in the first subsection of Section 8.1 were for only a hundred emergency room visits, perhaps chosen at random, or perhaps representing a single day's visits or several day's visits. But even if time of day is mathematically independent of arrival for an emergency, we might not always find the results we did. If we had examined a different sample, a larger or smaller sample, for example, or one taken at a somewhat different time, we might have found that the conditional and marginal frequencies were very close but were not exact matches. What, then, might we conclude?

FIGURE 8.4. DIFFERENT CONDITIONAL PROBABILITIES.

	A	B	C	D
1	*Frequencies*	Day	Night	Total
2	Emergency	17	13	30
3	Other	43	27	70
4	Total	60	40	100
5				
6	*Probabilities*	Day	Night	Total
7	Emergency	0.283	0.325	0.3
8	Other	0.717	0.675	0.7
9	Total	60	40	100
10				

Let us posit that the data in Figure 8.4 represents a sample of a hundred emergency room visits taken from among those visits that occurred in the month following the one in which the data in Figure 8.2 were taken. Cells A1:D4 give the actual frequencies for the hundred visits, which are divided, as before, into thirty visits for emergencies and seventy for other reasons, with sixty visits occurring during the day and forty visits occurring at night. Cells A6:D9 show the conditional and marginal probabilities by columns. Now, the conditional probability, for example, of coming for an emergency, given that one came during the day $(p(E|D) = .283)$, is not exactly the same as the marginal probability of coming during the day $(p(D) = .3)$. So one might conclude that the two variables are no longer independent mathematically, but are they close enough to be considered independent *statistically*, and what might that mean?

Statistically, if we took many samples of size 100 of people who came to an emergency room, we would expect that the conditional probabilities would not match exactly the marginal probabilities for every sample. This would be true even if the variables, time of arrival, and arrival for an emergency were truly mathematically independent of one another. So we would like to have a statistical test to determine whether the two variables can be considered statistically independent of one another, even if they cannot be considered strictly mathematically independent for every sample we may examine. The test of statistical independence is the chi-square, or χ^2 test.

The chi-square test is a test of independence between two variables. It is calculated as given in Equation 8.1. In Equation 8.1, r is the number of rows in the table and c is the number of columns. O is the observed frequency in each cell and E is the expected frequency in the cell. The squared difference between each observed frequency and each expected frequency is divided by the expected frequency. These values are then summed across all r × c cells in the table. The result is the chi-square value. If the chi-square value is greater than some predetermined value, the two variables will be considered statistically independent.

$$\chi^2 = \sum_{i=1}^{rc} \frac{(O_i - E_i)^2}{E_i} \tag{8.1}$$

Consider the data shown in cells B2:C3 in Figure 8.4 as the observed values. Based on the conditional probabilities shown in cells B7:C8, we know that the two variables shown in that table are not mathematically independent. But if we calculate the chi-square, will they be found to be statistically independent? To determine this, we need to know the expected values. But what are the expected values? It turns out that the expected values are the values we would expect to get if the marginal probabilities and the conditional probabilities are the same, or what we decided should be the values in cells B2:C3 in Figure 8.2, based on the distributions of the marginal values. Given these expected and marginal values, the calculation of the chi-square statistic for the data shown in cells B2:C3 in Figure 8.4 is as shown in Equation 8.2. The calculated chi-square value is .1984. The question then would be, what is the likelihood of finding a chi-square value that large if the null hypothesis that arriving for an emergency is independent of time of arrival is actually true?

$$\chi^2 = \frac{(17 - 18)^2}{18} + \frac{(13 - 12)^2}{12} + \frac{(43 - 42)^2}{42} + \frac{(27 - 28)^2}{28} = .1984 \tag{8.2}$$

The probability of a chi-square value as large as .1984, given that the null hypothesis of independence is true, is found with the =CHIDIST() function. The =CHIDIST() function takes two arguments: the value of the chi-square statistic and the number of degrees of freedom. The calculation of the =CHIDIST() function shown in Equation 8.3 is .656, which means that there is about a 66 percent probability of finding a chi-square value as large as .1984 under the null hypothesis that arrival for an emergency is independent of time of arrival. In general, we would reject the null hypothesis only if the probability of the chi-square value was less than .05; so, in this case, we would conclude that the observed frequencies in the cells B2:C3 in Figure 8.4 are not different enough from the expected frequencies that we would say that time of arrival and arrival for an emergency are *statistically independent* of one another.

$$p = \text{CHIDIST}(.1984,1) = .656 \tag{8.3}$$

But how large must a chi-square be before one can conclude that the two events are statistically independent? The value of the chi-square required, referred to as the critical value of the chi-square, can be found using the =CHIINV()

function. This function takes two arguments: the probability at which we will reject the null and the degrees of freedom. The critical value for the chi-square for a table with one degree of freedom (any table with two rows and two columns) is given in Equation 8.4. According to that equation, it is necessary to have a chi-square value of at least 3.84 before the null hypothesis of statistical independence is rejected at the 95 percent level of confidence.

$$\text{Chi-square} | \text{crit} = \text{CHIINV}(.05,1) = 3.84 \tag{8.4}$$

What kind of difference would be necessary between observed and expected values in the table in Figure 8.4 before the critical value of chi-square would be reached? Figure 8.5 shows a template for the calculation of chi-square as well as one of the smallest differences in the distribution of observed versus expected values that result in a chi-square that exceeds the critical value. Figure 8.5 deserves substantial explanation.

First, consider cell B2 of Figure 8.5. The value of 13 in the cell (thirteen people came for emergencies during the day) is the closest value to the expected (shown in cell B7) that can appear in that cell and produce a chi-square greater

FIGURE 8.5. TEMPLATE FOR THE CHI-SQUARE.

B7	▼	=	=B$4*$D2/$D$4		
A	**B**	**C**	**D**	**E**	**F**
1 Observed	Day	Night	Total		
2 Emergency	13	17	30		
3 Other	47	23	70		
4 Total	60	40	100		
5					
6 Expected	Day	Night	Total		
7 Emergency	18	12	30		
8 Other	42	28	70		
9 Total	60	40	100		
10					
11 Chi-square	Day	Night	Total		
12 Emergency	1.388889	2.083333	30	Chi-square	4.960317
13 Other	0.595238	0.892857	70	Prob	0.025935
14 Total	60	40	100	Crit	3.841455
15					
16 Probabilities	Day	Night	Total		
17 Emergency	0.217	0.425	0.3		
18 Other	0.783	0.575	0.7		
19 Total	60	40	100		
20					

than the critical value. Because there is one degree of freedom in this example, 13 in cell B2 fixes all three other cells in B2:C3, given the marginal values in column D and row 4. The expected values for the given marginal values (cells B7:C8) are shown in Figure 8.2, but here, a simple way of calculating those expected values is given. The formula for cell B7 is shown on the formula line above the spreadsheet. The formula uses the $ convention to fix appropriate rows and columns so that it can be copied to all four cells in which expected values are desired. To explain the formula, B$4 fixes the first term in row 4, which allows the formula to be moved to cell B8 without changing the reference to cell B4. $D5 fixes the second term in the equation in column D so that it is possible to move the equation to cell C7 without changing the reference to cell D2. Finally, $D$4 fixes the cell D4 so that it is possible to move the equation to any of the cells without changing the reference to cell D4. With this formula in B7, it is possible to click on the lower right corner of the cell and drag the formula across to cell C7, and then to drag both cells down to row 8. This produces the expected values for the marginal values observed.

The values shown in cells B12:C13 are the calculations of the chi-square statistic. Each cell represents one of the calculations—$(O - E)^2/E$, shown in Equation 8.1. The chi-square value itself is shown in cell F12 and is the sum of the cells B12:C13. The probability of the chi-square value is shown in F13 as .0259. Since this value is less than .05, we would reject the null hypothesis that the two variables—arrival for an emergency and time of arrival—are independent of one another.

The last table in Figure 8.5 shows the conditional probabilities of reason for arrival, given arrival during the day or during the night. These conditional probabilities show that about 22 percent of the people arriving during the day came for an emergency, whereas about 43 percent of those coming at night came for an emergency. In general, one of the best ways to interpret the results of a chi-square applied to any contingency table is to form the conditional probabilities by columns and interpret them by comparing rows. So the comparison of the conditional probabilities for those who came for an emergency during the day or during the night gives a succinct way of describing the differences in the observed values that produce the chi-square value large enough to reject the null hypothesis of independence.

Using the =CHITEST( ) Function

Excel does not include a Tools/Data Analysis add-in to do the chi-square test, but it does include a function that will carry out the chi-square analysis. This function is =CHITEST(). The =CHITEST() function takes two separate arguments: the range represented by the observed data and the range represented by the expected

FIGURE 8.6. THE =CHITEST( ) FUNCTION.

	D11	▼	=	=CHITEST(B2:C3,B7:C8)	
	A	B	C	D	E
1	Observed	Day	Night	Total	
2	Emergenc	13	17	30	
3	Other	47	23	70	
4	Total	60	40	100	
5					
6	Expected	Day	Night	Total	
7	Emergenc	18	12	30	
8	Other	42	28	70	
9	Total	60	40	100	
10					
11			CHITEST	0.025935	
12			Chi Square	4.960316	

data. The table in Figure 8.6 reproduces the observed and expected frequencies from Figure 8.5, but it now shows the calculation of the =CHITEST() function, in cell D11. The formula line in Figure 8.6 shows the two range—B2:C3 and B7:C8, which are included as arguments of the =CHITEST() function. The =CHITEST() function produces not the chi-square value but the probability of finding that value, given the null hypothesis of independence. The actual chi-square value can be reproduced by using the =CHIINV() function with the value of the probability and one degree of freedom. This reproduced chi-square value is shown in cell D12. The =CHIINV() function will not always reproduce the chi-square value, however. If the probability of the chi-square is less than 3.0E-7, the =CHIINV() function returns #NUM!.

The Chi-Square and Type I and Type II Errors

Chapter Seven introduced the notion of type I and type II errors with regard to the t distribution. A few comments should be made about type I and type II errors with regard to the chi-square distribution. The chi-square distribution is not a "normal" distribution as the t distribution is, in the sense that it is symmetrical about some mean value. In fact, the chi-square distribution tends to be heavily skewed to the right. Figure 8.7 shows the chi-square distribution with one degree of freedom. This is the most extremely skewed chi-square distribution. As degrees of freedom increase, the distribution begins to take on a less skewed

FIGURE 8.7. THE CHI-SQUARE DISTRIBUTION FOR ONE DEGREE OF FREEDOM.

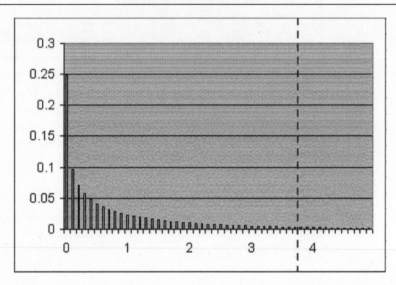

appearance, and if the degrees of freedom increase to forty or fifty, the distribution begins to look more and more normal. But most chi-square applications, particularly in regard to contingency tables, are limited to degrees of freedom in the range 1 (a two-by-two table) to less than 10 or 12 (a four-by-five table).

With one degree of freedom, the point in the distribution at which the null hypothesis of no relationship between two variables (as previously discussed) would be rejected at alpha = .05 would be at approximately 3.8 (as shown by the vertical dashed line in the figure). Any chi-square value that resulted in a probability to the right of the dashed line (that is, any value greater than 3.8) would be expected to occur less than 5 percent of the time when the null hypothesis is true. Thus, any value in that range would lead to the rejection of H0 (no relationship between or independence of the two variables) and the acceptance of the alternative—that the two variables are not independent. The area to the right of the dashed line, then, which is usually set at .05, is the area of type I error, or alpha.

Let us consider type I error in another way. In the example analysis shown in Figure 8.5, the expected joint probability 'and' for Day and Emergency is 18/100, or .18. Since the other probabilities in the table are fixed by .18, given the marginal values (the table has one degree of freedom), the expected probabilities for the other three cells are .12 for Night and Emergency, .42 for Day and Other, and .28 for Night and Other. If we were to generate many samples—say, a thousand samples of size 100—from a population in which these proportions were true, the distribution of chi-square values for these samples would be such that approximately 5 percent (about fifty out of the thousand) would have chi-square values that exceeded 3.8. So even though the null hypothesis of independence would be true, there would be some proportion of the samples for which we would reject H0.

But what now of beta or the type II error? How can we conceive of the type II error with this same example? To see this, consider the possibility that the true proportion of Day and Emergency visits is not .18 but .15 in the larger population (the other proportions change at the same time). If we again took many samples (a thousand samples of size 100) from a population in which the true proportion of Day and Emergency was .15, we would discover that about 70 percent of these samples had values of the chi-square that did not exceed 3.8 (the .05 level of significance). Thus, in the case of a true proportion for Day and Emergency of .15, we have about a 70 percent chance of making the type II error (accepting the null hypothesis of independence, or Day and Emergency equals .18) when it is false. What of an even greater variation from ,18? Suppose the actual probability of Day and Emergency in the population was .11. Do we now have any chance of making the type II error? The answer is yes. If we took many samples (a thousand samples of size 100) from a population in which the true proportion of Day and Emergency was .11, we would discover that about 10 percent of those samples would have values less than 3.8; so, in this case, we would have about a 10 percent chance of making the type II error.

As with the type II error associated with a normal or t distribution, we can reduce the type II error associated with the chi-square by increasing the sample size. If we were to take a large number of samples of a larger size (a thousand samples of size 200) from a population in which the true proportion of Day and Emergency was .15, we would discover that only about 50 percent of the samples would lead us to falsely accept H0 (type II error), whereas the other 50 percent would lead us correctly to reject H0. The larger the sample we take, the lower the level of beta will be for any given divergence of the true value from that hypothesized by H0.

Exercises for Section 8.1

1. Calculate expected values for the following two-by-two tables:

    a.

		25
		42
34	33	67

b.

		125
		230
200	155	355

c.

		33
		230
200	63	263

2. Calculate chi-square values for the following tables:

a.

18	7	25
16	26	42
34	33	67

b.

47	78	125
153	77	230
200	155	355

c.

21	12	33
179	51	230
200	63	263

3. Determine whether you would accept or reject the hypothesis of independence for the two variables in each of the tables in a, b, and c of Exercise 2.

4. Calculate conditional and marginal probabilities for the cross tabulations in a, b, and c of Exercise 2 and give them an interpretation.

Section 8.2 Examples of Chi-Square Analyses

Thus far the discussion has focused solely on contingency tables with one degree of freedom (two-by-two tables). This section will consider several examples of chi-square calculations taken from examples that have appeared in various journals and includes not only further discussion of two-by-two contingency tables, but of larger contingency tables as well.

An Example of a Two-by-Two Table

To better understand the chi-square test and its interpretation, consider the example shown in Figure 8.8. That figure shows data taken from an article by

FIGURE 8.8. EXAMPLE FROM THE LITERATURE.

	A	B	C	D	E	F	
1	*Observed*	Male	Female				
2	Violence	1130	1239	2369			
3	No Violence	2275	2849	5124			
4		3405	4088	7493			
5							
6	*Expected*	Male	Female				
7	Violence	1076.531	1292.469	2369			
8	No Violence	2328.469	2795.531	5124			
9		3405	4088	7493			
10							
11	*Chi-Square*	Male	Female				
12	Violence	2.655715	2.212014	2369	Chi-Square	7.118246	
13	No Violence	1.227828	1.022689	5124	Prob	0.00763	
14		3405	4088	7493	Crit	3.841455	
15							
16							
17	*Probabilities*	Male	Female				
18	Violence	33%	30%	32%			
19	No Violence	67%	70%	68%			
20		100%	100%	100%			

Halpern and others (2001), and the data shown in the table were taken from the second table in the article (p. 1682). The data shown in Figure 8.8 address the question of whether an adolescent's having experienced either physical or psychological violence from a partner in an opposite-sex romantic relationship is independent of whether the respondent is male or female. The implied null hypothesis is independence; the implied alternative is nonindependence.

Cells A1:D4 show the observed cell values and marginal values. Cells A6:D9 show the expected values based on the calculations shown in cell B7 in Figure 8.6. Cells A11:D14 show the calculation of the chi-square values for each cell and cell F12 shows the total chi-square value. The probability of this chi-square value under the null hypothesis of independence is shown in F13 as .0076. Because this value is less than .05, we reject the null hypothesis of independence and conclude that experiencing violence is not independent of sex.

Saying that experiencing violence is not independent of sex implies that either male adolescents or female adolescents are more likely than the other gender to experience violence when in an opposite-sex romantic relationship. But by looking at the observed values in A1:D4, it is difficult to tell which sex is more likely to experience such violence. In consequence, the easiest way to interpret the results of a chi-square test is by looking at the conditional probabilities of experiencing violence, given that the respondent was male or given that the respondent was female. Cells A17:D20 show the conditional probabilities of having experienced violence, given sexual identity. Perhaps somewhat surprisingly, 33 percent of males said that they had experienced violence, whereas 30 percent of females said the same. These percentage differences are not large, but the fact that there are 7,493 respondents in the study gives this relatively small percentage difference statistical significance.

Having seen the results from Figure 8.8, it is useful to say a few words about the difference between statistical significance and practical significance. The notion of statistical significance is associated with the rejection of the null hypothesis, whether that hypothesis is explicit or implied. So, in the case of the data examined in Figure 8.8, statistical significance refers to the fact that the chi-square value is large enough to reject the null hypothesis. But practical significance refers to the importance of a result found in a statistical test. Because the number of respondents is relatively large, as shown in Figure 8.8, a relatively small percentage difference results in statistical significance. Whether this relatively small percentage difference has practical significance or not is not a question that can be addressed by statistics. It is only a question that can be addressed by knowledge of the subject, experience, and understanding. Consequently, statistics can address statistical questions, but the value placed on the results of statistical analysis remains with the observer who must assess the importance of these results.

An Example of *n* by Two and Two by *n* Tables from the Literature

The extension of the chi-square statistic to tables with more than four cells is direct. The original data reported in the article referenced for Figure 8.8 were presented for the experiencing of physical violence, psychological violence, or no violence. The tables in Figure 8.9 show the data in both categories of violence or no violence. Cells A1:D5 are the observed values for the data, whereas cells A7:D11 are the expected values. Again, the expected values are calculated by multiplying the row total for each cell times the column total for the cell and dividing by the grand total. The formula used and replicated by dragging to each cell, B8:C10, is shown in the formula bar in Figure 8.9. The cells B14:C16 are the chi-square values for each individual cell, and the overall chi-square value is shown in F14. The probability of the chi-square value in F14, under the implied null hypothesis of independence, is given in F15. The value in F15 is now determined

FIGURE 8.9. AN *n*-BY-2 CHI-SQUARE.

B8		=	=B$5*$D2/$D$5		
	A	B	C	D	E	F
1	*Observed*	Male	Female			
2	Psychological	708	742	1450		
3	Physical	422	497	919		
4	No Violence	2275	2849	5124		
5		3405	4088	7493		
6						
7	*Expected*	Male	Female			
8	Psychological	658.91	791.09	1450		
9	Physical	417.62	501.38	919		
10	No Violence	2328.47	2795.53	5124		
11		3405	4088	7493		
12						
13	*Chi square*	Male	Female			
14	Psychological	3.6565	3.0456	1450	Chi-Square	9.0370
15	Physical	0.0460	0.0383	919	Prob	0.010905
16	No Violence	1.2278	1.0227	5124	Crit	5.991476
17		3405	4088	7493		
18						
19	*Probabilities*	Male	Female			
20	Psychological	21%	18%	19%		
21	Physical	12%	12%	12%		
22	No Violence	67%	70%	68%		
23		100%	100%	100%		

with =CHIDIST() with two degrees of freedom. The critical value for a chi-square with two degrees of freedom is given in F16.

Notice that the critical value is 5.99, which is very close to six. The data being analyzed in Figure 8.9 are presented in a three-by-two table, which results in six internal cells in the tables. The data analyzed in Figure 8.8 were in a two-by-two table. A two-by-two table has four cells and the critical value was 3.8. A three by two table has six cells and the critical value is about 6. In general, one can be fairly certain that if the chi-square value is as large as the number of cells in a table, it is likely that the null hypothesis of independence will be rejected at the .05 level.

Again, the question of how the interpretation of the data is to be made arises. The interpretation is best based on the conditional probabilities of experiencing different types of violence or no violence, given that the recipient is male or female. Cells B20:C22 shows these differences. The major difference in the experiencing of violence between males and females is that 21 percent of males reported experiencing psychological violence, whereas 18 percent of females reported such violence. There is no difference in the percentages for physical violence.

An example of a 2-by-n variable is also available from the literature. The data in Figure 8.10 came from a study of 3,158 women in the Sudan with at least one child that was reported in Studies in Family Planning. The women were asked if they wanted another child, and their answers were tabulated with the number of children they currently had in categories from 1 to 5 and 6 or more. The observed

FIGURE 8.10. NUMBER OF CHILDREN AND DESIRE FOR MORE.

B7		= =B$4*$H2/$H$4									
	A	B	C	D	E	F	G	H	I	J	K
1	Observed	1 Child	2	3	4	5	6+	Total			
2	Want More	512	426	398	320	233	482	2371			
3	Do not want more	21	37	54	104	114	457	787			
4	Total	533	463	452	424	347	939	3158			
5											
6	Expected	1 Child	2	3	4	5	6+	Total			
7	Want More	400.172	347.617	339.358	318.336	260.525	704.993	2371			
8	Do not want more	132.828	115.383	112.642	105.664	86.4753	234.007	787			
9	Total	533	463	452	424	347	939	3158			
10											
11	Chi square	1 Child	2	3	4	5	6+	Total			
12	Want More	31.2504	17.6746	10.1336	0.0087	2.90801	70.534	2371	Chi-Square	531.7207	
13	Do not want more	94.1481	53.2483	30.5295	0.02622	8.76099	212.498	787	Prob	1.1E-112	
14	Total	533	463	452	424	347	939	3158	Crit	11.07048	
15											
16	Probabilities	1 Child	2	3	4	5	6+	Total			
17	Want More	96%	92%	88%	75%	67%	51%	75%			
18	Do not want more	4%	8%	12%	25%	33%	49%	25%			
19	Total	100%	100%	100%	100%	100%	100%	100%			

frequencies are given in cells A1:H4. The expected frequencies are given in A6:H9 with the formula for the calculation of expected frequencies shown for cell B7 in the formula line at the top of the figure. The chi-square values for the individual cells are shown in A11:H14 and the overall chi-square, 531.72, is given in J12. The probability of the chi-square is given in J13. You should recognize that the chi-square value in this case is very large and the probability is very small. Because the number of cells in the table is 12, the critical value of the chi-square is about 12 (actually 11.07). Any value of the chi-square larger than this would lead us to reject the implied null hypothesis of independence between the number of children and the desire for an additional child. In short, we reject that implied null.

The conditional probabilities of wanting an additional child, given the number of children a woman already has, are shown in A16:H19. Ninety-six percent of women with only one child want an additional child. Only 51 percent of women with six or more children want an additional child. Between these two extremes there is a monotonic decrease in the percentage of women who want another child. The conclusion is quite clear. Among these women from the Sudan, the more children a woman has, the less likely she is to desire an additional child. Although this is not unexpected, the data from this study confirm the expectation.

An *n*-by-*n* Example from the Literature

The extension of the chi-square statistic from *n*-by-2 or 2-by-*n* to *n*-by-*n* tables is also direct. Consider, for example, the data shown in Figure 8.11. These data represent the results of a study carried out by Brook and Appel (1973) on the assessment of the quality of medical care. Each of three physicians reviewed 296 case records for patients who had been treated for urinary tract infection (UTI), hypertension (Hyper), or ulcer. The treatment of the case was judged adequate or inadequate by each of the three physicians. On the adequacy dimension the data are displayed in three categories, judged adequate by two or three physicians (Adequate by 2+), judged adequate by one (Adequate by 1), or judged adequate by none (Adequate by 0).

The cells A1:E5 show the observed data for the 269 cases. The cells A6:E11 show the expected values for each of the cells by the convention—column total * row total/grand total. The chi-square calculations for each individual cell are shown in A13:E17 and the overall chi-square value of 19.49 is shown in G14. The actual probability of obtaining a chi-square value that large under the null hypothesis that adequacy of treatment is independent of diagnosis is given in G15 as .0006, or six times out of ten thousand. Because the probability is so small, we conclude that we must reject the null hypothesis, which is equivalent to saying that judged adequacy of treatment depends on the initial diagnosis.

FIGURE 8.11. ADEQUACY OF TREATMENT OF THREE CONDITIONS.

	B14 ▼	= =(B2-B8)^2/B8				
	A	B	C	D	E	F	G
1	*Observed*	UTI	Hyper	Ulcer	Total		
2	Adequate by 2+	13	31	25	69		
3	Adequate by 1	17	29	12	58		
4	Adequate by 0	77	54	38	169		
5		107	114	75	296		
6							
7	*Expected*	UTI	Hyper	Ulcer	Total		
8	Adequate by 2+	24.943	26.574	17.483	69		
9	Adequate by 1	20.966	22.338	14.696	58		
10	Adequate by 0	61.091	65.088	42.821	169		
11		107	114	75	296		
12							
13	*Chi-square*	UTI	Hyper	Ulcer	Total		
14	Adequate by 2+	5.718133	0.73705	3.2319		69	Chi-Squa	19.49331
15	Adequate by 1	0.750296	1.986961	0.494567		58	Prob	0.000629
16	Adequate by 0	4.142812	1.888834	0.542761		169	Crit	9.487728
17		107	114	75	296		
18							
19	*Probabilities*	UTI	Hyper	Ulcer	Total		
20	Adequate by 2+	12%	27%	33%	23%		
21	Adequate by 1	16%	25%	16%	20%		
22	Adequate by 0	72%	47%	51%	57%		
23		100%	100%	100%	100%		

To see which diagnosis is more likely to be judged to be treated adequately, it is useful to form the table of conditional probabilities shown in A19:E23. Here it can be seen that 12 percent of UTI cases are judged adequately treated by two or three physicians, whereas 27 and 33 percent of hypertension and ulcer are similarly judged. However, 72 percent of UTI cases are judged adequately treated by not a single one of the three physicians. Clearly, the dependence between judgement of adequacy and diagnosis rests primarily in the difference between UTI cases and the other two.

Exercises for Section 8.2

1. Use the data on worksheet Violence 1 of Chpt 8–1.xls to replicate the analysis given in Figure 8.8.
2. The data on the SWC worksheet of Chpt 8–1.xls show the countries of the World, with the countries of Africa indicated as 1 on the variable Africa, and

countries with under-five mortality less than 100 indicated by 1 on the variable Child Friendly.

   a. Use the Pivot Table capability of Excel and the chi-square to test the hypothesis of independence between being a country in Africa and being child friendly.

   b. Use conditional probabilities to provide an interpretation of the result.

3. The data on the Hospital Stay worksheet of Chpt 8–1.xls show a sample of a hundred hospital stays by Sex and length of stay. Stays longer than three days are coded Long (Stay) and those three days or less are coded Short.

   a. Use the Pivot Table capability of Excel and the chi-square to test the hypothesis of independence between Sex and Stay as coded long or short.

   b. Use conditional probabilities to provide an interpretation of the results.

4. Use the data on worksheet Violence 2 of Chpt 8–1.xls to replicate the analysis given in Figure 8.9.

5. The DRG worksheet of Chpt 8–1.xls shows Sex and four DRG categories (DRG Categ) for three hundred hospital admissions.

   a. Use the Pivot Table capability of Excel and the chi-square to test the hypothesis of independence between Sex and DRG category as coded in four categories.

   b. Use conditional probabilities to provide an interpretation of the results.

6. Use the data on worksheet Adequacy to replicate the analysis given in Figure 8.11.

7. The Late Delivery worksheet of Chpt 8–1.xls shows the reason for late delivery of the noon meal in three wards of a hospital to be problems with personnel, the facility, or the patient.

   a. Use the Pivot Table capability of Excel and the chi-square to test the hypothesis of independence between Ward and the reason for lateness.

   b. Use conditional probabilities to provide an interpretation of the results.

Section 8.3 Small Expected Values in Cells

The use of the chi-square statistic assumes relatively little about the data. There is no underlying assumption, for example, that the data need be normally distributed. Any data in a contingency table will be acceptable. There is one limitation, however, about the magnitude of the expected value in any cell in the contingency table. In general, small expected values in any table cell tends to inflate the value of the chi-square and increase the likelihood of rejecting the null when it should not be rejected. There are several ways of dealing with this possibility, and these alternatives depend, in part, on the number of cells in a table.

Small Expected Values When $df = 1$

If the expected value in any cell of a two-by-two table is less than about 10, one way of dealing with the small expected values is to apply what is known as Yates's correction. Yates's correction is applied using the formula shown in Equation 8.5. The formula in Equation 8.5 indicates that the *absolute value* of the difference between the observed and expected frequencies is reduced by .5 before the value is squared. To see how the application of this equation works, consider the example shown in Figure 8.12.

$$\chi^2 = \sum_{i=1}^{rc} \frac{(|O_i - E_i| - .5)^2}{E_i} \tag{8.5}$$

Figure 8.12 shows data comparable to that in Figure 8.2. Except in the case of Figure 8.12, there are only fifty observations rather than a hundred. The

FIGURE 8.12. YATES'S CORRECTION.

B12		=	=(ABS(B2-B7)-0.5)^2/B7		
A	**B**	**C**	**D**	**E**	**F**
1 **Observed**	Day	Night	Total		
2 **Emergency**	5	10	15		
3 **Other**	25	10	35		
4 **Total**	30	20	50		
5					
6 *Expected*	Day	Night	Total		
7 **Emergency**	9	6	15		
8 **Other**	21	14	35		
9 **Total**	30	20	50		
10					
11 *Yates'*	Day	Night	Total		
12 **Emergency**	1.361111	2.041667	15	Chi-square	4.861111
13 **Other**	0.583333	0.875	35	Prob	0.027469
14 **Total**	30	20	50	Crit	3.841455
15					
16 *Standard*	Day	Night	Total		
17 **Emergency**	1.777778	2.666667	15	Chi-square	6.349206
18 **Other**	0.761905	1.142857	35	Prob	0.011743
19 **Total**	30	20	50	Crit	3.841455
20					

consequence of this difference, given the same marginal probabilities, is that the expected values for cells B7 and C7 are less than 10. In this case, the chi-square formula given in Equation 8.1 is not strictly appropriate, because it produces a chi-square value larger than it should be. For the observed data seen in cells A1:D4, the chi-square using the Yates's correction (Equation 8.5) is shown in cells A11:F14. The comparison chi-square using the standard formula (Equation 8.1) is shown in cells A16:F19. Although the decision one would reach does not differ in either of these computations, it can be seen that the Yates's corrected chi-square is a more conservative test. It is less likely than the standard formula to result in a rejection of the null hypothesis when expected cell values are small.

When expected cell values fall below 5, the Yates's correction is also no longer considered appropriate. In such a case, the statistical test recommended is the Fisher exact test. The calculation of the Fisher exact test, although not difficult using Excel, is complicated and difficult to understand, and so it is not presented here. In general, the decision reached by the Fisher exact method, although statistically correct, will not be different from the decision reached using either the chi-square or the chi-square with Yates's correction. One reasonable approach to the issue of very small cells would be to base the decision on the probabilities derived from the Yates's correction. This will be, in general, more conservative than Fisher's exact test, in that the null hypothesis of independence is slightly less likely to be rejected. But, at the same time, the probability of making the type I error will not be greater than the probability level that has been set.

Small Expected Values When $df > 1$

When degrees of freedom are greater than one, tables that are larger than two by two, there is no equivalent to the Yates's correction or the Fisher exact method. In such tables, there are two strategies that might be used. One is to try to increase the number of observations in general, so that the expected cell frequencies in all cells are at least 5 and preferably 10. Another strategy is to collapse cells where this might make logical sense in order to increase the expected values in cells. To illustrate this latter approach, consider again the data shown in Figure 8.11. Those data were originally given in the form of the table shown in Figure 8.13. The two rows, adequate by 3 and adequate by 2, were collapsed into a single row, adequate by 2+, to avoid the small expected value in cell M9.

It is worth noting that in the case of the data shown in Figure 8.13, numerous researchers would not bother to collapse the two rows adequate by 3 and adequate by 2. This could be considered to be justified because the expected value in cell M9 is not all that small and there is only one such cell smaller than 10. If there had been several cells with expected values smaller than 10, or if any of the

FIGURE 8.13. SMALL EXPECTED VALUES IN $df > 1$.

	J	K	L	M	N
1	Assessment	UTI	Hypert	Ulcer	Total
2	adequate by 3	2	19	8	29
3	adequate by 2	11	12	17	40
4	adequate by 1	17	29	12	58
5	adequate by 0	77	54	38	169
6	Total	107	114	75	296
7					
8	Assessment	UTI	Hypert	Ulcer	Total
9	adequate by 3	10.483	11.169	7.348	29
10	adequate by 2	14.459	15.405	10.135	40
11	adequate by 1	20.966	22.338	14.696	58
12	adequate by 0	61.091	65.088	42.821	169
13	Total	107	114	75	296
14					

cells had been less than 5, it would have been most advisable from the standpoint of the appropriateness of the chi-square value to either collapse the number of cells or increase the overall number of observations in the study.

Exercises for Section 8.3

1. Use the Emergency worksheet in Chpt 8–1.xls to replicate the analysis in Figure 8.12.
2. The data in the Satisfaction worksheet in Chpt 8–1.xls represent the responses of a random sample of thirty-five people to a satisfaction question about a primary care clinic.
   a. Use the Pivot Table capability of Excel and the Yates's correction for the chi-square to test the hypothesis of independence between Sex and satisfaction.
   b. Use conditional probabilities to provide an interpretation of the results.

References

Brook, R. H., and Appel, F. A. "Quality of Care Assessment: Choosing a Method for Peer Review." *The New England Journal of Medicine, 288,* 1323–1329, June 21, 1973.

Halpern, C. T., and others. "Partener Violence Among Adolescents in Opposite-Sex Romantic Relationships: Findings from the National Longitudinal Study of Adolescent Health." *AJPH,* Oct. 2001, *91*(10), 1679–1685.

t TESTS FOR RELATED AND UNRELATED DATA

The chi square discussed in Chapter Eight provides a means of assessing whether two or more categorical variables are statistically independent of one another. This chapter takes up the *t* test, which is a means of assessing whether a numerical variable—either continuous or discrete—is independent of a categorical variable that takes on only two values. The *t* test provides another capability, which is the ability assess whether a value found from a sample could have come from a population in which a hypothesized value is true. This chapter addresses both of these issues, beginning with the latter.

Section 9.1 What Is a *t* Test?

To begin with a discussion of the *t* test, recall the question addressed by the hospital financial officer in Chapter Seven, who wished to know the true average cost of a hospital discharge. He decided to take a sample of a hundred discharge records, calculate the true cost of each hospital stay, and use the mean cost of this sample of discharges as the mean cost for all twelve thousand hospital stays. Suppose that before the financial officer had taken the sample and determined the cost of each, the chief executive officer of the hospital had said to him, "If the average cost of a discharge is $6,000, our charges schedule is fine. If the average cost is more than $6,000, we are going to have to renegotiate our charge schedule with all our payers, and that will be a big hassle. On the other hand, if our cost is less than $6,000, our payers are going to demand that we renegotiate our charge schedule, and that is going to be a hassle also. So I want you to use your sample to determine if our average cost per discharge is $6,000 or not. But I want your best estimate of the true situation, because if it is not $6,000, we need to get to work."

If the financial officer has had some statistics in graduate school (which, of course, he has), he could tell the CEO that there is no way to tell from a sample if the average cost per discharge is exactly $6,000. He can only get an estimate of the average cost. But the financial officer decides to try to answer the CEO's question in the best way he can, using statistical analysis.

The financial officer posits the CEO's concern in the following two hypotheses:

H0: The average cost per discharge is $6,000.

Or,

H0: c = $6,000.

And

H1: The average cost per discharge is not $6 000.

Or,

H1: c ≠ $6,000.

The financial officer knows that the sample mean that he obtains for the cost of hospital discharges will be only one of many means he could have gotten, had he taken other samples instead of the one he took. He also knows that the distribution of the means from all those other samples will be approximately a t distribution, with degrees of freedom equal to the sample size minus 1. Can he use this information to test whether the mean cost he discovers from the one sample he gets would lead him to accept or reject H0? The answer is yes. The way this test is carried out is given in Equation 9.1.

$$t = \frac{\bar{x}_s - \mu_H}{S.E._{\bar{x}_s}} \tag{9.1}$$

where $\bar{x}_s$ is the sample mean, μ_H is the population value hypothesized by H0, and $S.E._{\bar{x}_s}$ is the standard error of the sample mean.

Chapter Seven discussed a sample of a hundred discharges drawn from the hospital discharge records, for which the average cost per discharge was exactly $6,586.30. Although not mentioned there, the standard deviation for the sample was $5,262.73, so the estimate of the standard error of the means, based on a sample size of 100, was \$5,262.73/sqrt(100), or \$526.27. Using this sample information, the *t* test can be used to assess the probability that the true cost per case is \$6,000, as shown in Equation 9.2.

$$t = \frac{6586.30 - 6000}{526.27} = 1.11 \tag{9.2}$$

The value of $t = 1.11$ can now be assessed using the =TDIST() function in Excel. The =TDIST() function takes three arguments: the *t* value, the number of degrees of freedom, and a 1 or 2, depending on whether the test is a two-tail test or a one-tail test. Because the CEO is interested in whether the true population mean cost per case is either greater or less than \$6,000, a two-tail test is appropriate. If the CEO had only cared if the true cost per case was greater than \$6,000, we would have conducted a one-tail test. The result of the =TDIST() function is shown in Equation 9.3.

$$=\text{TDIST}(1.11,99,2) = .268 \tag{9.3}$$

where 1.11 is the value of *t*, 99 is the degrees of freedom $(100 - 1)$, and 2 indicates the two-tailed test.

The result found in Equation 9.3 indicates that there is a .268 probability that H0 is true (that is, the true cost per case is \$6,000), given that the sample mean was \$6,586.30 with a standard error of the mean of \$526.27. Stated another way, there is a .268 probability that we could have gotten a sample value of \$6,586.30 from a population in which the true average cost per case is \$6,000. As was discussed in Chapter Seven, it is usually the case that we are interested in having a small type I error—or the likelihood of rejecting H0 when it is true. In this case, we would want a small likelihood of rejecting the belief that the cost per case average is \$6,000 if that belief is true. Usually, we would want the result of the *t* test to produce a probability of .05 or less before we would reject H0. And this is exactly what we will do in this case. Because the probability that H0 is true is as large as .268, we will not reject it (even though, having all the data, we know that the true mean is \$5,905 and change). This is a *t* test.

The *t* test can produce a result that may range from $-\infty$ to ∞, although practically speaking it is usually in a more finite range. The =TDIST() function works only with positive values of *t*, so that when using the =TDIST() function to determine the true probability of a negative *t* value, it is necessary to change the negative value to a positive one. Since the *t* distribution is symmetrical with regard to the probability of being at $-t$ or t, the conversion makes no difference. Consequently, if the two tail probability of a value of -2.3 was desired, the way to determine this would be by using =TDIST(2.3,*df*,2)

Where Does a *t* Test Come From?

Why have we used a *t* test, what does it mean, and where does it come from? To try to answer these three questions, all posed in one sentence, let us consider another example. Suppose the CEO had said that if the true cost per case is not $5,905.75, change must occur in the hospital. Now, since we know the true mean, we know that it is $5,905.75. But the financial guy doesn't know this. He still has to take a sample, calculate the true average cost of the sample, and run a *t* test to see if the sample mean was likely to have come from a population in which the true mean is $5,905.75. But it is highly unlikely that he will find the sample mean equal to $5,905.75. As was discussed earlier, one possible sample outcome is $6,586.30.

Now, it is essential to remember that in real life, one only ever takes a single sample and one must be satisfied, in general, with the results of that single sample. But this is a book, and in a book we are not constrained by the limits of real life. Instead of taking a single sample, let us propose to take a large number of samples—say, 250. We can do this by using the Tools/Data Analysis add-in in Excel. Having done this, we can calculate estimates of the mean and standard error for each of these samples and conduct a *t* test by the formula in Equation 9.1.

It was indicated earlier that the *t* test results are distributed as a *t* distribution. If we examine the results of 250 *t* tests, we would expect a large number of those to produce values in the range of −1 to 1. (Which corresponds to 1 standard deviation on each side of 0, the value that would be generated if there were no difference between the sample mean and H0.) In fact, we would expect that 68 percent of the results of the *t* tests from our 250 samples would lie between −1 and 1. Furthermore, we would expect 95 percent to lie between −2 and 2, for the same reason. Figure 9.1 shows a graph of the distribution of the 250 *t* tests, based on the samples taken from the twelve thousand hospital discharge records. Exactly 68 percent of the *t* tests provide results in the range −1 to 1. Ninety-three percent (rather than the expected 95 percent) of *t* tests provide results in the range −2 to 2. Seven percent of the results are outside the range −2 to 2 for the means of these 250 samples *when H0 is the true mean*. This means that when H0 is the true mean, there is about a 5 percent probability (in this example, 7 percent) of rejecting H0 when it is true. But, in general, the probability of rejecting H0 when it is true is small. The consequence of this is that if the *t* test produced a value outside the range −2 to 2, we would typically conclude that the sample *did not* come from a population in which H0 was true (even though we recognize that there is a small likelihood that it could have).

Let us look at this result from another perspective. Suppose H0 had been $4,500. That is, the CEO had said, "If the average cost of a hospital stay is not $4,500, we are going to have to make some changes." Now, when we draw the 250 samples and carry out the *t* tests, the distribution of the *t* values is as shown

FIGURE 9.1. DISTRIBUTION OF 250 *t* TESTS WHEN H0 = $5,905.

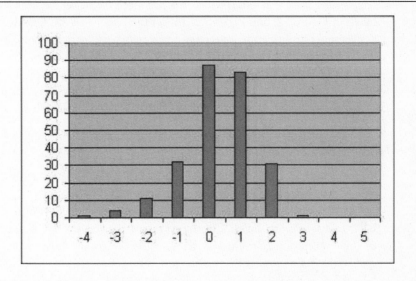

FIGURE 9.2. DISTRIBUTION OF 250 *t* TESTS WHEN H0 = $4,500.

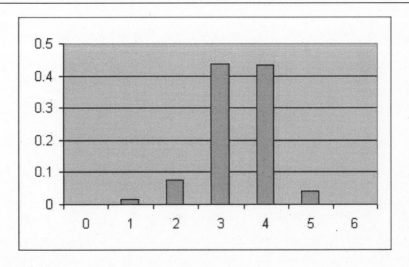

in Figure 9.2. This figure shows that the distribution of *t* values is centered on 3.5. A *t* value greater than 2 would lead us to reject H0 and accept the alternative. Thus, we would (correctly) conclude that the population mean is not $4,500.

But the calculation of the 250 *t* tests and their distribution as shown in Figure 9.2 also gives us one other type of information that is of interest. In general, we would accept H0 for any value of t within the range -2 to 2. Looking at Figure 9.2, it is possible to see that some of the t tests produced t values of less than 2 (the column labels in Figure 9.2 and Figure 9.1 reflect the Excel =FREQUENCY() function convention of putting the frequency between two values at the point of the higher value). In fact, about 9 percent of the 250 t tests produced values of less than 2. In testing the null hypothesis, H0: $c = \$4,500$, that 9 percent of samples would have led us to accept H0, producing the type II error of accepting H0 when it is false. So, in this case (where cost is posited to be $4,500), beta is about .09.

One-Tail and Two-Tail t Tests

The test that is discussed previously is a two-tailed test. As was discussed in Chapter Seven, assessments of hypotheses can be one-tailed or two-tailed. In a two-tailed test, the region of rejection of H0 can be at either end of the continuum of possible t values. In a one-tailed test, the region of rejection of H0 is in only one end of the continuum. In regard to the question of cost per hospital stay discussed earlier, the discussion is of a two-tail test. This is because the CEO indicated that he was concerned about the possibility that the mean value might be either more or less than H0 (in either case, adjustments would have to be made).

But, for example, suppose the CEO is not interested in knowing whether the true cost is less than $6,000. His only concern is that if the true costs are greater than $6,000, he will have to take steps to renegotiate charges to bring them into line with true costs. So, in this case, the hypotheses posed by the financial officer would be:

H0: The average cost per discharge is $6,000 or less.

Or,

H0: $c = <\$6,000$.

And

H1: The average cost per discharge is greater than $6,000.

Or,

H1: $c > \$6,000$.

Now the initial hypothesis and the alternative hypothesis are stated in such a way that the null will be rejected only if the sample mean is greater than $6,000. Any sample mean less than $6,000 produces a t test value that will NEVER be in the region of rejection of H0. This is logical, because any sample value less than $6,000 cannot be used to reject H0. The t test to assess H0 and H1 is as that given in Equation 9.1. But, now, the number of standard deviation units required for rejection of H0 will not be approximately 2 (depending on sample size) but will be closer to 1.7.

FIGURE 9.3. REGION OF REJECTION FOR TWO-TAIL TEST.

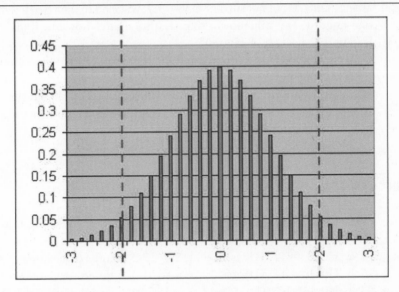

FIGURE 9.4. REGION OF REJECTION FOR ONE-TAIL TEST.

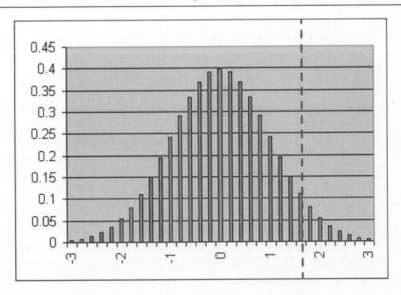

Figure 9.3 and Figure 9.4 show the comparative regions of rejection for a two-tail test (Figure 9.3) and a one-tail test (Figure 9.4). The region of rejection for the two-tail test is outside the two vertical dashed lines at −2 and 2. If the *t* test result falls outside −2 and 2, H0 will be rejected. The region of rejection for the one-tail

test is to the right of the dashed line in Figure 9.4 at about 1.7. Any t value larger than 1.7 (but not smaller than -1.7) will lead to the rejection of H0. In the one-tail test, any value lower than 1.7, no matter how low it may be, will not lead to the rejection of H0.

It is important to keep in mind the direction of H0 when interpreting the result of a one-tail t test. In the case of the hypothesis H0: c $= <\$6,000$, any value of t in the negative range will not lead to the rejection of H0. However, if H0 had been stated as c $= >\$6,000$, then any value of t in the positive range would not lead to the rejection of H0.

Exercises for Section 9.1

1. Calculate the t value for the following hypotheses, given the sample outcomes indicated.
   a. H0: $\mu = 11$, H1: $\mu <> 11$, $\bar{x} = 12.2$, standard deviation $= 8.9$, $n = 40$.
   b. H0: $\mu = 11$, H1: $\mu <> 11$, $\bar{x} = 14.0$, standard deviation $= 8.9$, $n = 40$.
   c. H0: $\mu = 11$, H1: $\mu > 11$, $\bar{x} = 13.7$, standard deviation $= 8.9$, $n = 40$.
   d. H0: $\mu = 234$, H1: $\mu <> 234$, $\bar{x} = 228.4$, standard deviation $= 40.53$, $n = 120$.
   e. H0: $\mu = 234$, H1: $\mu <> 234$, $\bar{x} = 226.4$, standard deviation $= 40.53$, $n = 120$.
   f. H0: $\mu = 234$, H1: $\mu > 234$, $\bar{x} = 226.4$, standard deviation $= 40.53$, $n = 120$.

2. Determine the probability of t in each example in Exercise 1 and decide for each whether you would accept or reject H0.

3. Use the Hospital charges worksheet in Chpt 4–1.xls. Assume that the hundred records represent a random sample from all hospital discharges for a year and test the hypothesis H0: Charges $= \$6,000$ against the alternative H1: Charges $<> \$6,000$, and indicate your conclusion.

4. Use the BP worksheet in Chpt 6–2.xls and the Uniform distribution option in Tools/Data Analysis with a random seed of 7375 to draw a sample of sixty blood pressure readings. Test the hypothesis H0: BP $= 83$ mmhg against the alternative H1: BP $<> 83$ mmhg, and indicate your conclusion.

5. Use the ER Wait worksheet in Chpt 6–2.xls and Uniform distribution option in Tools/Data Analysis with a random seed of 2538 to draw a sample of forty waiting times. Test the hypothesis H0: waiting time $=$ thirty-five minutes against the alternative H1: waiting time < 35 minutes, and indicate your conclusion.

Section 9.2 A *t* Test for Comparing Two Groups

Thus far, we have discussed a *t* test concerned with comparing a sample mean with an a priori hypothesized value. With that in mind, we tested whether the result of a sample could have been taken from a population in which the true mean was H0. But *t* tests can be used also to compare samples from two potentially different groups to determine if, statistically, they can be seen as different or not.

For example, suppose the financial officer of our hypothetical hospital was asked by the CEO to determine whether the costs of a hospital discharge differed between males and females. Although it may not be possible to negotiate differing charges on the basis of sex, it might still be important for the CEO to know if actual costs differed. So now, the financial officer might be addressing the following two hypotheses:

H0: The average cost per discharge is equal between men and women.

Or,

H0: $c_m = c_w$.

And

H1: The average cost per discharge is not equal between men and women.

Or,

H1: $c_m \neq c_w$.

Now, the financial officer must be somewhat careful about how he selects his sample of discharges. If the selection is done strictly randomly, there is a small possibility that either no men or no women might be selected for the sample, making it impossible to assess the hypotheses. Luckily, the financial officer knows that he can divide the total twelve thousand records into those for men and those for women, so that he can take a sample of each group. This is what is known as a stratified sample, because he will be stratifying the population into men and women before taking a sample from each group.

In general, with a stratified sample, it is best to take samples of equal size from each strata if the desire is to compare the two strata and if there is no perception that the variances of the two strata differ. Since there is no particular reason, a priori, for the financial officer to expect that the costs for men are more or less variable than the costs for women (even though the means may differ), the best decision is to take equal-sized samples of men and women. Since the financial officer believes he can still muster the manpower to ascertain the true costs of hospital stays for a total of a hundred discharges, the decision is to take a sample of discharges for fifty men and another for fifty women.

To determine if the cost for men and women is the same (the assessment of H0), it will first be necessary to determine the average cost for each sample of fifty. It will then be necessary to use the appropriate t test to determine whether the means of the two samples could have come from two populations in which the true mean of costs was the same. The t test that will be used to determine this *when sample sizes are the same* is given in Equation 9.4.

$$t = \frac{\bar{x}_1 - \bar{x}_2}{\sqrt{\dfrac{s_1^2 + s_2^2}{n}}} \tag{9.4}$$

where $\bar{x}_1$ is the sample mean for men, $\bar{x}_2$ is the sample mean for women, s_1^2 is the sample variance for men, s_2^2 is the sample variance for women, and n is equal to the sample size *in either group.*

Assume that the financial officer has taken a sample of fifty men and fifty women and has recorded an average cost of \$6,460.04 for men and \$6,177.30 for women, with variances (the square of the standard deviation or s^2) of 23837156 and 24477861. The t test to compare men and women is then found by the formula in Equation 9.5.

$$t = \frac{6460.04 - 6177.30}{\sqrt{\dfrac{23837156 + 24477861}{50}}} = .288 \tag{9.5}$$

The t value of .288 given in Equation 9.5 will not lead to rejection of H0. In general, if the level of the type I error (α) is set at .05, H0 will be rejected only when the absolute value of t is approximately 2 or greater. (Recall that t can be a negative or a positive number.) However, the exact probability of finding a t as large as .288 can be found by using the =TDIST() function. For this t test, because there are actually a hundred ($2n$) observations, and because one degree of freedom is used up for each sample, there are $2n - 2$ degrees of freedom. With $2n - 2$ degrees of freedom, the exact probability of finding a t value as large as .288 or larger is given by Equation 9.6. The interpretation of the probability given in Equation 9.6 is as follows: if the population mean for cost per discharge were exactly the same for both men and women, the t value calculated for a large number of samples of discharges for fifty men and fifty women would be as large as .288 in about 77 percent of the samples selected. Because the probability of getting a *t* value as large as .288 is very high, H0 is accepted and the financial officer reaches the conclusion that there is no cost difference between men and women.

$$p_t = \text{TDIST}(.288, 98, 2) = .774 \tag{9.6}$$

Type I and Type II Errors in Comparing Means

Let us consider further what it means to say that there is no difference in the cost between men and women. For the twelve thousand hospital discharges, there are 4,560 men and 7,440 women. The true mean of cost for men is $5,825.63 and for women it is $5,954.85. So, in fact, there is a real difference in the mean cost between men and women, although the difference is only $129.22. This is a real difference, but is it an important difference? Such a question is not one that statistics can answer. The question of what may be an important difference must be left to the CEO to decide.

But suppose there was truly no population level difference between the cost for men and the cost for women. Suppose the true mean for men was exactly equal to the true mean for women, which would then both be equal to $5,905.75. If we were to select a large number of samples of size 50 for men and 50 for women from these two populations and calculated the *t* value for each sample by using Equation 9.4, the distribution of those mean values would be a *t* distribution with 98 degrees of freedom. Furthermore, the distribution would look identical to that shown in Figure 9.3. Similarly, we would expect that about 5 percent of all *t* values calculated by using Equation 9.4 would have values outside the range −2 to 2. These would be the *t* values that would lead us to reject H0, *even when it was true* and would represent type I error.

Consider now type II error. Rather than looking at the real average difference between the two populations, which is only $129.22, assume that the true population mean for men was $5,000 and the true population mean for women was $7,000. If we assume the same variance as that which is true of the actual data, the distribution of the *t* test values from a large number of samples would look very much like the distribution shown in Figure 9.5. In Figure 9.5, about half the distribution is to the left of the dashed vertical line. That is the region in which we would reject H0 and conclude, in fact, that the true cost is different between men and women. To the right of the dashed vertical line, which also includes about half the distribution, is the region in which we will erroneously accept H0, even when the true average difference between the two groups is as large as $2,000. In this case, then, the type II error is about .5. The only way to reduce the type II error in this setting is to increase the size of the sample.

FIGURE 9.5. TYPE II ERROR FOR TRUE MEANS OF $5,000 AND $7,000.

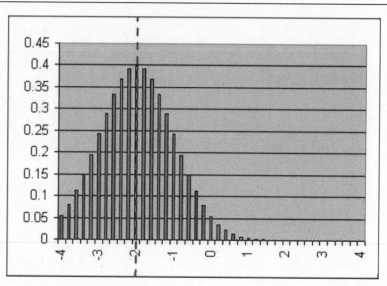

If we had the resources to increase the sample size to, for example, 150 for men and 150 for women, then the pooled standard error would be reduced considerably over a sample of 50 each. That would produce a graph of all possible *t* test values as shown in Figure 9.6. In this figure, the bulk of the *t* distribution is to the left of the vertical dashed line and only about 7 percent of the distribution is to the right of the dashed line. Thus, in this case, the probability of making the type II error has been reduced to about .07.

Comparing Unequal Size Samples

Thus far, the discussion has centered on equal sample sizes. This section, expands the *t* test for two groups to unequal sample sizes, and, in addition, introduces the notion of an experimental design.

A new resident physician has been asked by the senior physician with whom she is working to assist in a study of the effect of physician interaction with patients on the degree of knowledge gained by the patients on breast cancer. When the patients come to the clinic, they will be given a brochure about breast cancer with information about its etiology, detection, treatment, and prognosis. They will all have waiting time adequate to read the brochure if they wish to do so. They will then be randomly divided into two groups. One group (the

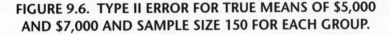

FIGURE 9.6. TYPE II ERROR FOR TRUE MEANS OF $5,000 AND $7,000 AND SAMPLE SIZE 150 FOR EACH GROUP.

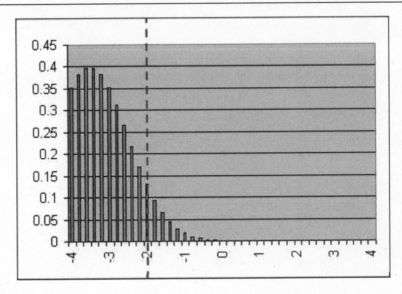

control group) receives no further information unless they ask for it. The second group (the experimental group) will have a five- to ten-minute one-on-one discussion with the physician about breast cancer, providing the same information as was contained in the brochure. At the end of their visit, all patients will be given a short questionnaire that assesses their knowledge of breast cancer on a 20-point scale. The purpose of the study is to determine if the patients who have the one-on-one discussion with the physician score higher on the questionnaire than those who do not.

This is a classic experimental design (although not a double-blind random clinical trial). But we will introduce one modification in the classic design. The study will be carried out over a one-month period. During that time, the physicians expect to have about sixty-five women come to the clinic who are appropriate for the study. But because of the time that is involved in interacting with the experimental group, they do not feel that they can include more than twenty-five women in the experimental group. One decision, then, would be to say that only twenty-five women would be included in the control group. But this may not be the best decision. Since the control group costs no extra resources (the space required to take the brief test and its scoring is not a significant resource drain), it is a better strategy to include all women who are not in the experimental group as controls. Given that the physicians expect sixty-five women in total, the projected control group will consist of forty women.

Let us now assume that the month has passed, the experiment has taken place, and postintervention knowledge tests have been obtained for sixty-five women. How do we conduct the t test that will determine whether the two groups are different? Since the two group (or sample) sizes are different, we cannot use the t test as given in Equation 9.4. Instead, we need a formula for the t test that takes into account the fact that the two sample sizes are not the same. The appropriate t test is as given in Equation 9.7.

$$t = \frac{\bar{x}_1 - \bar{x}_2}{\sqrt{s_p^2\left(\frac{1}{n_1} + \frac{1}{n_2}\right)}} \tag{9.7}$$

where $s_p^2 = (n_1 - 1)s_1^2 + (n_2 - 1)s_2^2/(n_1 - 1) + (n_2 - 1)$, and s_1^2 is the sample variance for group 1, s_2^2 is the sample variance for group 2, n_1 is the sample size for group 1, and n_2 is the sample size for group 2.

The complete data set from this experiment (wholly fictional) is given in Chpt 9–1.xls. Using those data, the results of the experiment are those shown in Figure 9.7. The figure shows, in columns A and B, some of the data from the study for both the Experimental group (the one that received the intervention) and the Control group (the one that did not). Columns E and F give the sample sizes, the mean, and the variance for each group, as well as the degrees of freedom

FIGURE 9.7. RESULTS OF A BREAST CANCER EXPERIMENT.

	A	B	C	D	E	F
	E10		=(E2-F2)/E9			
1	Experimenta	Control		n	25	40
2	11	10		Xbar	10.04	7.525
3	12	3		s^2	7.123333	10.05064
4	13	5				
5	14	11		n-1	24	39
6	8	10		n-1*s^2	170.96	391.975
7	13	9				
8	11	4		s pooled	8.935476	
9	9	11		SE pooled	0.762106	
10	8	5		t	3.300065	
11	12	8		df	63	
12	12	4		Prob	0.001594	
13	7	8				

for each group [n–1] and [n–1*s^2]. Cells E8 through E12 give the actual results of the *t* test. The value in E8 is the pooled variance following the formula for
s_p^2 given in Equation 9.7. Cell E9 gives the pooled standard error, which is the
denominator of the equation for *t* in Equation 9.7. The *t* value in cell E10 is
calculated by using the formula in Equation 9.7. The degrees of freedom in cell
E11 are the sum of cells E5 and F5 but are also $n_1 + n_2 - 2$. Cell E12 is the
95 percent confidence limit probability of finding a *t* value as large as 3.3 when
there is actually no difference between the experimental and the control group.
Since this probability, at approximately two chances in a thousand, is very small,
the conclusion is drawn that there is a difference between the two groups. Furthermore, because the mean for the experimental group is larger than the mean
for the control group, the conclusion is extended to say that the one-on-one
discussion with the physician made a difference in the amount of knowledge that
the women have.

The two *t* tests discussed thus far have different implications for what is actually known. The first *t* test, which compared discharges for men with discharges
for women, was only concerned with whether there was a difference. The test
does not and cannot say anything about the source of that difference. The difference might be due to differences in age between the men and women who
were discharged, differences in their diagnoses or severity of illness, differences
in length of stay, or other factors that have not been considered in the test. Other
statistical procedures might shed light on the source of difference, but the *t* test
cannot identify those possible differences. Conversely, if the assignment to the
experimental and the control groups for the second *t* test was adequately carried
out, the *t* test does have the capability of indicating whether or not the experimental intervention has the ability to affect the knowledge women have about
breast cancer (although this conclusion, too, must be tempered by the lack of
blindness). However, the ability of the *t* test to allow that conclusion to be drawn
depends entirely on the adequacy of the random assignment process.

An Assumption of Equal Variance

The *t* tests discussed thus far carry with them an assumption that the variances
of the two groups being compared are equal. With regard to the test for the difference between costs for men and women, the variances of the two groups (shown
as the denominator in Equation 9.5) differ only by about 3 percent. With regard to
the variances in the experimental setting, the values, shown as cells E3 and F3, differ by about 41 percent. Is there a statistical test for the equivalence of variance between the two groups, and if they are not equal, what can be done about it?

First, a test does exist for equivalence of variance in the *t* test setting. To
examine this test, we will use the data from the experimental setting discussed in

the second subsection of Section 9.2, where the variances differ by about 41 percent. The test of equivalence of variance is an F test. Whereas a t test is typically a test comparing mean values, an F test is typically a test comparing variances. The F test for the equivalence of variance for two groups in a t test setting is given in Equation 9.8.

$$F = \frac{s_1^2}{s_2^2} \tag{9.8}$$

where s_1^2 is the variance for one sample and s_2^2 is the variance for the other.

In the example discussed in the second subsection of Section 9.2, the experimental group of twenty-five women has a variance of 7.12 (see Figure 9.7), whereas the control group has a variance of 10.05. So the F test for the difference between these two variances is as that given in Equation 9.9 and has the value of .71. Whereas a t test has a single number representing degrees of freedom, an F test has two numbers representing degrees of freedom—one number for the numerator and one for the denominator. In this case, the degrees of freedom are 24 and 39 ($n_1 - 1$ for the experimental group and $n_2 - 1$ for the control group).

$$F = \frac{7.12}{10.05} = .71 \tag{9.9}$$

The F test is a test of equality of the variances, or $s_1^2 = s_2^2$. The F distribution is a nonsymmetrical distribution that generally looks like the picture shown in Figure 9.8. Figure 9.8 represents the F distribution for 24 and 39 degrees of freedom, but other F distributions are quite similar in appearance. The two dashed vertical lines indicate the lower and upper 95 percent limits. For 24 and 39 degrees of freedom, the F value must be approximately .5 or less (if the smaller variance is divided by the larger) or 2 or greater (if the larger variance is divided by the smaller) before the difference between the two variances is considered large enough to have come from populations in which the true variances are not equal. The actual value of the F test in Equation 9.9 (.71) has a probability of occurrence of about .18. Because this probability is relatively high, the conclusion that we would reach is that the two variances are equal.

In the case discussed earlier, the conclusion was drawn that the variances were equal. But what happens if the two variances prove not to be equal? In the case of unequal variances, the pooled variance formula in Equation 9.7 is no longer appropriate. Instead, the t test is conducted not by pooling the variance but by simply adding the variances divided by the sample sizes. In that case, the

FIGURE 9.8. *F* DISTRIBUTION.

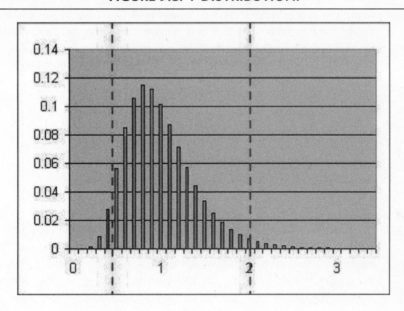

appropriate *t* test is given by Equation 9.10. It might be noted that when sample sizes are the same, the formula in Equation 9.10 will be exactly the same as the formula in Equation 9.4. The value of this is that *if sample sizes are the same,* the formula in Equation 9.4 can be used, whether variances are equal or not. But if the sample sizes are not the same, the formula given in Equation 9.7, or that given in Equation 9.10, will produce generally the same decision (although not the same numerical result for the *t*) most of the time. That is, if the decision to reject H0 was produced by Equation 9.7, it is highly likely that the same decision would be reached by using Equation 9.10.

$$t = \frac{\bar{x}_1 - \bar{x}_2}{\sqrt{\left(s_1^2/n_1\right) + \left(s_2^2/n_2\right)}} \tag{9.10}$$

To see the effect of the changes in the computation of the *t* test for unequal variance and unequal sample size, the *t* test as indicated in Equation 9.10 would produce the results shown in Equation 9.11 for the data from the breast cancer education study.

$$t = \frac{10.04 - 7.53}{\sqrt{(7.12/25) + (10.05/40)}} = 3.43 \tag{9.11}$$

If variances are known to be unequal and sample sizes are either equal or unequal, the appropriate degrees of freedom for the t test are reduced by the degree to which the variances differ. This reduction in the degrees of freedom for the t test may be carried out by several different formulas, all of which give approximately the same answer. But the most widely accepted method—the one most likely used by Excel—is given by the formula in Equation 9.12.

$$f = \frac{f_a f_b}{f_b c^2 + f_a (1 - c)^2}$$ (9.12)

where f is the adjusted degrees of freedom, $f_a = n_a - 1$, $f_b = n_b - 1$, and $c = \frac{s_a^2/n_a}{(s_a^2/n_a) + (s_b^2/n_b)}$.

The formula in Equation 9.12 gives 57.48 as the degrees of freedom for the t test in Figure 9.7. Although we have already concluded that there is no difference in the variance of the two samples, a more conservative test would be to use 57 degrees of freedom (the nearest whole integer to the calculated value) to make the test. In that case, we would conclude that the probability of a t value as large as 3.43 would be .0011.

An important question with regard to the presumed unequal variance is the question of how much difference it makes if variances are unequal. First, it is useful to note that if sample sizes are equal, using the equal or unequal variance formulas will generally result in the same decision. In only rare situations—when the t test value was right around 2, calculated using either formula (and for equal sample size, the t from either formula is the same)—would the unequal variance formula lead to a different decision. And in this situation, the unequal variance t test will always be less likely to reject H0. This is because the lower degrees of freedom for the unequal variance t test require a slightly larger value of t for statistical significance.

However, with both unequal variance and unequal sample sizes, it is essential to use the unequal variance t test. If the smaller sample also has the larger variance, the unequal variance t test is more likely to result in the acceptance of H0 than the equal variance t test. But if the smaller sample also has the smaller variance, the unequal variance t test is more likely than the equal variance t test to result in the rejection of H0. Thus, it is important, with the case of unequal sample sizes, to use the appropriate t test.

The Excel t Test Add-In

Excel provides two add-ins for t test of two groups. These are found under Tools/Data Analysis and are called t Test: Two Sample Assuming Equal Variance,

FIGURE 9.9. WINDOW FOR *t* TEST FOR EQUAL VARIANCE.

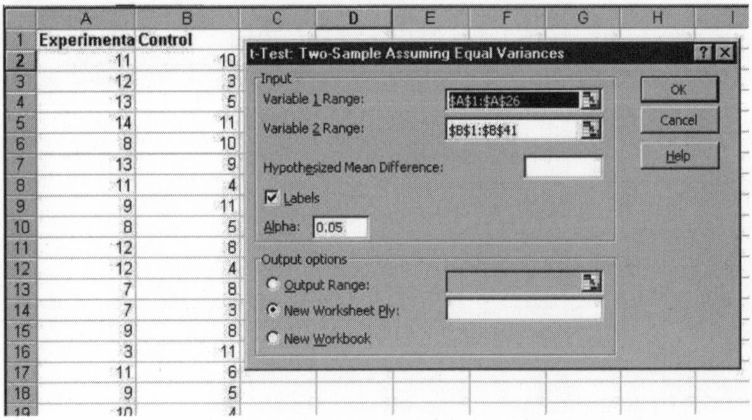

and *t* Test: Two Sample Assuming Unequal Variance. Let us look at each of these with the data from the breast cancer education experiment as the example. After selecting Tools/Data Analysis, it is necessary first to select *t* Test: Two Sample Assuming Equal Variance. The window that comes up for this procedure is shown in Figure 9.9. In this window, it can be seen that the data for the experimental group are included as variable 1 range, whereas the data for the control group are included as variable 2 range. Leaving the hypothesized mean difference blank is equivalent to putting in the value of zero. The labels box is checked because the first row contains the labels for the two data streams. The output will go on a new worksheet.

Pressing OK or hitting return will produce the result of this *t* test on a new worksheet. It can be seen, by comparing Figure 9.10 and Figure 9.7, that the results computed by the formula in Equation 9.7 and the results of the Excel add-in Figure 9.10 are identical. The Excel add-in also provides some additional information, particularly the level at which H0 would be rejected for one- and two-tail tests (*t* Critical one tail and *t* Critical two tail).

Consider, now, the add-in for a *t* test assuming unequal variance. That, too, is found under Tools/Data Analysis. Then select *t* Test: Two Sample Assuming Unequal Variance. When this option is selected, the window that appears is exactly the same as the window in Figure 9.9, except the title is *t* Test: Two Sample Assuming Unequal Variance. When the add-in is invoked, it produces a result—for the experimental data under consideration here—as shown in Figure 9.11.

There are three differences between the results shown in Figure 9.10 and those shown in Figure 9.11. The first is in the calculated value of the *t* test. It is 3.30 in

FIGURE 9.10. RESULTS OF EXCEL *t* TEST FOR EQUAL VARIANCE.

	A	B	C
1	t-Test: Two-Sample Assuming Equal Variances		
2			
3		Experimenta	Control
4	Mean	10.04	7.525
5	Variance	7.12333	10.05064
6	Observations	25	40
7	Pooled Variance	8.93548	
8	Hypothesized Mean Difference	0	
9	df	63	
10	t Stat	3.30006	
11	P(T<=t) one-tail	0.0008	
12	t Critical one-tail	1.6694	
13	P(T<=t) two-tail	0.00159	
14	t Critical two-tail	1.99834	
15			
16			

FIGURE 9.11. RESULTS OF THE EXCEL *t* TEST FOR UNEQUAL VARIANCE.

	A	B	C
1	t-Test: Two-Sample Assuming Unequal Variances		
2			
3		Experimenta	Control
4	Mean	10.04	7.525
5	Variance	7.123333	10.05064
6	Observations	25	40
7	Hypothesized Mean Difference	0	
8	df	57	
9	t Stat	3.43459	
10	P(T<=t) one-tail	0.000556	
11	t Critical one-tail	1.672029	
12	P(T<=t) two-tail	0.001113	
13	t Critical two-tail	2.002466	

Figure 9.10 and 3.43 in Figure 9.11. As noted previously, the value of 3.30 was calculated using Equation 9.7, whereas the value of 3.43 was calculated using Equation 9.10. A second is the absence of a pooled variance (s_p^2) value in Figure 9.11. This is because no pooled variance is calculated for the unequal variance *t* test. Finally, there is a difference in the degrees of freedom between the two figures. The equal variance degrees of freedom is simply $n_1 + n_2 - 2$, whereas the unequal variance degrees of freedom is found by using Equation 9.12.

Exercises for Section 9.2

1. Assume the following information for equal-sized samples and make the appropriate *t* tests.
   a. Group 1: $\bar{x} = 25$, $s^2 = 27.8$, $n = 15$; Group 2: $\bar{x} = 23$, $s^2 = 27.8$, $n = 15$.
   b. Group 1: $\bar{x} = 25$, $s^2 = 27.8$, $n = 15$; Group 2: $\bar{x} = 29$, $s^2 = 27.8$, $n = 15$.
   c. Group 1: $\bar{x} = 125$, $s^2 = 92.6$, $n = 40$; Group 2: $\bar{x} = 121$, $s^2 = 92.6$, $n = 40$.
   d. Group 1: $\bar{x} = 125$, $s^2 = 92.6$, $n = 40$; Group 2: $\bar{x} = 131$, $s^2 = 92.6$, $n = 40$.
   e. Group 1: $\bar{x} = 11$, $s^2 = 15$, $n = 130$; Group 2: $\bar{x} = 11.5$, $s^2 = 15$, $n = 130$.
   f. Group 1: $\bar{x} = 11$, $s^2 = 15$, $n = 130$; Group 2: $\bar{x} = 12.5$, $s^2 = 15$, $n = 130$.

2. Determine the probability of the *t* test result in a through *f* of Exercise 1 and decide whether you would accept or reject the hypothesis of no difference between the two groups in each case.

3. Assume the following information for unequal size samples and make the appropriate *t* tests.
   a. Group 1: $\bar{x} = 25$, $s^2 = 27.8$, $n = 30$; Group 2: $\bar{x} = 23$, $s^2 = 27.8$, $n = 15$.
   b. Group 1: $\bar{x} = 25$, $s^2 = 27.8$, $n = 30$; Group 2: $\bar{x} = 29$, $s^2 = 27.8$, $n = 15$.
   c. Group 1: $\bar{x} = 125$, $s^2 = 92.6$, $n = 40$; Group 2: $\bar{x} = 121$, $s^2 = 92.6$, $n = 25$.
   d. Group 1: $\bar{x} = 125$, $s^2 = 92.6$, $n = 40$; Group 2: $\bar{x} = 131$, $s^2 = 92.6$, $n = 25$.
   e. Group 1: $\bar{x} = 11$, $s^2 = 15$, $n = 130$; Group 2: $\bar{x} = 11.5$, $s^2 = 15$, $n = 90$.
   f. Group 1: $\bar{x} = 11$, $s^2 = 15$, $n = 130$; Group 2: $\bar{x} = 12.5$, $s^2 = 15$, $n = 90$.

4. Determine the probability of the *t* test result in a through *f* of Exercise 3 and decide whether you would accept or reject the hypothesis of no difference between the two groups in each case.

5. Use the data on the Cost worksheet of Chpt 9–1.xls that show the hospital cost for a randomly selected sample of thirty-four women and thirty-four men, and do the following:
   a. Calculate a *t* test of the hypothesis that cost for women is equal to cost for men, against the alternative that they are not equal, assuming equal variance.
   b. Decide whether to accept or reject the hypothesis of equality.

6. Use the data on the Breast C worksheet of Chpt 9–1.xls that show the data used for the analysis in Figure 9.7 and replicate the analysis shown in that figure.

7. Use the data on the Wait worksheet of Chpt 9–1 that represents the waiting time of a randomly selected group of people at an urgent care clinic and a randomly selected group of people at an emergency clinic.
   a. Calculate a *t* test of the hypothesis that wait time in the urgent care clinic is no different from wait time in the emergency clinic, assuming equal variance.
   b. Decide whether to accept or reject the hypothesis of equality.

8. Test the hypothesis of equality of variance for the following sets of data and determine whether to accept or reject the hypothesis.
   a. For group 1: $s^2 = 9$, $n = 20$; for group 2: $s^2 = 5$, $n = 20$
   b. For group 1: $s^2 = 9$, $n = 50$; for group 2: $s^2 = 5$, $n = 50$
   c. For group 1: $s^2 = 9$, $n = 50$; for group 2: $s^2 = 5$, $n = 100$
   d. For group 1: $s^2 = 21$, $n = 20$; for group 2: $s^2 = 33$, $n = 20$
   e. For group 1: $s^2 = 21$, $n = 50$; for group 2: $s^2 = 33$, $n = 50$
   f. For group 1: $s^2 = 21$, $n = 50$; for group 2: $s^2 = 33$, $n = 100$

9. Test the hypothesis of equality of variance and indicate the conclusion you reach.
   a. For the data on the Cost worksheet of Chpt 9–1.xls
   b. For the data on the Breast C worksheet of Chpt 9–1.xls
   c. For the data on the Wait worksheet of Chpt 9–1

10. Use the unequal variance formula (Equation 9.10) for the t test to test the hypothesis of equality of wait time for the data on the Wait worksheet of Chpt 9–1.

11. Use the Excel add-in for the equal variance t test and conduct a t test for the data on the Cost worksheet of Chpt 9–1.xls. Do the results replicate those found in Exercise 5.

12. Use the Excel add-in for the equal variance t test and conduct a t test for the data on the Breast C worksheet of Chpt 9–1.xls. Do the results replicate those found in Exercise 6?

13. Use the Excel add-in for the unequal variance t test and conduct a t test for the data on the Wait worksheet of Chpt 9–1. Do the results replicate those found in Exercise 10?

Section 9.3 A t Test for Related Data

Thus far, the discussion of t tests has focused either on a population value determined a priori or on the question of whether two groups or samples are the same or different. This section addresses a t test that can be used when two sets of data are related. In particular, this is a test of whether two measurements for the same group of people (or organizations, or any other identifiable entities) are similar or different.

Calculation of the Test

To examine this t test, consider a group of persons with adult onset diabetes who have come under the care of a diabetes clinic. The clinic is confident that the symptoms of diabetes—especially high blood sugar-can be controlled through a combination of exercise, weight loss, and diet and lifestyle changes. To assess this belief, the clinic has enrolled a group of forty volunteers, all with Hemoglobin A1c (HbA1c) measures above 7.8 (in general, HbA1c levels above 7.8 indicate some difficulties in controlling blood sugar levels). The average HbA1c level for this group of forty persons, at the time of enrollment in the study, was 8.49. The persons were counseled on diet, exercise, and lifestyle changes and had monthly meetings with their counselor to track progress toward agreed upon goals. At the end of a six-month period, the Hemoglobin A1c levels for these persons were again measured. The data for this study (entirely fabricated) are given in Chpt 9–2.xls. The mean HbA1c level for the entire group after the six-month study period was 8.25. The question is whether this reduction in HbA1c represents a statistically significant change.

The initial hypothesis for this study would typically be:

H0: The combination of exercise, weight loss, and diet and lifestyle changes has no effect on HbA1c levels, or,

H0: $HbA1c_b = HbA1c_a$, where b refers to before and a to after.

Because there is some expectation that the HbA1c levels will be lowered by the combination of exercise, weight loss, and diet and lifestyle changes, the alternative hypothesis is:

H1: HbA1c levels will be lower after the intervention than before, or,

H1: $HbA1c_b > HbA1c_a$.

The test of the hypothesis, H0, just given, is carried out using the formula in Equation 9.13.

$$t = \frac{\bar{d}_{x_b - x_a}}{S.E._{\bar{d}}} \qquad (9.13)$$

where $\bar{d}_{x_b - x_a}$ is the mean difference between the before and after measures, $S.E._{\bar{d}}$ is the standard error of the differences, and the degrees of freedom are $n - 1$ where n is the number of difference scores.

A partial file of the data for this before and after *t* test is given in Figure 9.12. The figure shows the before-data measure in column A, the after-data measure in column B, and the difference between the before and after data measures in column C. The mean difference value is given in F2 as .24 and the standard error of the difference is given in F5. The *t* test is shown in F6 (its calculation is shown in the formula line at the top). The probability of the occurrence of a *t* value as large as that shown in F6 is given in F7, which is the =TDIST() function for the *t* value of 2.4, 39 degrees of freedom, and one tail (because the only result of interest is

FIGURE 9.12. CALCULATION OF BEFORE AND AFTER *t* TEST.

	F6	▼	= =F2/F5			
	A	B	C	D	E	F
1	Before	After	Difference			
2	7.97	8.10	-0.13		dbar	0.24
3	8.53	7.77	0.76		SD dbar	0.632652
4	8.27	8.20	0.07		n	40
5	8.40	8.67	-0.27		SE dbar	0.100031
6	8.23	7.72	0.51		t	2.406754
7	7.90	7.91	-0.01		Prob	0.010465
8	8.63	8.12	0.51			
9	8.56	7.48	1.08			
10	8.36	7.90	0.46			
11	7.92	8.84	-0.92			
12	8.86	8.46	0.40			

a result where after is less than before). The probability of getting a *t* value as large as 2.4 with a one-tail test is about .01, which means that we would reject the hypothesis that the HbA1c levels are equal before and after the intervention, and we would in fact accept the alternative, which is that HbA1c levels are lower after the intervention.

Excel Add-In for Related Data

Excel provides an add-in for a *t* test of the difference between related observations of this type. It is called *t* Test: Paired Two Sample for Means. The test is invoked precisely the same way as the *t* tests discussed in the fourth subsection of Section 9.2. When the test is invoked, the first screen that comes up is exactly like that shown in Figure 9.9. The *t* test that results from the data partially shown in Figure 9.12 is as that shown in Figure 9.13. That figure shows the mean before and the mean after, although these are not actually used in the calculation of the *t* test. It also shows the before and after variance, again not used in the *t* test. Also shown is a Pearson Correlation. The *t* statistic and the probability of *t* are the same as those given in Figure 9.12.

Exercises for Section 9.3

1. Use the data on the HbA1c worksheet in Chpt 9–2.xls.
   a. Replicate the results found in Figure 9.12.

FIGURE 9.13. EXCEL ADD-IN FOR BEFORE AND AFTER *t* TEST.

	A	B	C	D
1	t-Test: Paired Two Sample for Means			
2				
3		Before	After	
4	Mean	8.49075	8.25	
5	Variance	0.271474	0.196487	
6	Observations	40	40	
7	Pearson Correlation	0.146592		
8	Hypothesized Mean Difference	0		
9	df	39		
10	t Stat	2.406754		
11	P(T<=t) one-tail	0.010465		
12	t Critical one-tail	1.684875		
13	P(T<=t) two-tail	0.020929		
14	t Critical two-tail	2.022689		
15				

   b. Replicate the results in Figure 9.13 with the Excel add-in for before and after measures.

2. The data on the Weight spreadsheet of Chpt 9–2.xls represent the weight of twenty-five people who went on a prescribed diet at the beginning of a one-year time period. The Before weights are their weights at the start of the program and After are their weights one year later.

   a. Use the formula in Equation 9.13 to test the hypothesis that weight before equals weight after against the alternative that weight after is less than before, and indicate your conclusion.

   b. Use the Excel add-in for related data and replicate the results found in a.

3. A health payer is concerned about the time it takes a group of account assessors to process certain aspects of health care claims. They initiate a training program to reduce the time involved. Average processing time for a fixed set of claims is determined before and after the training program. The data are shown on the Time spreadsheet in Chpt 9–2.xls.

   a. Using the formula in Equation 9.13, test the hypothesis that processing time before and after training is the same against the alternative that processing time after is less than before, and indicate your conclusion.

   b. Use the Excel add-in for related data and replicate the results found in a.

CHAPTER TEN

ANALYSIS OF VARIANCE

The first chapter introduced several different questions that could be addressed using statistics. One of these was the question of whether eight hospitals in a hospital alliance differed from one another in length of stay, readmission rates, or cost per case. If we were interested in whether just two of the hospitals differed from one another, we could use a *t* test, which is a test of whether a numerical variable is independent of a categorical variable that takes on only two values. But in this case, the question is whether a numerical variable is independent of a categorical variable that may take on more than two values—here, eight. One statistical test that can be used to determine if a numerical variable is independent of a multilevel categorical variable is analysis of variance, commonly referred to as ANOVA.

Section 10.1 One-Way Analysis of Variance

To simplify the example somewhat, we are going to assume that there are only four hospitals in the alliance, although the principles would be the same for essentially any number of hospitals. Now if we were to examine the question of whether the four hospitals in the hospital alliance differed on the measures of length of stay, readmission rates, or cost per case, we could use one-way analysis of variance. With length of stay, it is possible that we could obtain all the data for each hospital—for example, for the last month or the last year or the last ten years.

This would be an overwhelming amount of data for an example. For readmission rates, we might be able to get all the data for each hospital as long as the readmission was to the same hospital. Coordinating among hospitals in the alliance or with hospitals outside the alliance would be more difficult. So, in the case of length of stay, we might have too much information, and in the case of readmissions, we might have too little. But with regard to cost per case, we might be just right.

Recall that Chapter Seven discussed the likelihood that cost per case is not really known. But with a not insignificant amount of effort, it is possible for a hospital CFO, for example, to get a good idea of cost per case for a relatively small random sample of hospital discharges. Let us assume that the head of the hospital alliance has arranged an agreement with the hospital CFOs that they will each select a random sample of thirty hospital discharges, and then, using accounting procedures commonly agreed to, they will determine the cost of each of the thirty discharges for each hospital. When they have finished, they will have a cost figure assigned to each discharge. Before discussing these specific hospital discharges, it is useful to spend a little time discussing what analysis of variance means in relation to the *t* test, with the average cost of hospital discharges as the subject.

If we were examining only the average cost of the discharges from two hospitals, what we would actually be examining with a *t* test could be characterized as shown in Figure 10.1. Figure 10.1 shows two distributions: one around a mean discharge cost of $5,700 and one around a mean discharge cost of $9,400. For the sake of this discussion, each of these distributions is assumed to have a standard

FIGURE 10.1. AVERAGE COST DISTRIBUTION FOR TWO HOSPITALS.

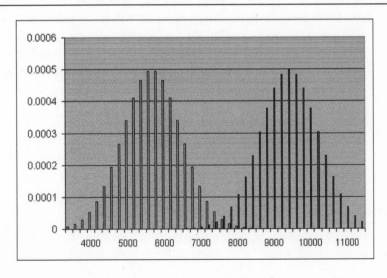

FIGURE 10.2. AVERAGE COST DISTRIBUTION FOR FOUR HOSPITALS.

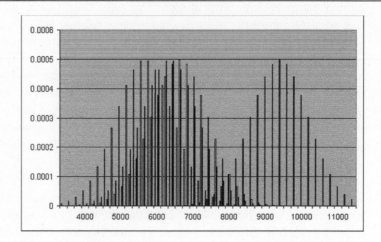

error of $800. The *t* test is a test of whether the two mean values, given their respective distributions, can be thought of as being different from one another. In the case of Figure 10.1, the *t* test would definitely indicate that these two means are different—or, more specifically, that the mean discharge cost is not independent of the hospital of discharge—because the two distributions overlap only slightly.

Analysis of variance examines essentially the same question, but for more than two levels of a categorical variable. Consider, for example the graph shown in Figure 10.2. Figure 10.2 shows the distribution around the average discharge cost for four hospitals, the lowest being $5,700, the next lowest being $6,300, the next lowest after that being $6,600, and the one with the largest average cost being $9,400. All of these hospitals are assumed to have equal standard errors of $800. Analysis of variance addresses the question of whether the average cost per discharge of any of the four hospitals can be seen as being different from any of the others, given the distributions of each of the average discharge rates. In the case of these four hospitals, it is quite likely that analysis of variance would show that their average costs per discharge are not all the same, particularly because there is little overlap between the distribution of the hospital with the highest average costs and that of the other three hospitals.

Equations for One-Way Analysis of Variance

So how is analysis of variance carried out? Analysis of variance depends on two pieces of information. The first of these is the *between group variance,* sometimes referred to as the explained variance, because it is associated with the differences between the groups—in this case, hospitals. The second is the *within group variance*, often referred to as the error variance, because it is a measure of the difference between the observations within the groups—in this case, hospitals—and cannot be accounted for by any information available to the analysis.

The between group variance (designated SS_B) is calculated as shown in Equation 10.1. Equation 10.1 indicates that the between group variance requires that the grand mean for all observations—in this case, the 120 observations from all four hospitals—be subtracted from the mean for each group—in this case, for each hospital, and then squared. The result for each hospital is then multiplied by the sample size from each hospital and summed across all m hospitals—here, four hospitals.

$$SS_B = \sum_{j=1}^{m} n_j (\bar{x}_j - \bar{\bar{x}})^2 \tag{10.1}$$

where m represents the number of separate groups, n_j designates the number of observations in each group, $\bar{x}_j$ designates the sample mean for group j, and $\bar{\bar{x}}$ designates the mean for all observations across all groups.

The within-group variance (designated SS_W) is calculated as shown in Equation 10.2. Equation 10.2 says that the mean cost for the sample from each hospital is subtracted from each separate observation for a specific hospital and squared. This result is summed over all observations for each group—hospital— and these results are then summed across all hospitals.

$$SS_W = \sum_{j=1}^{m} \sum_{i=1}^{nj} (x_{ij} - \bar{x}_j)^2 \tag{10.2}$$

Although the between-group variance SS_B and the within-group variance SS_W are all that are required for the calculation of the analysis of variance, it is useful to know the formula for the total variance (SS_T). This is useful because $SS_T = SS_B + SS_W$. If there is ever any doubt about whether your calculations have been carried out correctly, it is possible to calculate all three values and be sure that, in fact, $SS_T = SS_B + SS_W$. The formula for SS_T is shown in Equation 10.3. Equation 10.3 indicates that the grand mean for all observations is subtracted from each individual observation and that each of these results is squared. Then these are summed across all observations in each group and then across all groups.

$$SS_T = \sum_{j=1}^{m} \sum_{i=1}^{nj} (x_{ij} - \bar{\bar{x}})^2 \tag{10.3}$$

Calculation of One-Way Analysis of Variance for Four Hospitals

So, now, let us look at an example of the analysis of variance calculation, using Excel. The CFOs of four hospitals in the alliance—let us call them Albemarle Community, Beaufort Municipal, Catawba County, and Dare Regional—have agreed to select a random sample of thirty discharges and determine actual costs for these discharges. The data that they generated are contained in the file Chpt 10–1.xls, and the first fourteen observations are shown in Figure 10.3.

As should be clear from Figure 10.3, all of the first cost records (column C) are for a single hospital: Albemarle Community. The cost data for the other three hospitals are contained in the rows from 31 to 121. A discussion of the presentation in Figure 10.3 should begin with the Pivot Table in H2:I8. This Pivot Table shows the average cost for each hospital (cells I4:I7) and for all hospitals taken together (cell I8). The average cost per hospital and for all hospitals is obtained by changing Sum to Average in the Layout window for the Pivot Table (see Figure 4.22 in Chapter Four).

The computation of SS_T is contained in column D, which is labeled (C-Xbarbar)^2. This indicates that the overall average (designated $\bar{\bar{x}}$ in Equation 10.1 and Equation 10.3 and given as Xbarbar in the figure) is subtracted from the discharge cost figure in column C and then squared. The value of Xbarbar is taken from cell I8 in the pivot table. Each of the values in column D is summed in cell H11, labeled SS_T in cell G11. The formula for H11 is =SUM(D2:D121). Although SS_T is not part of the test of whether the four hospitals differ from one another, it is an important check of MS_B and MS_W.

The between-group variance, SS_B, is calculated in cells J4:J7 and summed in cell H12. The values in cells J4:J7 are calculated by subtracting the grand total mean in I8 from each of the hospital means in cells I4:I7, squaring the result, and

FIGURE 10.3. ANALYSIS OF VARIANCE FOR FOUR HOSPITALS.

	E2		=	=(C2-$I$4)^2							
	B	C	D	E	F	G	H	I	J	K	L
1	Hospital	Costs	(C-Xbarbar)^2	(C-Xbar^2)							
2	Albemarle	$5,342.61	2740146.377	1685779			Average of Costs				
3	Albemarle	$7,237.59	57427.9287	355936.7			Hospital ▼	Total	nj*(Xbar-Xbarbar)^2		
4	Albemarle	$11,801.95	23078428.01	26635553			Albemarle	6640.99	3822679		
5	Albemarle	$1,082.36	34994190.26	30898319			Beaufort	6253.90	16608450		
6	Albemarle	$2,379.59	21329237.54	18159493			Catawba	9380.71	1.7E+08		
7	Albemarle	$8,469.39	2165139.352	3343062			Dare	5716.21	49286011		
8	Albemarle	$4,453.55	6473964.999	4784875			Grand Total	6997.95			
9	Albemarle	$4,745.26	5074606.604	3593776							
10	Albemarle	$11,963.80	24659678.64	28332352			SS	df	MS	F	p
11	Albemarle	$5,294.96	2900170.683	1811785	SST	2726170568	119			
12	Albemarle	$2,965.55	16260239.68	13508827	SSB	240043485	3	80014495	3.7334	0.01323
13	Albemarle	$3,896.16	9621093.45	7534068	SSW	2486127083	116	21432130		
14	Albemarle	$6,074.21	853293.2783	321234.7		2726170568				
15	Albemarle	$7,217.18	48062.34098	331999.9							

multiplying by the number of observations for each hospital—in this case, thirty for each. The result is then summed in cell H12, the formula for which is =SUM(J4:J7). It might be mentioned that the 1.7E+08 in cell J6 is simply Excel's way of designating a number too large to display in the cell.

The within-group variance, SS_W, is calculated in column E and summed in H13. The formulas used by Excel to calculate the values in column E are shown in the formula bar. The individual hospital averages, given in cells I4:I7, are subtracted from the cost of the discharges for each hospital and squared to get the values in column E. The first thirty values in column E use the average for Albemarle Community; given in I4, the next thirty use the average for Beaufort Municipal, given in cell I5, and so on for the other two hospitals. The results of all these operations are summed in cell H13, labeled SS_W. The formula for cell H13 is =SUM(E2:E121). The value shown in H14 is the sum of cells H12 and H13, to verify that, indeed, SS_B and SS_W actually sum to SS_T.

The *F* Test for Differences in ANOVA

The test of whether hospital costs (a numerical variable) are independent of hospitals (a categorical variable that takes on four values) is an *F* test. The *F* test was discussed initially in Chapter Nine, where question was raised as to whether the variance of the numerical variable associated with a categorical variable that took on only two values was different for the two levels of the categorical variable. You will recall that if it was, then the *t* test assuming equal variance was not strictly appropriate (although in the case of equal-sized groups for each level of the categorical variable, it was probably adequate).

The use of the *F* test to determine the independence of hospital costs and hospital categories is similarly a test of variances. But, in this case, it is a test of whether the between-group variance—the variance that can be attributed to the differences between the hospitals—is large relative to the within-group variance. The within-group variance is variance that cannot be explained by information about the different hospitals, and it is considered error variance. But the *F* test of whether the between-group variance is large relative to the within-group variance is not directly a test of the relative size of SS_B and SS_W. If there are *m* different groups (in this case, four hospitals), then there are $m - 1$ degrees of freedom in SS_B. If there are n_j separate observations in each group (in this case, thirty cost figures for each hospital, although the number could be different for each hospital), then there are $n_1 - 1 + n_2 - 1 + \cdots + n_j - 1$ degrees of freedom in SS_W. In Figure 10.3, the degrees of freedom for SS_B and SS_W are shown in cells I12 and I13, respectively. The degrees of freedom for SS_T are given in cell I11. It is the total number of observations minus one, and it should always equal the sum of the degrees of freedom for SS_B and SS_W.

Cells J12 and J13 in Figure 10.3 show what is known as the mean square between groups and the mean square within groups, respectively. The mean square is found by dividing the between-group variance and the within-group variance by their respective degrees of freedom. The F test of whether the between-group variance is large relative to the within-group variance is actually calculated on the mean square values rather than on SS_B and SS_W. The formula for the F test is shown in Equation 10.4.

$$F = \frac{SS_B/df_{SS_B}}{SS_W/df_{SS_W}} = \frac{MS_B}{MS_W} \tag{10.4}$$

As Equation 10.4 shows, the F test is the mean square between groups divided by the mean square within groups. The result of this operation is shown in cell K12 in Figure 10.3. The value of the F is given as 3.7334. Now, of course, there arises the question of whether this F value is large or small. The probability of obtaining an F value as large as 3.7334 can be found with the =FDIST() function, which takes three arguments: the F value itself and the degrees of freedom in the numerator and in the denominator. The actual probability of this F value is given in cell L12 as .01323. The Excel function statement for that value is =FDIST(3.7334,3,116) but in the figure is actually stated as cell references K12, I12, and I13. What the probability value of .01323 says is that there is a very low probability of getting an F value as large as 3.7334 (actually, only about one time in a hundred sets of samples) if cost and hospital are actually independent of one another. In consequence, we would conclude that cost is not independent of the hospitals and that the hospitals do, in fact, differ in their costs.

Excel Add-In for One-Way Analysis of Variance

Now that we have examined one-way analysis of variance as calculated with the Excel spreadsheet operations, we can turn to the calculation of analysis of variance by using the Excel ANOVA Single-Factor Data Analysis add-in. The data for the Excel single factor ANOVA must be arranged differently from the data shown in Figure 10.3. The data must be arranged in columns, each column representing a single group-in this case, a single hospital. The first fourteen discharge costs for each of the four hospitals is shown in Figure 10.4, arranged in four columns. You will note that the data for Albemarle shown in the figure are the same as those shown in Figure 10.4.

By selecting Tools/Data Analysis and ANOVA: Single-Factor, the window shown in Figure 10.5, will come up. This window requests the same type of

FIGURE 10.4. DATA ARRANGEMENT FOR EXCEL SINGLE-FACTOR ANOVA ADD-IN.

	A	B	C	D
1	Albemarle	Beaufort	Catawba	Dare
2	$5,342.61	$6,844.89	$5,455.73	$1,035.75
3	$7,237.59	$6,283.80	$4,448.48	$6,130.58
4	$11,801.95	$5,206.09	$8,996.80	$2,584.28
5	$1,082.36	$22,030.51	$4,734.98	$2,635.85
6	$2,379.59	$5,372.86	$13,055.10	$5,371.03
7	$8,469.39	$2,197.14	$10,194.42	$14,433.99
8	$4,453.55	$13,472.69	$16,229.83	$2,283.88
9	$4,745.26	$8,486.18	$7,099.69	$3,630.39
10	$11,963.80	$2,447.01	$5,948.36	$4,775.36
11	$5,294.96	$19,182.24	$4,155.38	$6,084.66
12	$2,965.55	$10,021.34	$14,470.90	$1,414.80
13	$3,896.16	$1,594.57	$4,957.09	$6,630.33
14	$6,074.21	$4,412.80	$5,040.75	$5,139.11
15	$7,217.18	$7,000.21	$4,113.04	$16,346.71

FIGURE 10.5. WINDOW FOR ANOVA: SINGLE-FACTOR.

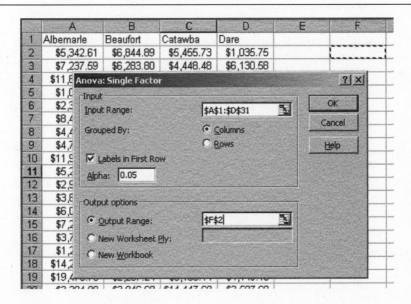

FIGURE 10.6. ANOVA: SINGLE-FACTOR OUTPUT.

	F	G	H	I	J	K	L
1							
2	Anova: Single Factor						
3							
4	SUMMARY						
5	Groups	Count	Sum	Average	Variance		
6	Albemarle	30	199229.6	6640.99	21757799		
7	Beaufort	30	187616.9	6253.90	24442189		
8	Catawba	30	281421.3	9380.71	23920882		
9	Dare	30	171486.2	5716.21	15607649		
10							
11							
12	ANOVA						
13	Source of Variation	SS	df	MS	F	P-value	F crit
14	Between Groups	240043485	3	80014495	3.73339	0.0132334	2.68281
15	Within Groups	2486127083	116	21432130			
16							
17	Total	2726170568	119				

information that most of the data analysis add-in windows do. The Input range is the data to be used in the analysis and includes all cells A1:D31. This includes all 120 observations. Because the data are arranged in columns by hospital, the Grouped by Columns circle is selected. The Labels in the first row box is checked to indicate that the names of the hospitals are in cells A1, B1, C1, and D1. The circle in Output Range indicates that the output will be in the same spreadsheet, beginning in cell F2.

Figure 10.6 shows the output of the ANOVA: Single-Factor data analysis add-in. As indicated in the output range in Figure 10.5, the analysis output begins in cell F2. Cells F6:F9 show the four hospitals. C6:G9 is the number of observations for each hospital. H6:H9 is the sum of costs for each hospital, and I6:I9 is the average cost for each. The variance in cells J6:J9 is calculated by the standard variance formula given in Chapter Six, Equation 6.3. An alternative way of calculating the within-group variance would be to multiply each of the variance numbers by the degrees of freedom for each hospital (29) and sum them. This produces the same number as that shown in cell G15 as the within groups sums of squares. Cells G14, G15, and G17 show the between groups, within groups, and total sums of squares, respectively. You may note that these are the same values obtained in Figure 10.3 by our calculations. The mean square values in cells H14 and H15, which represent the sums of squares divided by the appropriate degrees of freedom, are also the same as those calculated in Figure 10.3, as are the F test value and the probability of the F.

The additional information in Figure 10.6 is the number in cell L14 titled F crit, which stands for F critical. F crit is the value that must be reached by the F test (the division of MS_B by MS_W) in order to be at the .95 level of confidence. The value of F crit can be obtained with the Excel function =FINV(). The function =FINV() takes three arguments, the level of significance (in this case, .05), and the degrees of freedom in MS_B and MS_W. The F crit statement that produces the value in cell L14 is =FINV(.05,3,116).

The F test as discussed thus far provides a way to determine if a numerical variable treated as dependent is actually independent of a categorical variable that takes on more than two values. Why could the same F test not be used if the categorical variable takes on only two values, thus eliminating the need for the t test? The answer is that it could, but the t test has at least one advantage over the F test. The F test is always a two-tail test. There is no equivalent to the one-tail t test for the F test. In consequence, the t test remains useful if the categorical variable in question takes on only two values.

Where Do the Differences Lie in ANOVA?

The interpretation of the F test in either Figure 10.3 or Figure 10.6 is that at least one among the four hospitals under consideration is different from at least one other hospital in average cost. This is not a conclusion about the thirty sample observations from each hospital but rather a conclusion about all the discharges from the hospitals, assuming that the thirty discharges studied were drawn at random from all discharges. But determining that at least one hospital differs from at least one other is not the most satisfactory outcome. It might be pretty easy to decide that Catawba County hospital has higher costs (an average of $9,380.71 per discharge) than Dare Regional (an average of only $5,716.21). But what do we decide about Beaufort Municipal (at $6,253.90)? Does it have lower costs than Catawba, or higher costs than Dare? These questions cannot be answered directly by ANOVA, but they can be answered by several different statistical tests. Unfortunately for the users of Excel, most of these tests rely on something called the studentized range statistic, which is often designated q_r. Excel does not provide probability distributions for the studentized range statistic, so this section will discuss a technique provided by Winer (1962). This technique can provide a direct comparison between each hospital and every other hospital, and the result can be interpreted using the F distribution for which Excel does provide exact probabilities.

In discussing this statistical technique, it will be referred to as the test of differences between two means in ANOVA. It could equally be used to test one mean in comparison with all other means or two means in comparison with two others, but this discussion will concentrate only on the test of two means at a time. The formula for this test is given in Equation 10.5.

$$F = \frac{(\bar{x}_1 - \bar{x}_2)^2 / \left(\dfrac{1}{n_1} + \dfrac{1}{n_2}\right)}{MS_W}$$

(10.5)

where $\bar{x}_1$ is the mean of the first group to be compared, $\bar{x}_2$ is the mean of the second, and n_1 and n_2 are the respective sizes of the two samples. MS_W is the mean square within groups taken from the original F test.

Equation 10.5 results in an F test with 1 degree of freedom in the numerator and degrees of freedom for MS_W (the mean square error) in the denominator. We can use this F test to determine which of the four hospitals is different from the others. If we do so, there will be six comparisons, as shown in Figure 10.7. Figure 10.7 shows each hospital in cells F22:F25. They have been reordered with the lowest-average-cost hospital listed first. Cells G22:G25 give the average cost per discharge for each hospital. The hospitals have been listed again in cells H20:K20, with their average costs given in H21:K21. Incidentally, the hospitals and their costs in cells H20:K21 were generated by copying F22:G25 and the using Paste Special/Transpose in cell H20. The six meaningful hospital costs comparisons are given in the cells above and to the right of the main diagonal of the resulting table. These six comparisons contrast each hospital with every other hospital.

FIGURE 10.7. TEST OF DIFFERENCES BETWEEN TWO MEANS IN ANOVA.

I22		=	=((I$21-$G22)^2/(1/30+1/30))/$I$15		
	F	G	H	I	J	K
20			Dare	Beaufort	Albemarle	Catawba
21			5716.21	6253.90	6640.99	9380.71
22	Dare	5716.21		0.202344	0.598554	9.3984502
23	Beaufort	6253.90			0.10487	6.8427353
24	Albemarle	6640.99				5.2533851
25	Catawba	9380.71				
26						
27			Dare	Beaufort	Albemarle	Catawba
28			5716.21	6253.90	6640.99	9380.71
29	Dare	5716.21		0.653675	0.440704	**0.002702**
30	Beaufort	6253.90			0.746645	0.0100837
31	Albemarle	6640.99				0.0237078
32	Catawba	9380.71				
33						
34		F Prob	0.008512			

The data in the first table represent the calculation of the formula given in Equation 10.5. The formula bar gives the calculation for the cell I22, which is a comparison between Dare Regional and Beaufort Municipal. The dollar sign convention as given in the formula bar allows the formula for cell I22 to be copied to the other five cells to produce the result for each comparison. The fact that the sample size is the same for each hospital makes the term $(1/30 + 1/30)$ appropriate for each comparison. The last term, \$I\$15, refers to the mean square within groups (MS_W), given in cell I15 in Figure 10.6.

The second table in Figure 10.7 is the probability of the F value given in the first table. As you can see, the probability of an F as large as the .2023 in I22 is given in that table as .6537. This means that if the average cost for Dare Regional and Beaufort Municipal were actually the same, an F value as large as .2023 would be obtained from the formula in Equation 10.5 about 65 percent of the time. Since our alpha level throughout this book is assumed to be 5 percent, we would clearly not reject the null hypothesis that costs per discharge for Dare and Beaufort are the same. But what do we conclude, for example, about Beaufort Municipal and Catawba County hospitals? In that case, the probability of the F value as large as 6.843 is about .01. Should we reject the null hypothesis that the two hospitals are no different in average costs per discharge? The answer is probably not, which needs a little explanation.

In comparing each of the hospitals with every other hospital, six comparisons are made. And when a large number of comparisons are made following a significant overall F, the overall probability of alpha (α) increases. If we conduct six tests, the overall probability of alpha for all six tests will be $1 - (1 - \alpha)$.[6] If the initial alpha is .05, this produces an overall probability for all six tests of about .26. Thus, if we conduct six tests, there is about one chance in four that a difference large enough to reject the null hypothesis at the .05 level will occur *when we should not reject the null hypothesis*. We run the risk of making the type I error about one-fourth of the time.

To protect against this inflation in the true value of alpha over six tests, we can reduce the actual probability level at which we will reject the null hypothesis by the result of the formula shown in Equation 10.6. In that equation, α_{Adj} is the adjusted value of alpha, and c represents the number of comparisons being made. Whereas taking the cth root of $1 - \alpha$ would be a daunting task if it were being done with paper and pencil, happily, Excel can take a cth root with very little difficulty. The F probability that provides an overall .05 level for alpha for all six tests taken together is given in cell H34 in Figure 10.7. This value is calculated using the Excel formula statement $=1-(1-.05)\wedge(1/6)$, which is the Excel equivalent for Equation 10.6 when alpha is .05 and c is 6. Based on this adjusted alpha for all six tests, we would conclude that only one comparison leads us to reject the null hypothesis of no difference. This is the comparison shown in bold in Figure 10.7—namely, that between Catawba County and Dare Regional. In other words, Catawba's costs are different from those of Dare, but no other average discharge costs are different. With this in mind, the significant F value obtained in both Figure 10.3 and Figure 10.6 is a function of the difference between Catawba and Dare.

$$\alpha_{\text{Adj}} = 1 - \sqrt[c]{1 - \alpha} \qquad (10.6)$$

It would not always be necessary to make all possible two-group or two-hospital comparisons following a significant overall F. In some cases, it may be sufficient simply to know that there is an overall difference and that the test of differences between hospitals could be ignored. In other cases, it might be decided before the fact that if there are significant overall differences, it is because one group, such as Catawba County hospital, has greater costs than all the other three. In such a case, it would be reasonable to test Catawba against the other three only. This would result in only three comparisons, and the level of α_{Adj} would be, as expressed in Excel, $=1-(1-.05)^\wedge(1/3)=.017$.

Like the first t test discussed in Chapter Nine, the analysis of variance discussed here assumes equal variance across groups. There are several tests of the homogeneity of variance across groups, but the one discussed here is called the Bartlett test. The Bartlett test is a chi-square test and is carried out with the formula given in Equation 10.7. The formula in Equation 10.7 is somewhat imposing, but, in practice, it is easily calculated using Excel. The result of the calculation is shown in Figure 10.8.

$$\chi^2 = \frac{2.303}{c} \left(df_{MS_W} \log MS_W - \sum_{j=1}^{m} df_{G_j} \log s_{G_j}^2 \right) \qquad (10.7)$$

$$\text{where } c = 1 + \frac{1}{3(m-1)} \left(\sum \frac{1}{df_{G_j}} - \frac{1}{df_{MS_W}} \right)$$

Figure 10.8 replicates a part of the ANOVA output shown in Figure 10.6. The calculation of the Bartlett test is given in columns K and L. Cells K6:K9 represent the degrees of freedom in each group (cells G6:G9, respectively, minus 1, or 29) times the log of the variance (cells J6:J9). These results are summed in K10, which represents the term $\sum_{j=1}^{m} df_{G_j} \log s_{G_j}^2$ in Equation 10.7. Cells L6:L9 are 1 divided by the degrees of freedom in each group, and cell L10 is the sum of these, representing the term $\sum 1/df_{G_j}$ in the calculation of the term c. Cell K15 is cell H15, multiplied by the log of cell I15, and cell L15 is 1 divided by cell H15.

FIGURE 10.8. BARTLETT TEST FOR HOMOGENEITY OF VARIANCE.

	F	G	H	I	J	K	L
1							
2	Anova: Single Factor						
3							
4	SUMMARY						
5	Groups	Count	Sum	Average	Variance	df*log(Var)	1/df
6	Albemarle	30	199229.6	6640.99	21757799	212.79083	0.034483
7	Beaufort	30	187616.9	6253.90	24442189	214.25606	0.034483
8	Catawba	30	281421.3	9380.71	23920882	213.98454	0.034483
9	Dare	30	171486.2	5716.21	15607649	208.60679	0.034483
10						849.63822	0.137931
11							
12	ANOVA						
13	Source of Variation	SS	df	MS	F		
14	Between Groups	240043485	3	80014495	3.73339		
15	Within Groups	2486127083	116	21432130		850.40358	0.008621
16							0.111111
17	Total	2726170568	119			c	1.014368
18						Chi Square	1.737648
19						p	0.628596

Cell L16 is the result of the calculation of $1/(3 \times (m - 1))$, where m is the number of groups being compared. The calculated value of c is shown in L17 and the calculated chi-square value is shown in L18. This chi-square statistic has $m - 1$, or 3 degrees of freedom. The probability value for a chi-square of 1.738 is given in L19 and was found using the =CHIDIST() function. The actual Excel statement is =CHIDIST(1.738,3). The interpretation of the Bartlett test is this. If the variances of the four hospitals is in fact the same—that is, the null hypothesis is true, we would expect to find a chi-square value as large as 1.738 about 60 percent of the times we drew samples of size 30 from each of the four hospitals and conducted the Bartlett test. Since the likelihood of finding a chi-square value as large as 1.738 is so high, we will conclude that, in fact, the variances are the same.

The Bartlett test is one way of testing for the homogeneity of variance between the groups compared in ANOVA, but it is not an essential part of the ANOVA process. When variances differ across the groups in the order of magnitude—for example, of 1 to 3 (that is, the variance of one group is three times as large as the variance of a another), the results of ANOVA will not be greatly affected. Unless differences across the groups exceed the level of 1 to 3, ANOVA can be used with confidence.

Before leaving the one-way analysis of variance, it is important to comment on sample sizes. In the example given, all four hospitals contributed an equal number of observations—thirty—to the analysis. In many cases, it is not possible to obtain an equal number of observations for each group. In such a situation, everything that was discussed earlier in regard to ANOVA continues to apply. It is simply necessary to ensure that the appropriate number is used for n_j and for degrees of freedom for each group.

Exercises for Section 10.1

1. Use the data on the Costs worksheet of Chpt 10–1.xls and replicate the calculations in Figure 10.3.
   a. Use a pivot table and the formula in Equation 10.1 to calculate the between-group sums of squares (SS_B) for the costs in the four hospitals.
   b. Use the results of the pivot table from a and the formula in Equation 10.2 to calculate the within groups sums of squares (SS_W) for the costs in the four hospitals.
   c. Use the formula in Equation 10.3 to calculate the total sums of squares (SS_T) for the costs in the four hospitals.
   d. Determine the appropriate degrees of freedom and use the formula in Equation 10.4 to calculate the F value for a test of the null hypothesis that the mean costs in the four hospitals are all the same.
   e. Use the =FDIST() function to obtain the probability of the F value and draw the appropriate conclusion in regard to the null hypothesis.

2. The data on the Education worksheet of Chpt 10–1.xls represent the score received by three groups of women on a 20-point knowledge assessment of breast cancer risk following a visit to a breast cancer screening clinic. Persons 1 through 15 received no information, persons 16 through 30 received a pamphlet, and persons 31 through 45 received a brief face-to-face discourse on breast cancer risk from a physician. (The women were randomly selected— each to one of the three groups, and all received the face-to-face encounter with the physician following the experiment.)
   a. Use a pivot table and the formula in Equation 10.1 to calculate the between-group sums of squares (SS_B) for the three groups of women.
   b. Use the results of the pivot table from a and the formula in Equation 10.2 to calculate the within groups sums of squares (SS_W) for the three groups of women.
   c. Use the formula in Equation 10.3 to calculate the total sums of squares (SS_T) for the three groups of women.
   d. Determine the appropriate degrees of freedom and use the formula in Equation 10.4 to calculate the F value for a test of the null hypothesis that the mean knowledge score of the three groups of women are all the same.
   e. Use the =FDIST() function to obtain the probability of the F value and draw the appropriate conclusion in regard to the null hypothesis.

3. On a fresh spreadsheet, rearrange the data on the Costs worksheet of Chpt 10–1.xls into four columns, as shown in Figure 10.4.
   a. Use the Excel ANOVA: Single-Factor Data Analysis add-in to carry out the analysis of variance.
   b. Confirm that the results are the same as those obtained in Exercise 1.

4. On a fresh spreadsheet, rearrange the data on the Education worksheet of Chpt 10–1.xls into three columns, each column representing one of each of the three groups of women in Exercise 2.
   a. Use the Excel ANOVA: Single-Factor Data Analysis add-in to carry out the analysis of variance.
   b. Confirm that the results are the same as those obtained in Exercise 2.

5. Lay out a worksheet like the one shown in Figure 10.7 and replicate that figure for the data from the Costs worksheet of Chpt 10–1.xls.
   a. Use the formula in Equation 10.5 to calculate the F value for the difference between each hospital and every other.
   b. Use the formula in Equation 10.6 to calculate the adjusted value of alpha for the six comparisons.

6. Lay out a worksheet following the example in Figure 10.7 and make the comparison for the three groups from the Education worksheet of Chpt 10–1.xls
   a. Use the formula in Equation 10.5 to calculate the F value for the difference between each education group.
   b. Use the formula in Equation 10.6 to calculate the adjusted value of alpha for the three comparisons.

7. Lay out a worksheet like the one shown in Figure 10.8 and replicate the Bartlett test for homogeneity of variance, as shown in that figure, using the formula in Equation 10.7.

8. Lay out a worksheet following the example in Figure 10.8 and conduct the Bartlett test for homogeneity of variance, using the formula in Equation 10.7, and decide whether the null hypothesis of equal variance should be accepted or rejected.

Section 10.2 ANOVA for Repeated Measures

There were two essentially different types of t test discussed in Chapter Nine. The first of these was a t test for differences between two unrelated groups. One-way analysis of variance is the multiple group extension of that t test. The second was the t test for a single group measured two times. The extension of that test is ANOVA for repeated measures. In this case, there is one group of people, or of organizations, that are measured on some variable more than two times. The primary question is, is there is any difference between the several measurements?

One of the questions that is of concern to the hospital alliance has to do with the cost of readmissions. In particular, it is suspected that the later admissions in a string of readmissions for the same person are likely to be more expensive than the earlier admissions. Although it is not always easy to track readmissions, particularly if they are at different hospitals, one of the hospitals in the alliance has been able to put together a list of several hundred people who were admitted to any one of the hospitals at least three times in the last three years. They have selected a random sample of twelve of these people and have determined the actual cost of each admission. The question then is, do these costs differ from admission to admission? If we were considering only a single readmission, it would be possible to use the *t* test for related data, comparing the mean for the first admission with the mean for the second. Since we are considering three admissions, it is more appropriate to use analysis of variance for repeated measures. It might also be pointed out that twelve people is a very small sample. Thirty people would be better. But thirty people would make an example that would take up too much spreadsheet space to be easily shown in tables in this text.

In considering analysis of variance for repeated measures, the total variation in the data (SS_T) can be divided into the variation between people—or between groups—(SS_B) and the variation within people or groups (SS_W). In general, differences that may exist between people or groups (SS_B) are not of interest to us. Rather, we are interested in the differences within people or groups (SS_W). In the example discussed here, differences within people are differences that may reflect different costs of hospital stays, depending on which admission is being considered. But SS_W can also be divided into two sources of variation, variation due to the differences in costs of first, second, or third admissions (SS_A) and that variation cannot be explained by whether the admission is first, second, or third. This last variation is generally referred to as residual variation (SS_R).

The formula for the variation within people (or groups) is given in Equation 10.8. Equation 10.8 says that the mean for each person or group i, $\bar{x}_i$, is subtracted from each observation for the person or group. The result is squared and summed over all people. In the example under discussion here, each person was admitted three times to the hospital. The average cost of all three admissions is subtracted from the cost of each and is then squared. And then each of these three values is summed over all twelve people.

$$SS_W = \sum_{j=1}^{m} \sum_{i=1}^{n} (x_{ij} - \bar{x}_i)^2 \qquad (10.8)$$

where m is the number of different measurements.

FIGURE 10.9. DATA FOR ANOVA FOR REPEATED MEASURES.

D2			=	=(C2-$H$4)^2					
	A	B	C	D	E	F	G	H	I
1	Person	Admt	Cost	SSW	SST				
2	1	1	$2,319.69	1282669.50	4812620.72		Average of Cost		
3	1	2	$2,898.01	307170.89	2609674.22		Person	Total	
4	1	3	$5,139.02	2845226.77	391327.05			1	3452.24	1126185
5	2	1	$4,193.34	19032.04	102475.93			2	4331.30	33182.97
6	2	2	$3,243.61	1183062.28	1612515.50			3	5036.12	273171.4
7	2	3	$5,556.94	1502201.58	1088853.41			4	5491.03	955645.8
8	3	1	$2,508.31	6389806.54	4020620.95			5	2814.97	2884864
9	3	2	$4,244.97	625913.05	72086.13			6	2673.46	3385607
10	3	3	$8,355.07	11015451.23	14757978.06			7	6388.47	3515668
11	4	1	$7,088.50	2551910.40	6630838.15			8	4504.25	84.85992
12	4	2	$4,932.22	312268.62	175361.10			9	7099.32	6686679
13	4	3	$4,452.37	1078814.60	3731.82			10	5705.89	1421885
14	5	1	$1,786.17	1058429.44	7438103.17			11	3348.01	1358278
15	5	2	$3,140.76	106139.12	1884301.48			12	3316.46	1432798
16	5	3	$3,517.98	494223.06	990977.67		Grand Total	4513.46	
17	6	1	$4,413.98	3029421.47	9895.99				
18	6	2	$1,599.82	1152695.69	8489289.96		Average of Cost		
19	6	3	$2,006.57	444737.83	6284490.51		Admt	Total	
20	7	1	$6,767.15	143398.54	5079124.88			1	3898.89	377693.6
21	7	2	$2,713.24	13507315.55	3240787.05			2	3926.92	344022.7
22	7	3	$9,685.02	10867241.90	26745047.20			3	5714.56	1442647
23	8	1	$2,519.60	3938822.39	3975472.16		Grand Total	4513.46	
24	8	2	$7,210.54	7324023.61	7274248.02				

The initial calculation of SS_W can be seen in column D in Figure 10.9. Figure 10.9 shows an ID number for each person in the sample in column A and the number of the admission in column B. All admissions for the first seven people are shown in the figure. The data in the spreadsheet depicted in the figure actually occupy the first thirty-seven rows of the spreadsheet. Column C is the cost of each admission for each person. Column D is the initial calculation of SS_W.

The Excel formula used for the calculation is given in the formula bar in Figure 10.9. This formula indicates that the value in cell H4 was subtracted from C2. The value in H4 is the mean cost for person 1, which was obtained using the Pivot Table function and the average option. The dollar sign convention in D2 allows that formula to be copied to D3 and D4. Unfortunately, the calculation of SS_W is a little tedious, requiring that the $H$4 reference be changed to $H$5 for person 2, $H$6 for person 3, and so on. The result of the calculation of SS_W is shown in cell L4 in Figure 10.10. As the formula bar in that figure shows, SS_W is the sum of cells D2:D37 from Figure 10.9.

SS_A, which is the variation due to differences in admission costs, is calculated from the formula in Equation 10.9. Equation 10.9 indicates that SS_A is calculated by subtracting the grand mean from the mean for each admission

FIGURE 10.10. ANOVA REPEATED MEASURES RESULTS.

	L4	▼	= =SUM(D2:D37)		
	K	L	M	N	O	P
1						
2		SS	df	MS	F	p
3	SSB	69222144.55	11			
4	SSW	105175766.54	24			
5	SSA	25972353.07	2	12986177	3.607116	0.044168
6	SSR	79203413.47	22	3600155		
7						
8	SST	174397911.09	35			
9						
10		174397911.09				

(in this case, for example, as there are twelve people, there will be twelve first admissions averaged, and then twelve second and twelve third). Because this is a repeated measures ANOVA, n refers to the number of people or groups measured. There are n, or twelve, people observed in this case, but mn, or thirty-six, total admissions. The squared value for the m, or three, admissions is then summed and multiplied by the number of people in the study, or twelve. The result of this calculation is given in cell L5 in Figure 10.10.

$$SS_A = n \sum_{j=1}^{m} (\bar{x}_j - \bar{\bar{x}})^2 \tag{10.9}$$

The residual variation, SS_R, is the difference between SS_W and SS_A. It is shown for this example in cell L6 in Figure 10.10. In cell L6, SS_R was actually calculated by $SS_W - SS_A$. The formula for SS_R is somewhat complicated but is as shown in Equation 10.10. Equation 10.10 says that for each observation in the data set-in this case, twelve times three, or thirty-six, the mean across all three admission for each person $\bar{x}_i$, and the mean across all twelve people for each admission $\bar{x}_j$, are each subtracted from the individual observation corresponding to each of these means. The grand mean across all observations is added to this value and the result is squared. Then this figure is added across all thirty-six admissions.

$$SS_R = \sum_{j=1}^{m} \sum_{i=1}^{n} (x_{ij} - \bar{x}_i - \bar{x}_j + \bar{\bar{x}})^2 \tag{10.10}$$

The calculation of SS_R using the formula in Equation 10.10 is shown in Figure 10.11. The Excel statement for the term for SS_R corresponding to the first admission for the first person is shown in the formula bar for cell F2. D2 was taken from cell H4 in Figure 10.9 and E2 was taken from cell H20. The grand mean,

FIGURE 10.11. CALCULATION OF SS_R.

F2	▼	=	=(C2-D2-E2+$F$1)^2		
	A	B	C	D	E	F
	Person	Admt	Cost	Xbari	Xbarj	4513.46
1	Person	Admt	Cost	Xbari	Xbarj	4513.46
2	1	1	$2,319.69	3452.24	3898.89	268305.58
3	1	2	$2,898.01	3452.24	3926.92	1043.58
4	1	3	$5,139.02	3452.24	5714.56	235882.90
5	2	1	$4,193.34	4331.30	3898.89	227158.15
6	2	2	$3,243.61	4331.30	3926.92	251153.55
7	2	3	$5,556.94	4331.30	5714.56	602.27
8	3	1	$2,508.31	5036.12	3898.89	3660483.05
9	3	2	$4,244.97	5036.12	3926.92	41866.16
10	3	3	$8,355.07	5036.12	5714.56	4485293.33

which is given in cell F1, was taken from cell H16 in Figure 10.9. As the formula bar shows, the value in D2 and the value in E2 are each subtracted from C2. The grand mean in F1 is added to this total and the result is squared. The sum of column F (excluding the mean in F1) is not shown, but it is exactly equal to the value shown for SS_R in cell L6 in Figure 10.10.

Although the between-person variance SS_B and the total variance SS_T do not enter into the calculation of the F test, it is useful to know how they are derived. The formula for SS_T is exactly the same as the formula for SS_T for one-way ANOVA, which is shown in Equation 10.3, except that n_j will be only n, since, with repeated measures on the same people or groups, the number of observations for each measurement will always be the same. The formula for SS_B is shown in Equation 10.11.

$$SS_B = m \sum_{i=1}^{n} (\bar{x}_i - \bar{\bar{x}})^2 \qquad (10.11)$$

The initial steps in the calculation of both SS_T and SS_B are shown in Figure 10.9. SS_T is shown in column E and summed in cell L8 in Figure 10.10. The part within the parentheses for SS_B is calculated in cells I4:I115 in Figure 10.9, and the sum of those cells is multiplied by measurements (3) in cell L3 in Figure 10.10.

The degrees of freedom in repeated measures of ANOVA are given for this example in column M in Figure 10.10. The degrees of freedom for SS_B will always be $n - 1$. Degrees of freedom for SS_W will always be $n(m - 1)$. These, together, add to the degrees of freedom for SS_T, $nm - 1$. The degrees of freedom for SS_A,

FIGURE 10.12. DEGREES OF FREEDOM IN REPEATED MEASURES.

	K	L
16	SSB	n-1
17	SSW	n(m-1)
18	SSA	m-1
19	SSR	(n-1)(m-1)
20	SST	nm-1

$m - 1$, and the degrees of freedom for SS_R, $(n - 1)(m - 1)$, add together to the degrees of freedom for SS_W. These respective degrees of freedom are shown in Figure 10.12.

The F test for the differences between the costs of admissions is the mean square, due to admissions, MS_A, divided by the mean square residual MS_R. These are shown in cells N5 and N6, respectively, in Figure 10.10. The result of the division is shown in cell O5 in Figure 10.10. In cell P5 is given the probability of the F value. This figure, .044, says that if there were no difference in the cost of admissions across the three separate admissions considered, the probability of finding an F value as large as 3.6 would be about four chances out of one hundred samples. Because the likelihood is so small under the null hypothesis of no difference, it is concluded that the cost of admission is not independent of whether the admission is a first time, a first readmission (second admission), or a second readmission (third admission).

Where Do Observed Differences Lie?

Just as with the one-way analysis of variance, it is possible to consider, with the repeated measures design, where the differences between measures (in this case, admissions) might lie. The F test is again a test of the squared difference between two means—in this case, the mean cost of any admission. The formula for the F test is given in Equation 10.12. Equation 10.12 is a modification of Equation 10.5 that recognizes the fact that n is the same for each group and that the error mean square is designated mean square residual (MS_R). As with Equation 10.5, $\bar{x}_1$ refers to the mean of the first group in the comparison and $\bar{x}_2$ refers to the mean of the second. This F test has 1 degree of freedom in the numerator and degrees of freedom equal to that of MS_R in the denominator.

$$F = \frac{(\bar{x}_1 - \bar{x}_2)^2 / \frac{2}{n}}{MS_R}$$

(10.12)

FIGURE 10.13. COMPARISON ACROSS THREE ADMISSIONS.

J29	▼	=	=((J$28-$H29)^2/(2/12))/$N$6	
	G	H	I	J	K
27	Admission		1	2	3
28			3898.89	3926.92	5714.56
29		1	3898.89	0	0.00131	5.494192
30		2	3926.92		0	5.325845
31		3	5714.56			0
32					
33	Admission		1	2	3
34			3898.89	3926.92	5714.56
35		1	3898.89		0.971457	0.028519
36		2	3926.92			0.030798
37		3	5714.56			
38					
39	p		0.017		

In the case of the cost of the three admissions to the hospital, there could be three comparisons: that between admission 1 and admission 2, that between admission 1 and admission 3, and that between admission 2 and admission 3. The comparison across the three admissions is shown in Figure 10.13. The F test is shown as calculated in cells J29, K29, and K30. The formula for the F test as reproduced in Excel is shown in the formula bar for cell J29. Again, the use of the dollar sign convention, as given in the formula bar, allows the contents of the cell J29 to be copied to the other two cells directly. Cells J35, K35, and K36 show the probability of the F value given in the first three cells mentioned. Clearly, there is no difference between admission 1 and admission 2, with a p value of .971. However, admission 3 appears to be different in cost from both 1 and 2, with p values of .028 and .030. But since we have conducted three tests, the adjusted p value in H39 gives an overall level of .05 for all three tests, based on the formula in Equation 10.6. This says that for an overall level of .05 for all three tests, we have to have a level of .017 for any individual test. This leaves us with the anomalous result that we have found a significant overall F, but with any of the three individual comparisons, we do not find significant F values. Although this is anomalous, it is not uncommon, especially if one is using the stringent criteria of the adjusted alpha level. From a practical standpoint, since there is a significant overall F value, and as the third admission is clearly more costly that the first two, it is appropriate in this case to consider the statistically significant difference to lie with the difference between the first two admissions and the third.

Excel Add-In for Analysis of Variance with Repeated Measures

Excel does not provide a specific add-in for analysis of variance with repeated measures when there is only one group under consideration (in this case, the one group is the twelve people, each of whom was admitted to the hospital three times). Excel does provide a repeated measures ANOVA when there is more than one group and more than one measure on each group. This is later (in Section 10.3) discussed as what is known as a factorial design.

Exercises for Section 10.2

1. Use the data given on the Readmit worksheet of Chpt 10–1.xls to replicate the analysis of cost of readmissions shown in Figure 10.9 and Figure 10.10.
   a. Calculate SS_W—the variation within people, using the Pivot Table with person as the row variable (the pivot table should match that in cells G2:H16 in Figure 10.9) and the formula in Equation 10.8.
   b. Calculate SS_A—the variation due to differences in admission costs, using the Pivot Table with admission as the row variable (the pivot table should match that in cells G18:H23 in Figure 10.9) and the formula in Equation 10.9.
   c. Calculate SS_R—the residual variation—on a separate worksheet, using the formula in Equation 10.10, and confirm that it is equal to $SS_W - SS_A$.
   d. Calculate SS_B—the variation between people, using the Pivot Table in G2:H16 in Figure 10.9 and the formula in Equation 10.11.
   e. Calculate SS_T—the total variation, following the formula in Equation 10.3.
   f. Replicate the calculation of the F test statistic for the effect of readmission on cost, following the example in Figure 10.10.
   g. Use the formula in Equation 10.12 to replicate the results of the test of individual differences given in Figure 10.13.

2. The data on the HbA1c worksheet represent four measures of HbA1c for ten people on an exercise and diet regimen. The measures were taken at equal intervals over the course of a year. Replicate the analysis of repeated measures for these data by doing the following:
   a. Calculate SS_W—the variation within people, using the Pivot Table with person as the row variable and the formula in Equation 10.8.
   b. Calculate SS_A—the variation due to differences across measurements, using the Pivot Table with Measure as the row variable and the formula in Equation 10.9.
   c. Calculate SS_R—the residual variation—on a separate worksheet, using the formula in Equation 10.10, and confirm that it is equal to $SS_W - SS_A$.

    d. Calculate SS_B—the variation between people, using the formula in Equation 10.11.

    e. Calculate SS_T—the total variation, following the formula in Equation 10.3.

    f. Calculate the F test statistic for the effect of Measure, following the example in Figure 10.10.

    g. Use the formula in Equation 10.12 to replicate the results of the test of individual differences given in Figure 10.13.

Section 10.3 Factorial Analysis of Variance

Analysis of variance, like many special topics in statistics, is one to which entire books have been devoted. This chapter considers only one further application of analysis of variance, generally referred to as a factorial design. There are many different types of factorial designs, but the one considered here is one in which there is a single numerical variable as the dependent variable and two categorical independent variables. For example, suppose the hospital alliance was interested not only in differences between the four hospitals of the alliance but also in whether these differences were related to the sex of the patient. To simplify the calculations—and to present some variety in topics—instead of dealing with the cost of admission, this example will deal with the length of stay.

Consider that each hospital in the alliance has divided its admissions for the past year into those for males and those for females and each hospital randomly selects admissions for ten males and for ten females to include in the study. For each of these admissions, the length of stay is recorded and the data are submitted to analysis of variance. Figure 10.14 shows the entire analysis of variance for the data derived from the sample of ten males and ten females, taken from each of the four hospitals. Column A shows the name of the hospital. Only the first twenty-two of eighty admissions show in the figure—all for males—ten for Albemarle, ten for Beaufort, and two for Catawba. Column B shows the sex of the person admitted. Column C shows the length of stay. Columns D and E are used in the calculations and are discussed later.

The first step in the analysis of variance is to obtain the mean LOS by hospital, by sex, and by sex for hospitals. These values are given in the Pivot Table, beginning in cell G1. The values in this pivot table were obtained using the Average option in the Pivot Table, as was used in Figure 10.3 and Figure 10.9.

Column D shows the initial calculations for SS_T, the total sums of squares. SS_T is one of the least important calculations, but it is also one of the easiest and is therefore presented first. The formula for total sums of squares is given in Equation 10.13. Although the formula in Equation 10.13 appears complex with its triple summation signs, it is not. The symbols q and m in the formula refer to the number

FIGURE 10.14. ANOVA FACTORIAL ANALYSIS.

	H12	▾	=	=(H3-$J12-H$16+$J$16)^2						
	A	B	C	D	E	F	G	H	I	J	K	L
1	Hospital	Sex	LOS	SST	SSWC		Average of LOS	Sex ▾				
2	Albemarle	Male	4	4	0.16		Hospital ▾	Female	Male	Grand Total	SShosp	
3	Albemarle	Male	3	9	0.36		Albemarle	5.3	3.6	4.45	2.4025	
4	Albemarle	Male	5	1	1.96		Beaufort	6	4	5	1	
5	Albemarle	Male	4	4	0.16		Catawba	10.8	7.1	8.95	8.7025	
6	Albemarle	Male	8	4	19.36		Dare	6.2	5	5.6	0.16	
7	Albemarle	Male	6	0	5.76		Grand Total	7.075	4.925	6		
8	Albemarle	Male	3	9	0.36		SSsex	1.1556	1.1556			
9	Albemarle	Male	1	25	6.76							
10	Albemarle	Male	1	25	6.76		SShosp*sex	Sex				
11	Albemarle	Male	1	25	6.76		Hospital	Female	Male	Grand Total		
12	Beaufort	Male	3	9	1		Albemarle	0.0506	0.0506	4.45		
13	Beaufort	Male	1	25	9		Beaufort	0.0056	0.0056	5		
14	Beaufort	Male	3	9	1		Catawba	0.6006	0.6006	8.95		
15	Beaufort	Male	1	25	9		Dare	0.2256	0.2256	5.6		
16	Beaufort	Male	1	25	9		Grand Total	7.075	4.925	6		
17	Beaufort	Male	2	16	4							
18	Beaufort	Male	4	4	0			SS	df	MS	F	prob
19	Beaufort	Male	7	1	9		SShosp	245.3	3	81.77	4.53	0.0057
20	Beaufort	Male	13	49	81		SSsex	92.45	1	92.45	5.13	0.0266
21	Beaufort	Male	5	1	1		SShosp*sex	17.65	3	5.88	0.33	0.8064
22	Catawba	Male	2	16	26.01		SSWC	1298.6	72	18.04		
23	Catawba	Male	7	1	0.01		SST	1654	79			

of levels of the first factor and the second factor, respectively. If we consider hospitals as the first factor, then there are four of these, so $q = 4$. Sex, then, is the second factor, and there are obviously two levels for sex—so, $m = 2$. The formula says to begin with the first person for the first hospital and sex group, following the presentation in Figure 10.14 that would be Albemarle and a male. For that person, subtract the grand mean across all hospitals, sex groupings, and people (hence $\bar{\bar{x}}$), square the result, do this for every person in each sex group across all four hospitals, and sum it all up. Column D shows the first part of the calculation—that is, the square of the difference between each observation and the grand mean. The Excel formula for the first cell in the column that contains a number (cell D2) is =(C2-$J$7)^2. The dollar sign convention ensures that the grand mean is always used in the subtraction as the formula is copied to each cell in D. The sum of all eighty calculations in column D is given as SS_T in cell H23.

$$SS_T = \sum_{k=1}^{q}\sum_{j=1}^{m}\sum_{i=1}^{n}(x_{ijk} - \bar{\bar{x}})^2 \qquad (10.13)$$

The next sum of squares that may be discussed is SS_{WC}, which means sums of squares within cells. The sum of squares within cells is that portion of the variation in the data that cannot be attributed either to the hospital to which the patient was admitted or to sex of the patient. Consequently, in this example, SS_{WC} is the error variance. It is calculated using the formula in Equation 10.14. Equation 10.14 again indicates that a mean value is subtracted from every observation, squared, and summed across all eighty patients. But in this case, the mean value that is subtracted is the mean for each hospital and sex grouping. These mean values are those in cells H3:I6 in Figure 10.14. The initial calculation for SS_{WC} is carried out in column E. The Excel formula for cell E2 is =(C2-$I$3)^2. Cell I3, however, is in the terms given in Equation 10.14 only $\bar{x}_{11}$. It is the appropriate term to be subtracted only from the first ten observations (males in Albemarle). For males in Beaufort, the appropriate term changes to cell I4, and so on. This can be a little tedious, but is necessary for the calculation. The sum of all the calculations in column E is given in cell H22 as 1298.6.

$$SS_{WC} = \sum_{k=1}^{q} \sum_{j=1}^{m} \sum_{i=1}^{n} (x_{ijk} - \bar{x}_{jk})^2 \tag{10.14}$$

The sums of squares due to the differences between hospitals is given in Equation 10.15. The equation is given as SS_{rows}, because hospitals are the rows in the pivot table in Figure 10.14, and it should be clear that this is a general formula that applies to any two-factor factorial design, and not only to this specific one. The formula for SS_{rows} says that the overall average for all eighty observations is subtracted from the average for each hospital (this average is calculated across all people in a given hospital and both sex groups, hence the designation $\bar{\bar{x}}_q$), the result squared and added across all four hospitals. Then, since there are m times n, or twenty observations for each hospital, the resulting sum is multiplied by twenty. The first step in the calculation of SS_{rows}, or, in this case, SS_{hosp}, is given in cells K3:K6. The Excel formula for K3 is =(J3-$J$7)^2. The formula in K3 can then be copied to the other three cells. The sum of the cells K3:K6 is then multiplied by m times n in cell H19. The Excel formula for H19 is =20*sum(K3:K6).

$$SS_{rows} = mn \sum_{k=1}^{q} (\bar{\bar{x}}_q - \bar{\bar{x}})^2 \tag{10.15}$$

The sums of squares due to differences by sex is calculated in essentially the same way as the sums of squares due to hospitals. Because sex is the column designation in the Pivot Table in Figure 10.14, the formula for the sums of squares due to sex is given as SS_{cols} in Equation 10.16. It can be seen that Equation 10.15 and Equation 10.16 are quite similar. The initial computation of SS_{cols}—in this case—SS_{sex} is given in cells H8 and I8 in Figure 10.14. The Excel formula for cell

H8 is =(H7-$G$7)^2. The sum of H8 and I8 is multiplied by q times n, or forty in cell H20.

$$SS_{\text{cols}} = qn \sum_{j=1}^{m} (\bar{\bar{x}}_m - \bar{\bar{x}})^2 \qquad (10.16)$$

The only sums of squares left to calculate is what is known as the sums of squares due to interaction. In a factorial design, SS_{rows} and SS_{cols} (or the sums of squares due to the hospitals and the sums of squares due to sex) are known as *main effects*. But there may also be an effect that is due to what is called interaction. The computation of the sums of squares due to interaction is given in Equation 10.17. This equation says to take the mean for each sex and hospital ($\bar{x}_{jk}$), subtract the appropriate mean for sex ($\bar{\bar{x}}_j$) and the appropriate mean for hospital ($\bar{\bar{x}}_k$), add the grand mean ($\bar{\bar{x}}$), square the result, and add it across all sex and hospital groups. The initial calculation of $SS_{\text{rows·cols}}$—in this case, $SS_{\text{hosp·sex}}$—is carried out in cells H12:I15. The Excel formula for cell H12, following Equation 10.17, is given in the formula bar in Figure 10.14. The result of the calculations in H12:I15 are summed in H21. You can confirm that the sum of cells H19:H22 is equal to SS_T in cell H23.

$$SS_{\text{rows·cols}} = n \sum_{k=1}^{q} \sum_{j=1}^{m} (\bar{x}_{jk} - \bar{\bar{x}}_j - \bar{\bar{x}}_k + \bar{\bar{x}})^2 \qquad (10.17)$$

The degrees of freedom for this analysis are given in cells I19:I23. These degrees of freedom are calculated according to the equations shown in Figure 10.15. It should also be noted that the degrees of freedom shown in cells I19:I22 add to the total degrees of freedom in I23.

There are three F tests of interest in this analysis. There is an F test for the main effect of hospitals, an F test for the main effect of sex, and an F test

FIGURE 10.15. DEGREES OF FREEDOM IN TWO-FACTOR FACTORIAL ANOVA.

	N	O
1		
2	rows	q-1
3	cols	m-1
4	rows*cols	(q-1)(m-1)
5	within cells	qm(n-1)
6	total	qmn-1
7		

for the interaction between the two. The divisor in each of these F tests is the within cell variation SS_{WC}. The mean square values for each of these four elements are given in cells J19:J22, and are the SS values divided by degrees of freedom. The F tests are given in K19:K21 and the probabilities of these F values, based on =FDIST(), are given in L19:L21. The conclusion from these F tests and their probabilities is that there is a main effect due to hospitals (length of stay is not independent of hospital) and a main effect due to sex (length of stay is not independent of sex), but there is no effect due to interaction.

Excel Add-In for Factorial ANOVA

Excel provides two add-ins under Tools/Data Analysis for factorial analysis of variance. Only one of those, ANOVA: Two-Factor with Replication is discussed here. This is the analysis that will produce the results given in Figure 10.14. To carry out the analysis using ANOVA: Two-Factor with Replication, it is necessary first to rearrange the data in Figure 10.14 as they are shown in Figure 10.16. Only the observations for Albemarle and the first five observations for males and females, respectively, are shown for Beaufort in Figure 10.16. The remaining observations continue to row 41 of the spreadsheet. It should be clear that the observations for males are shown in column B and those for females are shown in column C. Also shown in Figure 10.16 is the ANOVA: Two-Factor with Replication window for carrying out the analysis. In that window, the input range is given as

FIGURE 10.16. DATA ARRANGEMENT FOR ANOVA: TWO-FACTOR WITH REPLICATION.

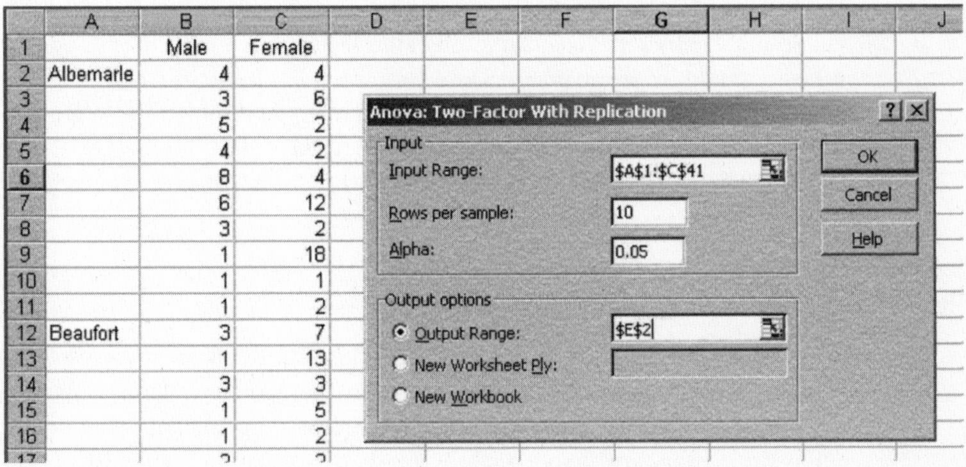

FIGURE 10.17. RESULTS OF ANOVA: TWO-FACTOR WITH REPLICATION.

	E	F	G	H	I	J	K	
36	ANOVA							
37	Source of Variation	SS	df	MS	F	P-value	F crit	
38	Sample	245.3	3	81.77	4.53	0.0057	2.73	
39	Columns	92.45	1	92.45	5.13	0.0266	3.97	
40	Interaction	17.65	3	5.88	0.33	0.8064	2.73	
41	Within	1298.6	72	18.04				
42								
43	Total	1654	79					
44								

$A$1:$C$41. This indicates that Excel recognizes that there will be a row of labels at the top of the data and a row of labels in the left column. Rows per sample is given as 10, which means Excel will appropriately treat each ten rows as a different set of observations. The output range is given as $E$2, which means the output will begin in that cell.

The results of the ANOVA: Two-Factor with Replication is given in Figure 10.17. Only the ANOVA table is shown in the figure, but there are several tables of averages that precede the ANOVA results. They take up rows 2 to 35 but are not shown in the figure. As the figure shows, the results of the Excel ANOVA add-in are the same as those calculated in Figure 10.16. The only difference is the values of F_{crit}, given in column K. Again, these are the levels that the F values would have to reach to be significant at the .05 level.

When one-way analysis of variance was discussed, it was indicated that both the formulas and the Excel add-in allowed for different sample sizes across the different groups. Neither the formulas given in this section (for a two-factor ANOVA) nor the Excel add-in permit unequal group sample sizes. It is possible to carry out two—or multifactor analysis of variance—with unequal sample sizes in groups, but the analysis becomes much more complicated and is often more easily performed using dummy variables in multiple regression, which is discussed in Chapter Thirteen.

Repeated Measures in a Factorial Design

The title of the Excel add-in, ANOVA: Two-Factor with Replication suggests that at least one of the factors is being measured more than one time. However, using the ANOVA: Two-Factor with Replication add-in for a repeated measure design is not as straightforward as one might wish. As performed in Figure 10.17, the

FIGURE 10.18. SIMPLE DATA FOR REPEATED MEASURES IN A FACTORIAL DESIGN.

	A	B	C	
1		Male	Female	
2	Admit 1	4	4	
3		3	6	
4		5	2	
5		4	2	
6		8	4	
7	Admit 2	3	7	
8		1	13	
9		3	3	
10		1	5	
11		1	2	
12	Admit 3	2	10	
13		7	7	
14		3	16	
15		14	4	
16		3	11	

results are not appropriate to repeated measures on the same set of persons or organizations. The results seen in Figure 10.17 are appropriate, as used in the figure, to a single measure on any included observation.

If the Excel add-in for ANOVA: Two-Factor with Replication is actually used to carry out analysis of variance in a factorial design where one variable is measured more than one time, some additional work must be done to get to the appropriate answers. To see that, let us consider a simple example. The data in Figure 10.18 show the length of stay for five men and five women for three different hospital admissions. This represents a factorial design with repeated measures on one variable: hospital admissions. The observation in cell B2, a four, represents a four-day stay for the first man on the spreadsheet, cell B7 represents the same person's length of stay for his second admission, and cell B12 represents his length of stay for his third admission. Similarly, the four in cell C2 represents the length of stay for the first woman on the spreadsheet. Her second stay is represented by cell C7 and her third stay is represented by cell C12. If we use the ANOVA: Two-Factor with Replication add-in to analyze these data, the result is as that shown in Figure 10.19. The conclusion that one would draw from this analysis is that there is a difference between the three admissions, but not between the two sexes, in length of stay. This would be based on the fact

FIGURE 10.19. ANOVA RESULTS FOR REPEATED MEASURES IN A FACTORIAL DESIGN.

	E	F	G	H	I	J	K
29							
30	ANOVA						
31	Source of Variation	SS	df	MS	F	P-value	F crit
32	Sample	89.26667	2	44.63333	3.735007	0.038705	3.402832
33	Columns	38.53333	1	38.53333	3.224547	0.085144	4.259675
34	Interaction	45.26667	2	22.63333	1.894003	0.172285	3.402832
35	Within	286.8	24	11.95			
36							
37	Total	459.8667	29				
38							

FIGURE 10.20. SOURCES OF VARIATION AND DEGREES OF FREEDOM IN FACTORIAL DESIGNS.

	N	O	P	Q	R	S	T
1	Two variable factorial design				Two variable factorial design		
2	No repeated measures				Repeated meaures on rows		
3	Variation		df		Variation		df
4	Total		qmn-1		Total		qmn-1
5	Between Cells		qm-1		Between Cells		qm-1
6	Columns		m-1		Columns		m-1
7	Rows		q-1		Rows		q-1
8	Columns*Rows		(m-1)(q-1)		Columns*Rows		(m-1)(q-1)
9							
10	Within Cells		qm(n-1)		Within Cells		qm(n-1)
11					Subjects within		m(n-1)
12					Groups		
13					Rows * Subjects		m(n-1)(q-1)
14					within Groups		
15							

that the probability for the F related to the samples (the three admissions) is less than .05, whereas the probability related to the columns (male and female) is not less than .05. We would also conclude no interaction effects.

But this conclusion would not take into account the fact that the three admissions were for the same group of people. In comparing what is given in the ANOVA printout with what is appropriate for a repeated measures design, the diagram in Figure 10.20 is useful. This diagram was adapted from Winer (1962). As the figure shows, the between-cell variation is the same for both repeated and nonrepeated measures. It can be divided into variation due to the columns, variation due to the rows, and the interaction between columns and rows. Where the nonrepeated measure design has only one error term, however—that being the within-cell variation, the repeated measures design has two error terms. The within-cell variation can be divided into variation due to subjects within groups (one source of error) and variation due to rows (the repeated measure) times subjects within groups (the second source of error). It turns out that the appropriate error term to construct the F test for differences between columns is subjects within groups, whereas the appropriate error term for differences between rows and for the column and row interaction is rows times subjects within groups. Thus, the F test for nonrepeated measures is not appropriate for the repeated measures case.

To find the values for subjects within groups and for rows times subjects within groups, it is necessary to have the mean value for each person across all measures, something not produced by the Excel add-in. Figure 10.21 shows the analysis for two factors when one is a repeated measure. The average for each person across all measures is obtained in cells E2:F6. As there are ten people, there are ten averages. The way in which the average is produced is shown in the formula bar. This can be copied directly to all the cells in E2:F6 to obtain the appropriate average values. Cells E14 and F14 contain the overall average for men and the overall average for women. The formula for the sums of squares for subjects within groups is given in Equation 10.18. This equation says to take the average for each person across all three measures (the designation $\bar{x}_{k(ij)}$ means that the ij observations are nested within the k measures), subtract the overall mean for each level of j, square the result, sum them all up, and multiply by the number of repeated measures.

The initial steps in this operation can be seen in cells E8:F12. Cells E14 and F14 contain the mean for each sex group ($\bar{\bar{x}}_j$). The Excel formula for cell E8 is =(E2-E$14)^2. The dollar sign convention allows this formula to be copied to every cell, E8:F12, to produce the terms to be summed for subjects within groups. The formula is completed in cell C21 by multiplying the sum of E8:F12 by 3, the number of repeated measures.

$$SS_{\text{subj }wG} = q\sum_{j=1}^{m}\sum_{i=1}^{n}(\bar{x}_{k(ij)} - \bar{\bar{x}}_j)^2 \qquad (10.18)$$

The appropriate analysis of variance table is shown in cells A18:G28. The sources of variation are divided into those that are between subjects and those that are within subjects. The three quantities in bold are those that came from the Excel analysis shown in Figure 10.19. Subjects within groups, plus the column variable—sex-adds to the total between subjects variation of 99.87. Subtracting the between subjects variation from the total variation (cell C28) provides the total for within-subjects variation. Subtracting the two values given in Figure 10.19 for

FIGURE 10.21. APPROPRIATE ANALYSIS FOR REPEATED MEASURES, TWO-FACTOR DESIGN.

	E2	▼		=	=AVERAGE(B2,B7,B12)		
	A	B	C	D	E	F	G
1		Male	Female				
2	Admit 1	4	4		3	7	
3		3	6		3.667	8.667	
4		5	2		3.667	7	
5		4	2		6.333	3.667	
6		8	4		4	5.667	
7	Admit 2	3	7				
8		1	13		1.284	0.360	
9		3	3		0.218	5.138	
10		1	5		0.218	0.360	
11		1	2		4.840	7.471	
12	Admit 3	2	10		0.018	0.538	
13		7	7				
14		3	16		4.133333	6.4	
15		14	4				
16		3	11				
17							
18	Source		SS	df	MS	F	p
19	Between Subj		99.8667	9			
20	Sex		**38.5333**	1	38.53333	5.026087	0.055262
21	Subj w G		61.3333	8	7.666667		
22							
23	Within Subjects		360	20			
24	Admissions		**89.2667**	2	44.63333	3.167357	0.069361
25	Admissions * Sex		**45.2667**	2	22.63333	1.60615	0.23138
26	Admissions*subj w G		225.467	16	14.09167		
27							
28	Total		459.867	29			
29							

admissions and the interaction term produces the term *admissions times subjects within groups*. The degrees of freedom appropriate to each of these sources of variation are given in column D. The appropriate F test for the difference between the sexes is the mean square for sex divided by the mean square for subjects within groups. The appropriate F test for both admissions and the interaction term requires the mean square for admissions times subjects within groups as the divisor. When these appropriate tests are carried out, we would no longer conclude that there is a difference across admissions, as we incorrectly concluded in Figure 10.19.

Exercises for Section 10.3

1. Use the data on the LOS worksheet in Chpt 10–1.xls and replicate the analysis given in Figure 10.14.
   a. Replicate the Pivot Table given in cells G1:J7 in Figure 10.14.
   b. Use the formula in Equation 10.13 to calculate SS_T as shown in column D in Figure 10.14.
   c. Use the formula in Equation 10.14 to calculate SS_{WC} as shown in column E in Figure 10.14.
   d. Use the formula in Equation 10.15 to calculate SS_{rows} (difference between hospitals) as shown in column K and cell H19 in Figure 10.14.
   e. Use the formula in Equation 10.16 to calculate SS_{cols} (difference between sexes) as shown in cells H8:I8 and H20 in Figure 10.14.
   f. Use the formula in Equation 10.17 to calculate $SS_{rows \cdot cols}$ (interaction between hospital and sex) as shown in cells H12:I15 and cell H21 in Figure 10.14.
   g. Determine the appropriate degrees of freedom, calculate the mean square values, and carry out the F tests as shown in I18:K23 in Figure 10.14.

2. The data on the Wait worksheet of Chpt 10–1.xls represent the waiting time in minutes for seventy-two emergency room visits. The visits were randomly selected with twelve taken from among true emergencies and twelve taken from among nonemergencies for each of three shifts. Use the factorial analysis of variance to determine whether there is a difference between shifts and between emergencies and nonemergencies in waiting time in the emergency room.
   a. Replicate the Pivot Table given in cells G1:J7 in Figure 10.14 for the Wait data.
   b. Use the formula in Equation 10.13 to calculate SS_T as shown in column D in Figure 10.14 for the Wait data.
   c. Use the formula in Equation 10.14 to calculate SS_{WC} as shown in column E in Figure 10.14 for the Wait data.
   d. Use the formula in Equation 10.15 to calculate SS_{rows} (difference by emergency status) as shown in column K and cell H19 in Figure 10.14 for the Wait data.
   e. Use the formula in Equation 10.16 to calculate SS_{cols} (difference between shifts) as shown in cells H8:I8 and H20 in Figure 10.14 for the Wait data.
   f. Use the formula in Equation 10.17 to calculate $SS_{rows \cdot cols}$ (interaction between shift and emergency) as shown in cells H12:I15 and cell H21 in Figure 10.14 for the Wait data.

g. Determine the appropriate degrees of freedom, calculate the mean square values, and carry out the *F* tests as shown in I18:K23 in Figure 10.14 to determine if there is a main effect of emergency status, a main effect of shift, or an interaction.

3. Rearrange the data for hospital LOS as given in Figure 10.16 and carry out the analysis of variance using the ANOVA: Two-Factor with Replication add-in. Confirm that the results are the same as those found in Exercise 1.

4. Rearrange the data for waiting time in the emergency room with Shift as the column variable (three columns) and emergency or other as the row variable (first twelve rows emergency, last twelve rows other), and carry out the analysis of variance using the ANOVA: Two-Factor with Replication add-in. Confirm that the results are the same as those found in Exercise 2.

5. Use the data on the worksheet Readmit2 in Chpt 10–1.xls and replicate the analysis given in Figure 10.21.

a. Generate the ANOVA: Two-Factor with Replication results for the data on the Readmit2 worksheet as the first step.

b. Generate the appropriate sums of squares for subjects within groups, using the formula in Equation 10.18.

c. Complete the analysis as shown in cells A18:H28 in Figure 10.21.

6. The data on the Test-Retest worksheet of Chpt 10–1 represent eighteen women who were randomly assigned to three educational formats at a breast cancer screening clinic. Six women received no educational intervention, six women received a pamphlet, and six received face-to-face information from a physician. The women were measured on a 20-point scale of knowledge at the beginning and at the end of the visit. Replicate the analysis in Figure 10.21 for these women.

a. Generate the ANOVA: Two-Factor with Replication results for the data on the Test-Retest worksheet as the first step.

b. Generate the appropriate sums of squares for subjects within groups, using the formula in Equation 10.18.

c. Complete the analysis as shown in the cells in Figure 10.21, using Figure 10.20 for the appropriate degrees of freedom.

Reference

Winer, B. J. *Statistical Principals in Experimental Design.* New York: McGraw Hill, 1962.

CHAPTER ELEVEN

SIMPLE LINEAR REGRESSION

L inear regression is a statistical method for determining the relationship between one or more *independent* variables and a single *dependent* variable. In this chapter we look at what is called simple linear regression. Simple linear regression refers to the relationship between a *single* independent variable and a single dependent variable.

Section 11.1 Meaning and Calculation of Linear Regression

To examine what is meant by the relationship between an independent variable and a dependent variable, consider the four graphs shown in Figure 11.1. This figure shows examples of four different possible relationships between two variables. The black points in each graph represent individual observations (there are actually fifty of these, but it may be difficult to count them). The horizontal axis (from 0 to 20) represents the value of any individual observation on the independent variable. This variable is commonly designated x. The vertical axis (from 0 to 20) represents the value of each individual observation on the dependent variable. The dependent variable is commonly designated y. So if one looks at the point farthest to the right in chart a), that individual observation has a value of approximately 15 on the variable x (the horizontal axis) and 15 on the variable y (the vertical axis). If we look at the point farthest to the right in chart b),

FIGURE 11.1. EXAMPLES OF RELATIONSHIPS.

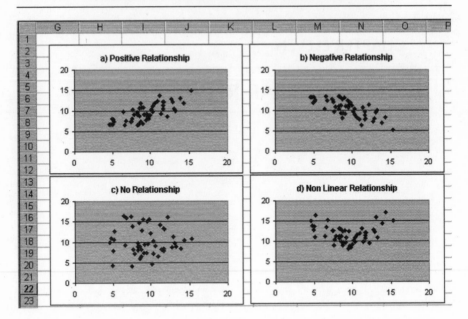

that observation has a value of approximately 15 on the variable *x*, but about 5 on the variable *y*.

Each of the charts in Figure 11.1 demonstrates a possible relationship between the variable *x* and the variable *y*, which is briefly described in the chart title. The chart a) shows a positive relationship between *x* and *y*. This means that observations with larger values of *x* tend also to have larger values of *y*. The chart b) shows a negative relationship between *x* and *y*. In this case, observations with larger values of *x* tend to have smaller values of *y*. In general, knowing something about *x* in either chart a) or chart b) will allow you to predict something about *y* even if you have no other knowledge of *y*.

Chart c) shows another type of relationship between *x* and *y*—in this case, no relationship at all. In chart c), observations with small values of *x* tend to have both large and small values of *y*, and observations with large values of *x* also appear to have both large and small values of *y*. In general, knowing something about the value of *x* is no better than knowing nothing about *x* in predicting values of *y* for data that conform to chart c). Chart d) shows yet a different type of relationship between *x* and *y*, one that is called a nonlinear relationship. In chart d), knowledge of *x* will provide a better prediction of *y* than no knowledge of *x*, but because the relationship is not linear, simple linear regression, as discussed in this chapter, will not be adequate to describe the relationship. Simple linear regression will provide us with no useful information about chart d). Chapter Thirteen discusses ways to

FIGURE 11.2. POSITIVE RELATIONSHIP WITH THE BEST-FITTING STRAIGHT LINE.

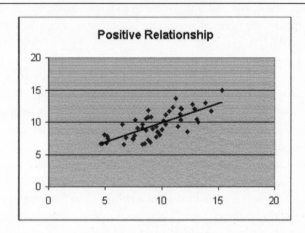

adapt regression analysis to deal with chart d), but, for now, nonlinear relationships will be ignored. One of the important things about being able to produce charts of data with Excel, however, is the ability to determine, through examination of the resulting charts, whether linear regression can adequately describe the relationship.

Linear regression can describe the data in chart a) and chart b) in Figure 11.1, but what does that mean? What it means is that the regression process will assign a best-fitting straight line to the data. What does best fitting mean? In a little while, a formal definition of best fitting will be produced, but for now, think of it as a line through the data that go through the means of both x and y and come as close as possible to all the points in the data set. Consider specifically chart a) in Figure 11.1. This chart is reproduced as Figure 11.2. In addition to the data points shown in Figure 11.1, Figure 11.2 shows the best-fitting straight line. This is the line that comes closest to all points in the data set while at the same time going through the true mean of both x and y.

A straight line in a two-dimensional space (the space defined by the values of x on the horizontal axis and y on the vertical axis) can be described with an equation as shown in Equation 11.1. Any point on the line is the joint graphing of a selected value of x and the value of y defined by Equation 11.1. If we knew that b_1 was .5 and b_0 was 2, then if x was 5, y would be 4.5. If x was 10, y would be 7. If x was 0, y would be 2.

$$y = b_1 x + b_0 \qquad (11.1)$$

In interpreting Equation 11.1, the two coefficients b_1 and b_0 have particular meanings. The coefficient b_1 is frequently referred to as the slope of the line. In concrete terms, b_1 is the distance the line rises in a vertical direction as x increases by one unit. So if x increases from 2 to 3, y increases by one half unit. The coefficient b_0 is frequently referred to as the intercept of the line. It represents specifically the point at which the line crosses the y axis, or the value of y when x is equal to 0.

If we are representing the points in Figure 11.2 with the best-fitting straight line, we must recognize that most of the points do not fall on the straight line (actually, perhaps none of them do). To account for this, the equation shown in Equation 11.1 is likely to be modified in one of two ways, both shown in Equation 11.2. The representation in Equation 11.2a indicates that the straight line equation is only an estimate of the true value of y. The designation $\hat{y}$ (pronounced y hat by statisticians) indicates that the value produced by the straight-line equation is an estimate of the true value of y. The representation in Equation 11.2b is the actual value of y rather than an estimate. The e at the end of the equation indicates that some value e (termed the error) must be added to the formula in order to produce the true value of y.

$$\hat{y} = b_1 x + b_0 \tag{11.2a}$$

$$y = b_1 x + b_0 + e \tag{11.2b}$$

What Does Regression Mean in Practical Terms?

To get a better understanding of what a straight-line prediction of y by x means in practical terms, let us consider twenty hospital admissions, the length of stay of each admission, and the charges for the stay. Figure 11.3 shows data on twenty hospital admissions that were randomly selected from a file of two thousand admissions. First, regression is a statistical test of the independence of the two variables—the length of stay and the total charges. The implicit null hypothesis is that the two variables are independent. If we reject that null hypothesis, we are left with the conclusion that the two variables are dependent on one another. But the nature of this dependence is very explicit. If we look back at Equation 11.2, either Equation 2a or Equation 2b indicates explicitly that the value of y is dependent on the value of x but not the other way around. In terms of the data shown for the twenty hospital stays in Figure 11.3, it is quite likely that total charges are dependent on the length of stay. However, it would make little logical sense to suggest that the length of hospital stay was dependent on what was charged for the stay.

Furthermore, what does it mean to reject the null hypothesis of independence? Because regression deals with linear relationships, rejecting the null hypothesis of independence would mean finding a linear relationship between, for example, the length of stay and the charges for which the slope of the line

FIGURE 11.3. TWENTY HOSPITAL STAYS.

	A	B	C
1	Stay	LOS	Charges
2	1	3	$2,614
3	2	5	$4,307
4	3	2	$2,449
5	4	3	$2,569
6	5	3	$1,936
7	6	5	$7,231
8	7	5	$5,343
9	8	3	$4,108
10	9	1	$1,597
11	10	2	$4,061
12	11	2	$1,762
13	12	5	$4,779
14	13	1	$2,078
15	14	3	$4,714
16	15	4	$3,947
17	16	2	$2,903
18	17	1	$1,439
19	18	1	$820
20	19	1	$3,309
21	20	6	$5,476

could be determined to be different from zero. To see if it is likely that we will be able to find such a straight line, consider the graph of the length of stay and the charges as shown in Figure 11.4. By looking at Figure 11.4, it is possible to see that the data from the twenty hospitals suggests that as the length of stay increases, total charges also increase. The short lengths of stay have the lowest costs and the longer lengths of stay have the highest costs. The single ten-day stay has the highest cost of all.

The data also appear to show a linear relationship. It is relatively easy to imagine a straight line that begins at about $2,000 when LOS is one day and then goes up to about $9,000 when LOS is ten days. Imagining such a straight line, we could say that its slope—that is, the change in the dollar value of total charges as LOS changes by one day—is the difference between $2,000 and $9,000, divided by the difference between one day of stay and ten days of stay. Accepting this logic, the slope of the straight line through the data in Figure 11.4 could be tentatively calculated as given in Equation 11.3. From a practical standpoint, then, we could conclude that for these hospitals (and the hospitals from which the sample of

FIGURE 11.4. GRAPH OF LENGTH OF STAY AND CHARGES.

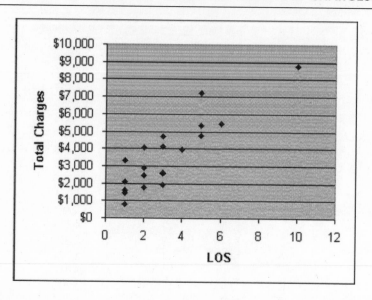

twenty was taken), as the length of stay increases by one day, the total charges increase by $777.78.

$$\text{Slope} = b_1 = (\$9{,}000 - \$2{,}000)/(10 - 1) = \$777.78 \qquad (11.3)$$

Furthermore, by finding the dollar value of the straight line at any point along its path, we can predict what the actual dollar value of any number of days of stay will be. Typically, the dollar value that is used as the reference point for setting the position of the line for all points is the dollar value of 0 on the X axis. Although a hospital stay of zero days may not actually exist, the straight line through the data will cross the Y, or vertical axis, at some point. That point, known as the intercept, could be calculated as $2,000 (the cost of a one-day stay) minus $777.78 (the slope of the line) or, as given in Equation 11.4, $1,222.22.

Based on the simple expedient of imagining where the straight line runs through the data in Figure 11.4, we come up with the predictor equation for charges, as shown in Equation 11.5.

$$\text{Intercept} = b_0 = \$2{,}000 - \$777.78 = \$1{,}222.22 \qquad (11.4)$$

$$\text{Charges} = \$777.78 \, \text{LOS} + \$1{,}222.22 \qquad (11.5)$$

Equation 11.5 matches the format of a straight line, as is given in Equation 11.1. What does this mean in practical terms? It means that if a hospital wishes to project the cost of any length of stay in the hospital, it can do so by multiplying the length of stay by $777.78 and adding a constant amount of $1,222.22.

Although this will not indicate precisely what the charges for any individual stay will be, it can be a good guideline on the average.

But before we can accept this result as a good guideline for anticipating the total charges, we must be able to reject the null hypothesis of independence between the charges and the length of stay. We have so far done nothing that would allow us to reject that null hypothesis, although we would feel, just by looking at the data in Figure 11.4, that we should reject that hypothesis in favor of the explicit hypothesis given in Equation 11.5, which is that charges are dependent on the length of stay. Furthermore, though we have found a line that may seem to fit the data, we may not necessarily have found the best-fitting straight line. Both of these issues are taken up in the next section.

Calculating Regression Coefficients

In the previous section we considered how we might estimate regression coefficients based on a simple examination of the plot of the data in a two-dimensional space. In this section we actually calculate the coefficients, using formulas that produce the exact coefficients b_1 and b_0, which represent the best-fitting straight line through the data. At this point, it is probably useful to formally define the best-fitting straight line. The best-fitting straight line is the line that minimizes the sum of squared differences between each individual data point and the line predicted by the coefficients. The formal definition of a best-fitting straight line can be seen in Equation 11.6.

$$\sum (y - \hat{y})^2 = \min \tag{11.6}$$

Given the formal definition of a best-fitting straight line, as shown in Equation 11.6, the two formulas for the coefficients b_1 and b_0 are as given in Equation 11.7 and Equation 11.8. The formulas in Equation 11.7 and Equation 11.8 are derived using calculus. Some discussion of the derivation is developed in Chapter Twelve, but there is no assumption that you need to understand calculus to proceed.

$$b_1 = \frac{\sum (x - \bar{x})(y - \bar{y})}{\sum (x - \bar{x})^2} \tag{11.7}$$

$$b_0 = \bar{y} - b_1 \bar{x} \tag{11.8}$$

Given the formulas in Equation 11.7 and Equation 11.8, it is possible to proceed to find the coefficients for the best-fitting straight line mathematically rather than relying on the eyeball method. The calculations for finding the coefficients are developed in Figure 11.5.

FIGURE 11.5. CALCULATION OF COEFFICIENTS.

	G2	▼	=	=E22/D22			
	A	B	C	D	E	F	G
1	Stay	LOS (x)	TC (y)	x-xbar	y-ybar		
2	1	3	$2,614	-0.15	-981.236	b1	$ 803.99
3	2	10	$8,769	6.85	5173.884	b0	$1,062.59
4	3	2	$2,449	-1.15	-1146.55		
5	4	3	$2,569	-0.15	-1026.45		
6	5	3	$1,936	-0.15	-1658.96		
7	6	5	$7,231	1.85	3635.564		
8	7	5	$5,343	1.85	1747.464		
9	8	3	$4,108	-0.15	512.984		
10	9	1	$1,597	-2.15	-1998.24		
11	10	2	$4,061	-1.15	466.134		
12	11	2	$1,762	-1.15	-1833.62		
13	12	5	$4,779	1.85	1184.044		
14	13	1	$2,078	-2.15	-1516.85		
15	14	3	$4,714	-0.15	1118.464		
16	15	4	$3,947	0.85	351.534		
17	16	2	$2,903	-1.15	-692.406		
18	17	1	$1,439	-2.15	-2156.3		
19	18	1	$820	-2.15	-2774.94		
20	19	1	$3,309	-2.15	-285.736		
21	20	6	$5,476	2.85	1881.184		
22		3.15	$3,595.15	94.55	76016.95		

In Figure 11.5, the means of the length of stay and the total charges are shown in B22 and C22, respectively. Each value of x minus the mean of x is shown in column D and each value of y minus the mean of y is shown in column E. Cell D22, which is the denominator in the formula in Equation 11.7, takes advantage of the Excel =SUMSQ() function that finds the sum of the squares of a stream of numbers. In this case, the function was invoked as =SUMSQ(D2:D21). Cell E22, which is the numerator in the formula in Equation 11.7, takes advantage of the Excel =SUMPRODUCT() function that finds the sum of the product of two streams of numbers. In this case, the function was invoked as =SUMPRODUCT(D2:D21,E2:E21). The value of b_1, shown in G2, was calculated, as the formula bar shows, by dividing the value in E22 by that in D22. The value of b_0, shown in G3, was calculated by subtracting B22*G2 from C22. The result of this calculation is the set of coefficients b_1 and b_0 for a best-fitting straight line through the data, as defined by Equation 11.6. Although the coefficients are not exactly the same as those estimated in the first subsection of Section 11.1, they are certainly of the same order of magnitude.

Exercises for 11.1

1. Use the data on the Hospital charges worksheet of Chpt 4–1.xls and generate the following *xy* charts. (The first variable in each case should be considered the independent variable.)
   a. Age with LOS
   b. Age with Charges
   c. Charges with Medicare

2. Which, if any, of the charts in a, b, or c (preceding) appear to be the best to fit a linear model and why? Which appear to be the worst?

3. Use the data on the HDI worksheet of Chpt 6–1.xls and generate the following *xy* charts. (The first variable in each case should be considered the independent variable.)
   a. AdLit99 with LifeEx99
   b. GrossEnrol99 with LifeEx99
   c. GDP/c (PPP99) with LifeEx99

4. Which, if any, of the charts in a, b, or c (preceding) appear to be the best to fit a linear model and why? Which appear to be the worst?

5. Use the following values of b_1 and b_0 and the values of the independent variable x to determine the values of y, and graph the resulting numbers.
   a. $b_1 = .5, b_0 = 3, x = 2, 5, 9, 14$
   b. $b_1 = 1.2, b_0 = -120, x = 225, 321, 452, 511$
   c. $b_1 = -.73, b_0 = 534, x = 150, 231, 344, 427$
   d. $b_1 = .0002, b_0 = 60, x = 40, 60, 80, 100$

6. Use the data on the Charges worksheet in Chpt 11–1.xls to replicate the calculation of b_1 and b_0, shown in Figure 11.5.

7. The data on the U5Mort worksheet in Chpt 11–1 represent female literacy (FemLit) and under-five mortality (U5Mort) for 114 countries of the world, each having more than one million inhabitants. The data were taken from the *State of the World's Children* (2001). Use these data to calculate b_1 and b_0 for FemLit as a predictor of U5Mort, following the example in Figure 11.5.

Section 11.2 Testing the Hypothesis of Independence

We have determined the coefficients for the straight-line equation that best fits the data in Figure 11.4 and Figure 11.5. The question now is, can we use this information to determine whether we will accept or reject the implicit null hypothesis of independence between the charges and the length of stay. In looking at the data, it appears clear that we should reject the null hypothesis, because the points so clearly show that as the length of stay increases, the charges increase. But we can calculate both a measure of the degree of this relationship and a statistical test for the null hypothesis.

Both the calculation of the degree of the relationship and the statistical test (an F test) for the null hypothesis depend on calculating variances. In this case, the variances are all with respect to the dependent variable, y. The total variance in y is as that shown in Equation 11.9, which is the mean of y subtracted from each value of y and the result squared and then summed across all values of y (thus, SS_T, which stands for sums of squares—total).

$$SS_T = \sum (y - \bar{y})^2 \tag{11.9}$$

The total variance in y can be considered as being divided into two portions. One portion is that which can be accounted for with the knowledge of the regression coefficients, termed sums of squares due to regression, or SS_R, and shown in Equation 11.10. The second portion is that which cannot be accounted for with the knowledge of the regression coefficients, termed sums of squares due to error, or SS_E, shown in Equation 11.11. In both Equation 11.10 and Equation 11.11, $\hat{y}$ is as that given in Equation 11.2. Also, $SS_T = SS_R + SS_E$.

$$SS_R = \sum (\hat{y} - \bar{y})^2 \tag{11.10}$$

$$SS_E = \sum (y - \hat{y})^2 \tag{11.11}$$

The calculation of the degree of the relationship between the length of stay and the charges is the calculation of a ratio of the amount of variation that can be accounted for by the regression line and the total variation. This ratio is sometimes called the coefficient of determination but is almost universally referred to as R^2. The formula for R^2 is as given in Equation 11.12.

$$R^2 = SS_R / SS_T \tag{11.12}$$

The calculation of the R^2 is given in Figure 11.6. Several of the calculations in Figure 11.6 deserve explanation. The values in column H, cells H2:H21, are calculated using the formula in Equation 11.2a. These are the predicted values of y ($\hat{y}$), based on the regression coefficients in G2 and G3. It should be noted that the average of the predicted values is exactly the same as the average of the actual values of y. This will always be true and is a way to check the accuracy of

FIGURE 11.6. CALCULATION OF R^2 AND F.

	A	B	C	D	E	F	G	H	I	J
1	Stay	LOS (x)	TC (y)	x-xbar	y-ybar			yhat	yhat-ybar	y-yhat
2	1	3	$2,613.91	-0.15	-981.236	b1	$ 803.99	$3,474.55	-$120.60	-$860.64
3	2	10	$8,769.03	6.85	5173.884	b0	$ 1,062.59	$9,102.46	$5,507.31	-$333.43
4	3	2	$2,448.60	-1.15	-1146.55			$2,670.56	-$924.58	-$221.96
5	4	3	$2,568.70	-0.15	-1026.45	SST	78485804.6	$3,474.55	-$120.60	-$905.85
6	5	3	$1,936.19	-0.15	-1658.96	SSR	61116626.0	$3,474.55	-$120.60	-$1,538.36
7	6	5	$7,230.71	1.85	3635.564	SSE	17369178.6	$5,082.52	$1,487.38	$2,148.19
8	7	5	$5,342.61	1.85	1747.464			$5,082.52	$1,487.38	$260.09
9	8	3	$4,108.13	-0.15	512.984	R^2	0.7787	$3,474.55	-$120.60	$633.58
10	9	1	$1,596.91	-2.15	-1998.24			$1,866.57	-$1,728.57	-$269.66
11	10	2	$4,061.28	-1.15	466.134	MSR	61116626.0	$2,670.56	-$924.58	$1,390.72
12	11	2	$1,761.53	-1.15	-1833.62	MSE	964954.4	$2,670.56	-$924.58	-$909.03
13	12	5	$4,779.19	1.85	1184.044			$5,082.52	$1,487.38	-$303.33
14	13	1	$2,078.30	-2.15	-1516.85	F	63.3363	$1,866.57	-$1,728.57	$211.73
15	14	3	$4,713.61	-0.15	1118.464	p	2.64E-07	$3,474.55	-$120.60	$1,239.06
16	15	4	$3,946.68	0.85	351.534			$4,278.53	$683.39	-$331.85
17	16	2	$2,902.74	-1.15	-692.406	S.E.	982.3209	$2,670.56	-$924.58	$232.18
18	17	1	$1,438.85	-2.15	-2156.3	S.E.b1	101.0235	$1,866.57	-$1,728.57	-$427.72
19	18	1	$820.21	-2.15	-2774.94			$1,866.57	-$1,728.57	-$1,046.36
20	19	1	$3,309.41	-2.15	-285.736	t	7.96	$1,866.57	-$1,728.57	$1,442.84
21	20	6	$5,476.33	2.85	1881.184	p	2.64E-07	$5,886.51	$2,291.36	-$410.18
22		3.15	$3,595.15	94.55	76016.95			$3,595.15	$ 0.00	$ 0.00

calculations. The values in column I, I2:I21, represent the difference between the predicted values of y and the mean of y ($\hat{y} - \bar{y}$). The mean of this column, shown in I22, should always be 0. The values in column J, J2:J21, represent the difference between each value of y and the predicted values of y ($y - \bar{y}$). Again, the mean of these data, shown in J22, will always be 0.

The total sums of squares (SS_T), shown in G5, were calculated using the =SUMSQ() function on cells E2:E21. The sums of squares that can be accounted for by the regression equation (SS_R)—typically called the sums of squares due to regression—were calculated using the =SUMSQ() function on cells I2:I21. R^2, shown in cell G9, was calculated by Equation 11.12. The value of R^2 can range from 0.00 to 1.00 and literally means the proportion of variation in the dependent variable y that can be predicted, knowing the values of the independent variable x and the coefficients for the best-fitting straight line through the data. In this case, 78 percent of the variation in charges can be accounted for by knowledge of the length of stay.

The sums of squares due to error (SS_E)—that proportion of the variation in y that cannot be accounted for by knowledge of x, shown in G7—is calculated using the =SUMSQ() function on cells J2:J21. The unexplained portion of the variation, SS_E, accounts for the 22 percent of the variation in charges that cannot

FIGURE 11.7. TOTAL VARIANCE, REGRESSION VARIANCE, AND ERROR VARIANCE.

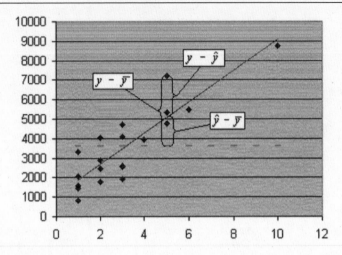

be accounted for by knowing the length of stay. That portion of the variation that can be accounted for by regression is known also as the explained variance, and the portion that cannot be accounted for is known as the unexplained variance.

It might be useful to consider again what the notion of explained variance and unexplained variance means in terms of the chart first shown in Figure 11.4. That chart is reproduced in Figure 11.7. There are several additions that have been added to Figure 11.7. The solid line sloping from the lower left to the upper right is the best-fitting straight line through the points, as defined by the regression coefficients calculated in Figure 11.6. The dashed horizontal line represents the mean of the points shown in cell C22 in Figure 11.6. There are three labeled brackets. The bracket labeled $y - \bar{y}$ represents the total variation for the length of stay of five days, shown in cell B7 in Figure 11.6. That bracket represents the value of charges for that stay—$7,230.71—minus the mean charges for all stays— $3,595.15, or $3,635.56. The bracket labeled $\hat{y} - \bar{y}$ represents the difference between the predicted value for that stay—$5,082.52—and the mean of all stays— $3,595.15, or $1,487.38. This is the portion of the variation in the charges for this stay that can be predicted using the regression equation. The bracket labeled $y - \hat{y}$ represents the difference between the actual charges for this particular stay— $7,230.71—and the predicted value of $5,082.52, or $2,148.19. This is the portion of the variation in the charges for this stay that cannot be predicted with the regression equation. When all these differences for each point are squared and summed, the values of SS_T, SS_R, and SS_E are generated.

The R^2 value tells us the degree of relationship between the length of stay and charges. In this case, the length of stay accounts for 78 percent of the variance in the charges. This would generally be considered a very high degree of relationship. But still not yet discussed explicitly is the resolution of the question of whether we can reject the null hypothesis of independence between the two variables. The resolution of that question is given formally by the F test shown in cell G14 in Figure 11.6. This F test is calculated by the formula given in Equation 11.13. The formula in Equation 11.13 is usually described as the division of the mean square due to regression by the mean square error. The mean square values are found by dividing SS_R and SS_E by their respective degrees of freedom.

$$F = MS_R/MS_E \qquad\qquad (11.13)$$

where
$$MS_R = SS_R/1$$
$$MS_E = SS_E/(n - 2)$$

The F value shown in G14 is 63.34, a relatively large value of F. The probability of this F is given in cell G14 as 2.64E-07. This indicates that the F value calculated would have been found approximately three times out of ten million different samples of twenty observations if charges were independent of the length of stay. Since this is an extremely small probability, we reject the null hypothesis of independence and conclude that the two variables are, in fact, not independent.

There are several additional values in Figure 11.6. These include the overall standard error of estimate ($S.E.$) in G17, the standard error of b_1 ($S.E.$ $b1$) in G18, a t test in G20, and the probability of the t in G21. Each of these deserves some discussion.

The standard error shown in G17 is the average error of the actual observations around the regression line shown in Figure 11.7. It is calculated using the formula given in Equation 11.14.

$$S.E._{\text{reg}} = \sqrt{SS_E/(n - 2)} \qquad\qquad (11.14)$$

The standard error of b_1 ($S.E.$ b_1 in cell G18) is the average variation of the coefficient, b_1. The coefficient b_1 in any regression analysis is a sample-based estimate of the true population coefficient β_1. As a sample mean value $\bar{x}$, an estimate of the true population mean μ has a range within which there is a probability of the true mean being found, so too the coefficient, b_1, has a similar range. That range is determined by the $S.E.$ b_1. But the $S.E.$ b_1 also serves another function. Just as a t test can be conducted by dividing appropriate mean values by their standard errors, a t test can be conducted to determine whether the coefficient b_1 is different from 0. If the t test does not produce a t value large enough to reject the implied null hypothesis that b_1 is 0, the conclusion would have to be that the null hypothesis of independence of the variables x and y would be rejected. The standard error of b_1 is calculated using the formula in Equation 11.15.

$$S.E.\ b_1 = S.E._{\cdot reg}\Big/\sqrt{\sum (x - \bar{x})^2} \qquad (11.15)$$

The t test to determine if b_1 is different from 0 is shown in Equation 11.16, and the value of the t test for the length of stay and the charges is shown in G20. The probability of the t test is shown in G21. You will note that it is exactly the same as the probability of the F test in cell G15. This is no accident. In simple linear regression with a single predictor variable, the probability of the F test will always be the same as the probability of the t test. This is because the F test of the general hypothesis of independence is exactly the same as the t test of the null hypothesis that the coefficient b_1 is zero. In multiple regression, which we will take up in a later chapter, the F test and the individual t tests for regression coefficients will not have the same probabilities, but in one independent variable linear regression, they do.

$$t = \frac{b_1}{S.E.\ b_1} \qquad (11.16)$$

It is useful to note that there is no comparable test in this analysis to determine whether the coefficient b_0 is different from zero. In this analysis no standard error for b_0 has been determined, but the primary reason that no test for b_0 is conducted is because whether b_0 is different from 0 has no bearing on the rejection or nonrejection of the null hypothesis of independence. The coefficient b_0 is simply an anchor for the left side of the regression line. Whether it is 0 or different from 0 is usually not central to the analysis. In the analysis discussed here, no value for b_0 has even been found. We will see when we move to multiple regression, however, that a value for the standard error of b_0 will be produced by the analysis.

Exercises for 11.2

1. Use the data from the Charges worksheet of Chpt 11–1.xls and the calculations of b_1 and b_0 carried out in Exercise 6 of Section 11.1 to replicate the calculations shown in Figure 11.6.
    a. Calculate the total sums of squares (SS_T) as given in Equation 11.9 and shown in cell G5 in Figure 11.6. (Use the =SUMSQ() function on the data in column E.)

b. Calculate the predicted values of TC $\hat{y}$ in column H by using the formula in Equation 11.1.

c. Calculate the difference between $\hat{y}$ and $\bar{y}$ in column I and the value of SS_R (sums of squares due to regression) by using Equation 11.10 and the =SUMSQ() function on the data in column I.

d. Calculate the values of $y - \hat{y}$ in column J and the value of SS_E (sums of squares due to error) by using Equation 11.11 and the =SUMSQ() function on the data in column J.

e. Calculate the value of R^2 by using Equation 11.12.

f. Calculate the degrees of freedom for SS_R and SS_E as shown in Equation 11.13 and the values of MS_R and MS_E, using the same formula. Calculate the value of F from the same formula.

g. Determine the probability of F with the =FDIST() function and the appropriate degrees of freedom.

h. Determine the standard error of regression by using the formula in Equation 11.14.

i. Determine the standard error of b_1 by using the formula in Equation 11.15.

j. Calculate the t value for b_1 by using the formula in Equation 11.16 and determine its probability with the =TDIST() function.

2. Use data on the U5Mort worksheet in Chpt 11–1 and the results of the calculation of b_1 and b_0 for FemLit as a predictor of U5Mort from Exercise 7 of Section 11.1 and replicate the complete analysis in Figure 11.6.

a. Calculate the total sums of squares (SS_T) as given in Equation 11.9. (Use the =SUMSQ() function.)

b. Calculate the predicted values of U5Mort ($\hat{y}$) in column H by using the formula in Equation 11.1.

c. Calculate the difference between $\hat{y}$ and $\bar{y}$ in column I and the value of SS_R (sums of squares due to regression) by using Equation 11.10 and the =SUMSQ() function on the data in column I.

d. Calculate the values of $y - \hat{y}$ in column J and value of SS_E (sums of squares due to error) by using Equation 11.11 and the =SUMSQ() function on the data in column J.

e. Calculate the value of R^2 by using Equation 11.12.

f. Calculate the degrees of freedom for SS_R and SS_E as shown in Equation 11.13 and the values of MS_R and MS_E, using the same formula. Calculate the value of F from the same formula.

g. Determine the probability of F with the =FDIST() function and the appropriate degrees of freedom.

h. Determine the standard error of regression by using the formula in Equation 11.14.

    i. Determine the standard error of b_1 by using the formula in Equation 11.15.

    j. Calculate the t value for b_1 using the formula in Equation 11.16 and determine its probability with the =TDIST() function.

Section 11.3 The Excel Regression Add-In

Now that we have worked through the steps of regression analysis, we can look at the capabilities of the Excel regression add-in. When Tools/Data Analysis is invoked, the window shown again in Figure 11.8 will come up. When regression is selected, the regression window shown in Figure 11.9 comes up. In Figure 11.9, several things should be noted. First, the box labeled Input Y Range contains the cell reference to the y variable, total charges, which is in cells C1:C21. The box labeled Input X Range contains the cell references for length of stay, which is in cells B1:B21. The box with the Labels label is checked, indicating that the first row in each column is a label. If the cells B1 and C1 were not included in the input range boxes, but the Labels box was checked, Excel would treat the values 3 for the length of stay and $2,613.91 as labels and would not include that observation in the analysis.

    The box labeled Constant is Zero should never be checked. There is an analysis known as weighted least squares that involves the assumption that the constant is 0, but, in general, that box should be left unchecked. The confidence level is given as 95 percent by default. It is possible to change this to another level by checking the Confidence Level box. The final thing in the regression window that must be checked is the place where the output is to go. It can go on the same sheet, on a new worksheet, or in a new workbook. By checking output range and then putting E1 in the output range box, the output will be placed on the same sheet

FIGURE 11.8. EXCEL DATA ANALYSIS ADD-IN WINDOW.

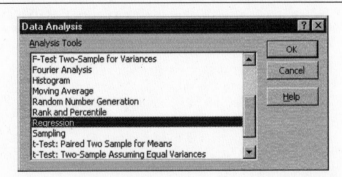

FIGURE 11.9. REGRESSION SETUP WINDOW.

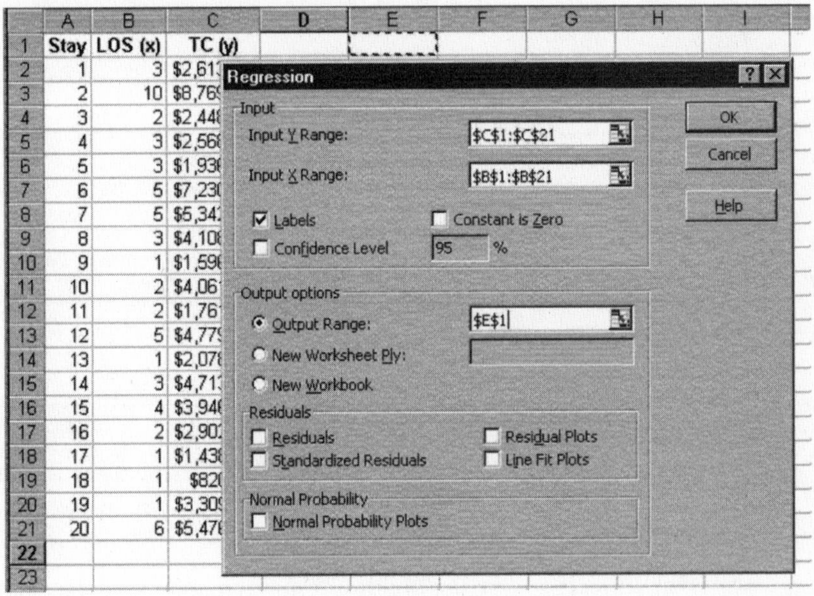

in cell E1. There are several other boxes in the Regression window that produce additional results, but in general we will not use these boxes in this book.

If we click the OK button with the regression setup window, as shown in Figure 11.9, the results shown in Figure 11.10 will be produced. The table shown in Figure 11.10 is exactly as it appears in the regression output for any set of data. The label—for example, Adjusted R in E6—is actually Adjusted R Square, but it cannot be completely seen because the column is not wide enough. Similarly, "andard Err" in G16 is really Standard Error, but the cell is too narrow for the entire title to show. It is possible to see the entire titles by putting the cursor between, for example, E and F at the top of the sheet and double-left-clicking the mouse. But after a little use, the absence of complete labels will not be a problem.

But let us look at the various different numbers that are produced by the Regression analysis add-in. The first number in the table is labeled Multiple R. This value, which is often called the correlation coefficient, represents the correlation between the two variables, x and y. The correlation coefficient can be calculated by the formula shown in Equation 11.17, but it can also be found by taking the square root of R square in cell G9 in Figure 11.6. One caveat to taking the square root of R^2 to find r, however, is that r may be negative or positive. If the value of b_1 is negative, the actual value of r in two-variable linear regression

FIGURE 11.10. RESULTS OF REGRESSION ADD-IN.

	E	F	G	H	I	J	K	L	M
1	SUMMARY OUTPUT								
2									
3	*Regression Statistics*								
4	Multiple R	0.882438							
5	R Square	0.778697							
6	Adjusted R	0.766402							
7	Standard E	982.3209							
8	Observatio	20							
9									
10	ANOVA								
11		*df*	*SS*	*MS*	*F*	*ignificance F*			
12	Regressior	1	61116626	61116626	63.33629	2.64E-07			
13	Residual	18	17369179	964954.4					
14	Total	19	78485805						
15									
16		*Coefficients*	*andard Err*	*t Stat*	*P-value*	*Lower 95%*	*Upper 95%*	*ower 95.0%*	*pper 95.0%*
17	Intercept	1062.588	386.6709	2.748042	0.013227	250.2216	1874.954	250.2216	1874.954
18	LOS (x)	803.9868	101.0235	7.95841	2.64E-07	591.744	1016.23	591.744	1016.23
19									

will be negative. However, the Multiple R shown in the Excel regression result will always be positive.

$$r = \frac{\sum (x - \bar{x})(y - \bar{y})}{\sqrt{\sum (x - \bar{x})^2 \sum (y - \bar{y})^2}} \tag{11.17}$$

The R^2 value shown in F5 is exactly the same value as that calculated for R^2 by using the formula shown in Equation 11.12 and as given in cell G9 in Figure 11.6.

The Adjusted R Square represents the reduction of the actual R^2 to reflect the number of independent variables in the prediction equation (as shown in Equation 11.2). In general, the more independent variables, or regressors or predictor variables (the three terms all apply to the same thing), that are included in the regression equation (with two-variable regression, there is always only one) the larger will be the R^2. This is because every additional independent variable reduces the size of SS_E. To counter this, the adjusted R^2 reduces the value of R^2 to reflect this decrease in SS_E. The formula for the adjusted R^2 is shown in Equation 11.18. More is said about the adjusted R^2 in Chapter Twelve.

$$R_{\text{adj}}^2 = 1 - (1 - R^2)\frac{n - 1}{n - 2} \tag{11.18}$$

The standard error, what we labeled *S.E.* in Figure 11.6 (cell G17), is shown in cell F7 of the Excel regression output (Figure 11.10). The number of observations—twenty—is confirmed in cell F8 in Figure 11.10. The ANOVA section of the Excel regression output also matches our previous calculations. *SS* Regression in Figure 11.10, cell G12 at 61, 116, 626, matches the value of SS_R in cell G6 in Figure 11.6. A brief examination of the two figures will show that all the *SS* values and *MS* values in Figure 11.10 match their corresponding values in Figure 11.6. The *F* test value of 63.336 is the same in both figures, as is the probability of F, 2.64E-07.

Similar results are found with regard to the coefficients themselves. The coefficients b_1 and b_0, shown as LOS(x) and Intercept, respectively, in Figure 11.10 are the same in both figures, as is the standard error of b_1. The standard error of b_0 was not calculated in Figure 11.6. In general, whether b_0, the intercept term, can be shown to be different from 0 or not is irrelevant to the decision to reject the null hypothesis of independence between the two variables in the analysis. The intercept represents no more than an anchor to establish the position of the regression line. But since the standard error of b_0 is given in the Excel regression output, it is useful to know how it can be calculated. The formula for the standard error of b_0 is given in Equation 11.19. Although Σx^2 is not calculated in Figure 11.6, it is easy to confirm with =SUMSQ(C2:C21) that it is 293, and the term in the denominator in Equation 11.19 is $\sqrt{6.4539}$, which gives a value for *S.E.* b_0 of 386.67.

$$S.E.\ b_0 = S.E._{\cdot reg} \Big/ \sqrt{n \sum (x - \bar{x})^2 \Big/ \sum x^2} \qquad (11.19)$$

The *t* statistic for the coefficient b_1 as shown in Figure 11.10, was calculated in cell G20 in Figure 11.6. These both match, as do their probabilities. The *t* statistic for b_0 was not calculated in Figure 11.6, but if it were, it would equal that found in the Excel regression output. The last four columns in rows 16 to 18 in Figure 11.10 give upper and lower 95 percent limits for the coefficients b_1 and b_0. If the user requests a level of confidence other than 95 percent, the upper and lower limits will then be given as the last two sets of cells. These values, though not found in Figure 11.6, can be found in exactly the same way that upper and lower 95 percent limits are found for a mean value. The lower value of 591.744, for example, which is shown in cell J18 (and L18) in Figure 11.10, is calculated exactly as shown in Equation 11.20. The other limits can be found in the same way.

$$\text{Lower} = b_1 - t_{18}\ S.E.\ b_1 = 803.987 - 2.101 \times 101.024 = 591.744 \quad (11.20)$$

Exercises for 11.3

1. Use the data from the Charges worksheet of Chpt 11–1.xls.
   a. Generate the regression analysis by using the Excel Tools/Data Analysis/ Regression add-in and replicate the analysis shown in Figure 11.10.
   b. Make sure that all the values in this result equal those found in Exercise 1 of Section 11.2.

2. Use the data from the U5Mort worksheet of Chpt 11–1.xls.
   a. Generate the regression analysis by using the Excel Tools/Data Analysis/ Regression add-in and replicate the analysis in Exercise 2 of Section 11.2.
   b. Make sure that all the values in this result equal those found in Exercise 2 of Section 11.2.

Section 11.4 The Importance of Examining the Scatterplot

The scatterplots shown in Figure 11.1 provide one example of data not appropriate for two-variable regression: example d. This relationship is curvilinear and, consequently, is not best described by using a straight line. This section looks at some other cases in which regression analysis must be used very carefully. The presentation in this section is inspired by a similar presentation in *Statistics for Managers Using Microsoft Excel* (Levine, Berenson, and Stephan, 1999).

Four different data sets are shown in Figure 11.11. For each of these data sets, the best-fitting straight line is defined by the equation, $y = .50x + 1.55$ (The best-fitting straight line for data set four is actually $y = .51x + 1.55$). If you calculate the regression coefficients b_1 and b_0 for each of these data sets, they will be

FIGURE 11.11. FOUR DATA SETS.

	A	B	C	D	E	F	G	H	I	J	K	L
1	Data set one			Data set two			Data set three			Data set four		
2	X	Y		X	Y		X	Y		X	Y	
3	5	5		5	4		5	7		5	3	
4	6	4		7	6		7	6		5	4	
5	6	6		9	5		9	6		5	5	
6	7	4		11	8		11	6		14	5	
7	7	5		13	7		13	6		14	9	
8	7	6		15	10		15	7		14	13	
9	8	4		17	9		17	8		22	5	
10	8	6		19	12		19	10		22	16	
11	9	5		21	11		21	13		22	20	
12	20	12		23	14		23	17		22	10	

FIGURE 11.12. SCATTER PLOTS OF FOUR DATA SETS WHERE $y = .5x + 1.55$.

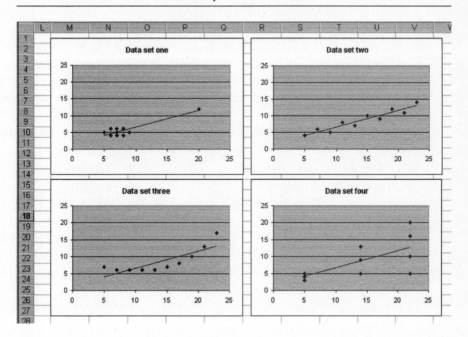

essentially equal for each data set. But only one of these data sets could be considered appropriate for simple linear regression with one predictor variable, x.

The xy scatter plots of these four data sets, along with the best-fitting straight line, are shown in Figure 11.12. Looking at Figure 11.12, it should be possible to see visually why only one of these data sets—data set two—is appropriate for simple linear regression analysis. Although the equation for the best-fitting straight line for data set one is exactly the same as that for data set two, that line depends entirely on the value at $x = 20$ and $y = 12$. If that value were not included, the coefficient of b_1 would have been 0 and there would be no relation between x and y at all. In essence, the entire relationship found between x and y in this case depends on a single data point. The single data point in this case is often called an *outlier*. When outliers are present, it is important to decide whether they are unduly affecting the regression results.

Data set three is inappropriate for simple linear regression because the data actually show a curved relationship between x and y. Regression can be used to describe the data in set three, but it must be curvilinear regression, which is taken up in Chapter Thirteen. In essence, a straight line relationship between x and y is not the correct model for describing the way the x variable affects the y variable in set three.

Data set four may be a little more difficult to see as being inappropriate for simple linear regression. The points do tend to lie along the straight line defined by the regression equation, they do not seem to picture a nonlinear relationship as in data set three, and the line is not defined by a single outlier as in data set one. The problem with the use of simple linear regression to analyze data set four is that the variance in the data is not the same at each point that a value of x is recorded. When x is 5, the three values taken on by y have an average variance (the difference between each value of y at $x = 5$ and the mean of the values of y at $x = 5$ divided by the number of values of y at $x = 5$) of .33. The three values taken on by y when $x = 14$ have an average variance of 5.33. The four values taken on by y when $x = 22$ have an average variance of 10.89.

One of the basic assumptions of simple linear regression is that the variance of y across all values of x is constant. In the case of the data in data set four, this is clearly not the case. As the value of x increases, the variance in y increases. Although most authors agree that the results of regression analysis are not greatly affected by violating this assumption of equal variance, in fact, the more appropriate analysis of the data in data set four would be an analysis called weighted least squares. Weighted least squares are discussed in Chapter Fourteen, but in a different context. For those interested in general treatment of weighted least squares, any good introductory text in econometrics will provide a discussion of its calculation and use.

Section 11.5 The Relationship Between Regression and the *t* Test

This section considers the relationship between regression and the *t* test. (Remember that *t* tests were discussed in Chapter Nine.) The one that is particularly examined here is the *t* test for two different groups. Consider the example given in Chapter Nine of the two groups of women, one of whom received information from a physician about breast cancer and the other having received only written information. Between the two groups, did this result in different knowledge about breast cancer? The results of the *t* test, with both equal and unequal variance assumptions, were shown in Figures 9.10 and 9.11 in Chapter Nine. The mean knowledge assessment score for the two groups were 10.040 for the women who received information from a physician and 7.525 for the women who received only a pamphlet. For the equal variance assumption, the pooled variance was .762 and the value of the *t* statistic $((10.040 - 7.525)/.762)$ was 3.3.

Figure 11.13 shows the data for the comparison between the two groups redone using regression analysis. The dependent variable in the regression is the score received by each woman, whether in the experimental or control group, on the knowledge test. The independent variable is a variable that is coded 1 if the woman is in the experimental group and 0 if she is not. Such a variable is called a dummy variable, probably because it does not actually represent a numerical variable but, rather, serves as a categorical variable that can be treated as a numerical variable.

In examining Figure 11.13, it is possible to see that the intercept term (7.525) is the mean of the control group. The coefficient indicated as Group is the coefficient on the dummy variable that takes on only the values 1 and 0. As such, the value of 2.515 is not a slope but is, rather, the value that is added to the intercept to get the mean of the experimental group. It is easy to see that 7.525 + 2.515 = 10.040. Furthermore, it is possible to see that the t test on the coefficient for group, which is precisely the difference between the control group and the experimental group divided by the pooled variance (.762), is exactly the same as the t test for two groups assuming equal variance. This will always be the case. Whenever a dummy variable is employed in regression, the coefficient will be the difference between the mean of the group coded 0 and the mean of the group coded 1. The t test for the coefficient will be exactly the same as the t test for the difference in means.

FIGURE 11.13. REGRESSION AS A t TEST.

	D	E	F	G	H	I
1	SUMMARY OUTPUT					
2						
3	*Regression Statistics*					
4	Multiple R	0.383909				
5	R Square	0.147386				
6	Adjusted R Sq	0.133853				
7	Standard Error	2.989227				
8	Observations	65				
9						
10	ANOVA					
11		*df*	*SS*	*MS*	*F*	*ignificance F*
12	Regression	1	97.31115	97.31115	10.89043	0.001594
13	Residual	63	562.935	8.935476		
14	Total	64	660.2462			
15						
16		*Coefficients*	*andard Err*	*t Stat*	*P-value*	*Lower 95%* *Upp*
17	Intercept	7.525	0.472638	15.92127	9.23E-24	6.580507	8.
18	Group	2.515	0.762106	3.300065	0.001594	0.992051	4.l
19							

An important thing to note when a variable is employed in a regression context is that a dummy actually defines two different regression equations. In this simple case of a single dummy variable, the original regression equation, shown in Equation 11.21, actually becomes two equations as shown in Equation 11.22. It should be clear that these values are just the mean of the group designated 0 and the group designated 1 by the dummy variable, respectively.

$$\hat{y} = b_1 x + b_0 \tag{11.21}$$

$$(\hat{y} \mid x = 0) = b_0, \text{ and}$$
$$(\hat{y} \mid x = 1) = b_1 + b_0 \tag{11.22}$$

Exercises for 11.5

1. Use the data on the Cost worksheet of Chpt 9–1.xls that show the hospital cost for a randomly selected sample of thirty-four women and thirty-four men.
   a. Rearrange the data so that they can be analyzed using regression and add an independent variable that is 1 for women and 0 for men.
   b. Test the hypothesis that the cost for women is equal to the cost for men, against the alternative that they are not equal using regression.

2. Use the data on the Breast C worksheet of Chpt 9–1.xls that show the data used for the analysis in Figure 11.13.
   a. Rearrange the data so that they can be analyzed using regression and add an independent variable that is 1 for the women in the experimental group and 0 for the women in the control group.
   b. Replicate the analysis shown in Figure 11.13.

3. Use the data on the Wait worksheet of Chpt 9–1 that represent the waiting time of a randomly selected group of people at an urgent care clinic and a randomly selected group of people at an emergency clinic.
   a. Rearrange the data so that they can be analyzed using regression and add an independent variable that is 1 for Emergency and 0 Urgent care.
   b. Test the hypothesis that waiting time is equal for both groups, against the alternative that they are not equal using regression.

References

Levine, D. M., Stephan, D., Krebbiel, T. C., and Berenson, M. L. Statistics for Managers Using Microsoft Excel. (2nd ed.) Englewood Cliffs, N.J.: Prentice Hall, 1999.
The State of the World's Children 2001, UNICEF, New York, Dec. 2000.
   [http://www.unicef.org/sowc01/tables/#].

CHAPTER TWELVE

MULTIPLE REGRESSION: CONCEPTS AND CALCULATION

Chapter Eleven considered simple linear regression, its calculation and its interpretation. This chapter extends the simple linear regression model to include more than one predictor variable. This is what is known as multiple regression. This chapter will consider the nature of multiple regression and the calculation of the basic multiple regression results.

Section 12.1 Introduction

As a means of introducing the multiple regression model, it will be contrasted to simple linear regression. In this contrast, the Excel regression add-in, considered in Chapter Eleven, will be extended to multiple regression.

The Extension of Simple Linear Regression

The simple linear regression model is as shown in Equation 12.1. In the simple linear regression model, the coefficient b_1 represents the slope of the regression line in an XY graph, and the coefficient b_0 represents the intercept of the regression line, or the value of dependent variable y when the independent variable x is equal to 0. The symbol e represents the error—the difference between the actual values of y and the predicted values of y.

$$y = b_1 x + b_0 + e \qquad (12.1)$$

The multiple regression model extends the simple linear regression model to include more than one independent variable. In the context of the presentation in Equation 12.1, the multiple regression model could be presented as shown in Equation 12.2. In Equation 12.2, the subscript m represents any number of independent variables, and the three dots in a row represent the b coefficients and x variables from 2 to m that are included in the equation but not shown.

$$y = b_1 x_1 + b_2 x_2 + \cdots + b_m x_m + b_0 + e \qquad (12.2)$$

The relationship in the simple linear regression model can be pictured visually as a line (the regression line) in a two-dimensional graph where, by convention, the horizontal axis is the x variable and the vertical axis is the y variable. This has been seen in Chapter Eleven on simple linear regression. In simple terms, the relationship of a single independent variable to a dependent variable can be pictured in a two-dimensional space. If there were two independent variables (x variables), it would be possible to picture this relationship as a plane in a three-dimensional space—although this is not easily shown on two-dimensional paper. If there are more than two independent variables, it becomes impossible to picture this either on two-dimensional paper, or even conceptually. If there are m independent variables, the logical extension is that we should be able to construct a model of all the variables at the same time by producing an m dimensional figure in an $m + 1$ dimensional space. Since human beings can easily deal with the notion of only three dimensions at a time, it becomes virtually impossible to picture graphically the simultaneous relationship of all x variables to the y variable. Happily, for the understanding of multiple regression, it is not necessary to form this mental picture. It should be enough simply to understand that each independent x variable may have some effect on y that is assessed simultaneously with the effect of all other x variables.

The purpose of multiple regression analysis is essentially the same as that of linear regression. We are trying to understand whether there is any relationship between each of the independent variables x and the dependent variable y, and if so, what that relationship may be. To do this for simple regression, we learned that there are two algebraic formulas that can be used to find directly the values of b_1 and b_0. Similarly, there is a direct algebraic strategy for finding all the coefficients b_m and b_0 in the multiple regression model. However, the use of this strategy is sufficiently mathematically complex that, until the advent of modern computers, the solution of multiple regression relationships beyond a very few

FIGURE 12.1. COST DATA FOR TEN HOSPITALS.

	B	C	D	
1	Y	X1	X2	
2	Cost	Size	Visibility	
3	2750	225	6	
4	2400	200	37	
5	2920	300	14	
6	1800	350	33	
7	3520	200	11	
8	2270	250	21	
9	3100	175	21	
10	1980	400	22	
11	2680	350	20	
12	2720	275	16	
13				

independent variables x was rarely attempted. Fortunately, the Excel add-in that easily allows us to do simple linear regression also allows us to do multiple regression with up to sixteen independent variables x. In general, few practical applications of multiple regression require this many independent variables.

To examine the way in which Excel can be used for multiple regression, let us consider the data shown in Figure 12.1. In Figure 12.1, the variable y is cost per hospital case for ten hospitals. The variable X1 is the size of the hospital in the number of beds. The variable X2 is a measure of the extent to which the administrator of the hospital can accurately compare his hospital with other hospitals, in terms of costs. An administrator who has a more accurate view of the competition receives a higher score on the visibility scale. Although the data shown in Figure 12.1 are wholly fabricated, they were fabricated with the recognition that larger hospitals are frequently thought to have lower case costs than smaller hospitals, and hospitals in which the administrator is knowledgeable about the competition are also likely to have lower case costs. Even though these data are for only ten hypothetical hospitals, they can be used to demonstrate both the regression capability of Excel and the calculation of the regression coefficients.

The first step in the description of the use of Excel for multiple regression is a discussion of how the Tools/Data Analysis/Regression add-in can be used to carry out multiple regression. Recall that the initial regression window is as shown in Figure 12.2. This figure also shows the entries needed to produce the regression results. As with simple linear regression, the dependent variable, which is cost, is shown in the Input Y Range box as $B$2:$B$12. The independent variable, however, shown in the Input X Range box, is now different from the simple linear regression model. For multiple regression, the entry for the X variable is given as

FIGURE 12.2. EXCEL REGRESSION WINDOW.

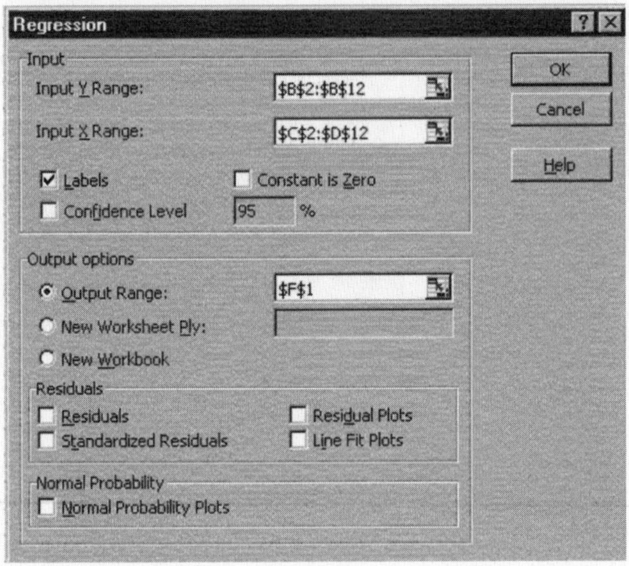

$C$2:$D$12. Excel has been instructed to select not a single column but two contiguous columns to be included as the independent variable data.

As was the case with single variable regression, the labels box has been checked to indicate that the first cell in each row of data is to be treated as a data label. The last important component in the regression window is the output range, which, in this case, is given as cell F1 in the spreadsheet in which the data appear. Checking OK in the regression window will carry out the multiple regression operation and show the results beginning in cell F1.

The results of the multiple regression are shown in Figure 12.3. This figure is quite similar to that for simple linear regression, except that now, instead of having one named variable (other than the intercept), there are two: Size and Visibility. The interpretation of the results given in Figure 12.3 is essentially the same as the interpretation that would be given for simple linear regression. The interpretation of the Regression Statistics section is essentially the same as that of simple linear regression, except that now the Adjusted R Square takes into account the two independent variables. The ANOVA is interpreted just as it was in simple linear regression, but it should be noted that there are now 2 degrees of freedom in the regression and $n - 3$ in the residual. The regression coefficients are also interpreted exactly as in simple linear regression except that there are now two slope coefficients rather than one.

FIGURE 12.3. MULTIPLE REGRESSION OUTPUT.

	F	G	H	I	J	K	L
1	SUMMARY OUTPUT						
2							
3	*Regression Statistics*						
4	Multiple R	0.8340336					
5	R Square	0.6956121					
6	Adjusted R Sq	0.6086441					
7	Standard Error	323.9537					
8	Observations	10					
9							
10	ANOVA						
11		*df*	*SS*	*MS*	*F*	*Significance F*	
12	Regression	2	1678818.023	839409	7.998485	0.015559511	
13	Residual	7	734621.9772	104946			
14	Total	9	2413440				
15							
16		*Coefficients*	*Standard Error*	*t Stat*	*P-value*	*Lower 95%*	*Upper 95%*
17	Intercept	4240.131	435.6084415	9.733813	2.56E-05	3210.081442	5270.18054
18	Size	-3.7623152	1.442783962	-2.60768	0.035032	-7.17395474	-0.3506757
19	Visibility	-29.895527	11.66297571	-2.56328	0.037372	-57.4740623	-2.3169913

There is an important point to consider when interpreting the slope coefficients. In simple linear regression we saw that the regression line could be graphed quite clearly as a straight line in a two-dimensional space (that is, with the *x* or independent variable on the horizontal axis and the *y* or dependent variable on the vertical axis). With two independent variables, a graph of the predicted values would have to be a plane (a two-dimensional figure) in a three-dimensional space. By extension, if we were to hope to graph the results of, for example, five independent variables, that would have to be a five-dimensional figure in a six-dimensional space. Since the average human cannot generate a mental image of any space with more than three dimensions, it should be apparent that it would be impossible to produce a visual image of the results of most multiple regression analyses. The useful visual aids are pretty much limited to simple linear regression.

There is another point to clarify when looking at the coefficients from multiple regression. These coefficients are computed simultaneously. If either coefficient were calculated independently (that is, in a simple linear regression), it would not be equal to the coefficients calculated in multiple regression, except in that unusual situation in which there was absolutely no relationship between the two independent variables. Furthermore, the *R* Square obtained from multiple regression is not the sum of the *R* Square that would be obtained from two simple linear regressions with the same two variables. In fact, either of the two independent variables may produce nearly as large an R Square as the two variables taken together.

The Solution to the Multiple Regression Problem

In Chapter Eleven we learned how to calculate the regression coefficients from original data and found that the results we obtained were exactly the same as those obtained by the Excel Data Analysis Regression package. In this chapter we are going to look at how the results of multiple regression can be found. In general, because the multiple regression coefficients are found simultaneously, the formula for the solution of the multiple regression problem is not so easily expressed as the solution for the simple linear regression.

To consider the formulas for finding the coefficients that best fit the data in a multiple regression situation, specifically this section examines the case of two independent variables as the simplest multiple regression case. Also this section introduce the use of some relatively elementary calculus. You don't have to understand the calculus involved to use the results or do anything else in this book, but those who do understand calculus should be able to see how it is possible to arrive at the equations necessary to solve the multiple regression problems. Recall that the criterion for a best-fitting regression result is as that shown in Equation 12.3. If there are two independent variables, as discussed earlier, in Section 12.1, then $\hat{y}$ in Equation 12.3 can be defined as shown in Equation 12.4, where b_0 represents the coefficient for the intercept.

$$\sum (y - \hat{y})^2 = \text{minimum} \tag{12.3}$$

$$\hat{y} = b_1 x_1 + b_2 x_2 + b_0 x_0 \tag{12.4}$$

If $\hat{y}$ is as that given in Equation 12.4, then the problem of multiple regression is to find the coefficients b_j that minimize the expression in Equation 12.5.

$$\sum (y - b_1 x_1 - b_2 x_2 - b_0 x_0)^2 = \text{minimum} \tag{12.5}$$

Calculus provides a direct solution to the problem of finding the formulas that provide the coefficients b_j that minimize the expression in Equation 12.5. The solution is to take the partial derivative of Equation 12.5, with respect to each of the three b_j coefficients. Although how this is done may not be clear to you if you don't understand calculus, don't despair. It is important to know that it can be done. And you will never have to know how to do it to understand anything else in this section of the book—or in the book in general.

Okay, if we use calculus and take the partial derivative of Equation 12.5, with respect to each of the three b_j coefficients, the result will be three new equations, as shown in Equation 12.6.

$$\frac{\partial}{\partial b_1} = -2\sum x_1(y - b_1x_1 - b_2x_2 - b_0x_0)$$

$$\frac{\partial}{\partial b_2} = -2\sum x_2(y - b_1x_1 - b_2x_2 - b_0x_0) \qquad (12.6)$$

$$\frac{\partial}{\partial b_0} = -2\sum x_0(y - b_1x_1 - b_2x_2 - b_0x_0)$$

It is the case that if we set the equations in Equation 12.6 equal to zero, we can solve for the regression coefficients that will best fit the original dependent variable data. After setting the three equations equal to zero, we can drop the partial derivative signs in the equations (the symbols in front of the equal signs) and, after a little algebra, we end up with the three formulations in Equation 12.7.

$$\sum x_1 y - b_1\sum x_1^2 - b_2\sum x_1x_2 - b_0\sum x_1x_0 = 0$$

$$\sum x_2 y - b_1\sum x_1x_2 - b_2\sum x_2^2 - b_0\sum x_2x_0 = 0 \qquad (12.7)$$

$$\sum x_0 y - b_1\sum x_1x_0 - b_2\sum x_2x_0 - b_0\sum x_0^2 = 0$$

or

$$b_1\sum x_1^2 + b_2\sum x_1x_2 + b_0\sum x_1x_0 = \sum x_1 y$$

$$b_1\sum x_1x_2 + b_2\sum x_2^2 + b_0\sum x_2x_0 = \sum x_2 y$$

$$b_1\sum x_1x_0 + b_2\sum x_2x_0 + b_0\sum x_0^2 = \sum x_0 y$$

The equations in Equation 12.7 represent a set of simultaneous equations. Since both the independent variables denoted by x and the dependent variable y are known values, all of the terms in Equation 12.7 that involve summations of x or y can be calculated; hence, they are known values. But the coefficients b_j are what we are interested in discovering. They are the unknown values. With that in mind, some of you might recognize the second three expressions in Equation 12.7 as being three equations with three unknowns. In general, a set of equations with an equal number of unknowns can be solved simultaneously for the unknown values, and thus, we should be able to solve this set of three equations for the coefficients b_j that we wish to find. If you remember ninth grade algebra, you know that you can solve this problem with something called successive elimination. The first step in the successive elimination process is to find the various summations involving x and y. Figure 12.4 shows the calculation of

FIGURE 12.4. CALCULATION OF SUMS.

	G6	▼	=	=SUMPRODUCT(B3:B12,C3:C12)		
	A	B	C	D	E	F	G
1	Y	X1	X2	X0			
2	Cost	Size	Visibility	Intercept			
3	2750	225	6	1		X1^2	794375
4	2400	200	37	1		X2^2	4833
5	2920	300	14	1		X0^2	10
6	1800	350	33	1		X1X2	55825
7	3520	200	11	1		X1X0	2725
8	2270	250	21	1		X2X0	201
9	3100	175	21	1		X1Y	6896750
10	1980	400	22	1		X2Y	497750
11	2680	350	20	1		X0Y	26140
12	2720	275	16	1			

the various known values required by the simultaneous equations in Equation 12.7 for the data on hospitals given originally in Figure 12.1 and repeated again here. The values in cells G6:G11 were found by using the =SUMPRODUCT() function that multiplies two separate strings of data together and sums the result of all the multiplication operations. The construction of the =SUMPRODUCT() statement can be seen in the formula line in Figure 12.4 for the variables X1 (Size) and X2 (Visibility). It can be seen in the formula line presentation that the =SUMPRODUCT() function takes two arguments: the data range for the first variable and the data range for the second variable. The values in cells G3:G5 could also have been produced by using the =SUMPRODUCT() function, with the same range entered for each argument. But they were actually produced by using the =SUMSQ() function, which takes one argument and acts by squaring each subsequent value and putting the sum of those operations into the appropriate cell.

With the various sums calculated that are called for in the three simultaneous equations given in Equation 12.7, it is possible to undertake the solution to the equations, and the solution for coefficient b_j is shown in Figure 12.5. Rows 15 to 17 in Figure 12.5 represent the three simultaneous equations. As shown, the b1, b2, and b3 designations in row 14 represent the coefficient by which each of the numbers in the corresponding row must be multiplied to produce the values in column E, which represent the sums of X1Y, X2Y, and X0Y, respectively.

Successive elimination for the solution of b_j proceeds by eliminating, successively, each of the other two coefficients. This is equivalent to finding the value of the equations when the values by which the other coefficients are multiplied are equal to 0. Rows 19, 20, and 21 show the result of finding an equation with two

FIGURE 12.5. SUCCESSIVE ELIMINATION FOR b_1.

	A	B	C	D	E	F
A20		▼	= =D15/D16			
	A	B	C	D	E	
14		b1	b2	b0		
15		794375	55825	2725	6896750	
16		55825	4833	201	497750	
17		2725	201	10	26140	
18						
19		794375	55825	2725	6896750	
20	13.55721	756831.5	65522.01	2725	6748103	
21		37543.53	-9697.01	0	148646.8	
22						
23		794375	55825	2725	6896750	
24	272.5	742562.5	54772.5	2725	7123150	
25		51812.5	1052.5	0	-226400	
26						
27		37543.53	-9697.01		148646.8	
28	-9.21332	-477365	-9697.01		2085895	
29		514908.5	0		-1937248	
30		-3.76232				
31						

variables and two unknowns with b_0 eliminated. Row 15 is replicated in row 19. To produce row 20, row 16 is multiplied by the value in A20, which is found by dividing cell D15 by cell D16. You will note that the result in D20 is exactly the value in D19. Row 20 is then subtracted from row 19 to produce row 21, which is essentially one equation with two rather than three unknown values, b_1 and b_2. The same process is repeated in rows 23 to 25. Row 15 is again copied to row 23, but, now to produce row 24, row 17 is multiplied by the value in cell A24, which is cell D15 divided by cell D17. Again, the result in D23 is the same as that in D24. Subtracting row 24 from row 23 produces a second equation with two unknowns in row 25.

The final step of this successive elimination is shown in rows 27 to 29. Row 21, the first of the two equations in two unknowns that were found, is copied to row 27. Row 28 is the result of multiplying row 25 by the value in cell A28, which is cell C21 divided by cell C25. Again, note that the values in cells C27 and C28 are equal. Now, subtraction of row 28 from row 27 leaves a single variable (b_1) with a nonzero value. The solution to the equation in row 29 is shown in B30. You can confirm that that is the same value that was found for the coefficient of Size in Figure 12.3, the Excel Tools/Data Analysis/Regression-produced result.

The other two coefficients can be found in much the same way. It should be clear that successive elimination is a tedious process involving a lot of division, multiplication, and subtraction. Because it is also what is known as an iterative process, it can be very difficult to set up in a systematic way on an Excel spreadsheet. Moreover, as the number of coefficients gets larger, the amount of work involved in the successive elimination approach to solving simultaneous equations grows geometrically. Basically, it is not a very efficient way to do multiple regression. Happily, there is a much more efficient way to solve simultaneous equations—essentially to solve the multiple regression problem, and Excel can deal with it quite effectively. But to understand that strategy for finding multiple regression coefficients, it is necessary to understand a little about matrix math, which is the topic of the next section.

Exercises for Section 12.1

1. Use the data shown in Figure 12.1 (also given on the Hospitals worksheet in Chpt 12–1.xls).
   a. Replicate the analysis given in Figure 12.3 by using the Tools/Data Analysis/Regression add-in.
   b. Replicate the analysis given in Figure 12.5 and find the coefficient for b_1 by using successive elimination.
   c. Find the other two coefficients by the same method and make sure they match those given in Figure 12.3.

2. The data on the SWC worksheet of Chpt 12–1.xls is taken from the *State of the World's Children 2001* (2000). It shows rates of under-five mortality (U5Mort), female literacy (FemLit), and access safe water (SafeW) for 113 countries of the world, each with over one million inhabitants. Use the data to do the following:
   a. Carry out an analysis such as that given in Figure 12.3 by using the Tools/Data Analysis/Regression add-in.
   b. Carry out an analysis such as that given in Figure 12.5 and find the coefficient for b_1 by using successive elimination to find the coefficient for FemLit.
   c. Find the other two coefficients by the same method.

Section 12.2 Multiple Regression and Matrices

In order to understand how the computer carries out regression analysis—which automatically leads to a better understanding of regression, it is necessary to understand something about matrix math. This section is a brief introduction to matrix math.

An Introduction to Matrix Math

A matrix is a set of numbers in a two-dimensional space. Matrices are almost always designated with capital letters in boldface type. In general, a matrix **X** has n rows and m columns, as shown in Equation 12.8, where the first subscript denotes the row and the second denotes the column.

$$\mathbf{X} = \begin{bmatrix} x_{11} & x_{12} & \cdots & x_{1m} \\ x_{21} & x_{22} & \cdots & x_{2m} \\ \cdot & \cdot & & \cdot \\ \cdot & \cdot & & \cdot \\ \cdot & \cdot & & \cdot \\ x_{n1} & x_{n2} & \cdots & x_{nm} \end{bmatrix} \tag{12.8}$$

A matrix is said to have *dimensions* equal to n and m so that the matrix **X** has dimensions $n \times m$ (rows first, columns second). The following is a typical example of a 2×3 matrix:

$$\begin{bmatrix} 2 & 5 & 7 \\ 1 & 14 & 11 \end{bmatrix}$$

A *vector* is a matrix with dimensions $n \times 1$ or $1 \times m$, as shown in Equation 12.9.

$$\mathbf{x} = \begin{bmatrix} x_1 \\ x_2 \\ \cdot \\ \cdot \\ \cdot \\ x_n \end{bmatrix}, \quad \mathbf{y} = \begin{bmatrix} y_1 & y_2 & \cdots & y_m \end{bmatrix} \tag{12.9}$$

The following are typical examples of a 3×1 vector and a 1×3 vector:

$$\begin{bmatrix} 3 \\ 15 \\ 6 \end{bmatrix}, \quad \begin{bmatrix} 9 & 27 & 52 \end{bmatrix}.$$

A *scalar* can be considered a matrix of dimensions 1×1. The individual entries of any matrix or vector are scalars, but scalars can stand alone. A scalar is simply a number.

The *transpose* of a matrix $\mathbf{X}$, designated $\mathbf{X}'$, is a matrix in which the first row of $\mathbf{X}$ becomes the first column of $\mathbf{X}'$, the second row of $\mathbf{X}$ the second column of $\mathbf{X}'$, and so on, so that if

$$\mathbf{X} = \begin{bmatrix} x_{11} & x_{12} & x_{13} \\ x_{21} & x_{22} & x_{23} \end{bmatrix}, \qquad \text{then} \qquad \mathbf{X}' = \begin{bmatrix} x_{11} & x_{21} \\ x_{12} & x_{22} \\ x_{13} & x_{23} \end{bmatrix};$$

Or if $\mathbf{X} = \begin{bmatrix} 7 & 3 & 2 \\ 1 & 9 & 5 \end{bmatrix},$ then $\mathbf{X}' = \begin{bmatrix} 7 & 1 \\ 3 & 9 \\ 2 & 5 \end{bmatrix};$

Addition and subtraction may be performed on matrices if each has equal rows and equal columns. The two matrices $\mathbf{X}$ and $\mathbf{Y}$ may be added, as shown in Equation 12.10.

$$
\begin{array}{ccccc}
\mathbf{X} & + & \mathbf{Y} & = & (\mathbf{X} + \mathbf{Y})
\end{array}
$$

$$\begin{bmatrix} x_{11} & x_{12} \\ x_{21} & x_{22} \\ x_{31} & x_{32} \end{bmatrix} + \begin{bmatrix} y_{11} & y_{12} \\ y_{21} & y_{22} \\ y_{31} & y_{32} \end{bmatrix} = \begin{bmatrix} x_{11} + y_{11} & x_{12} + y_{12} \\ x_{21} + y_{21} & x_{22} + y_{22} \\ x_{31} + y_{31} & x_{32} + y_{32} \end{bmatrix}; \qquad \text{or}$$

$$\begin{bmatrix} 7 & 1 \\ 3 & 9 \\ 2 & 5 \end{bmatrix} + \begin{bmatrix} 6 & 2 \\ 2 & 4 \\ 4 & 3 \end{bmatrix} = \begin{bmatrix} 13 & 3 \\ 5 & 13 \\ 6 & 8 \end{bmatrix} \qquad (12.10)$$

The matrix $\mathbf{Y}$ can also be subtracted from $\mathbf{X}$, as shown in Equation 12.11.

$$
\begin{array}{ccccc}
\mathbf{X} & - & \mathbf{Y} & = & (\mathbf{X} - \mathbf{Y})
\end{array}
$$

$$\begin{bmatrix} x_{11} & x_{12} \\ x_{21} & x_{22} \\ x_{31} & x_{32} \end{bmatrix} - \begin{bmatrix} y_{11} & y_{12} \\ y_{21} & y_{22} \\ y_{31} & y_{32} \end{bmatrix} = \begin{bmatrix} x_{11} - y_{11} & x_{12} - y_{12} \\ x_{21} - y_{21} & x_{22} - y_{22} \\ x_{31} - y_{31} & x_{32} - y_{32} \end{bmatrix}; \qquad \text{or}$$

$$\begin{bmatrix} 7 & 1 \\ 3 & 9 \\ 2 & 5 \end{bmatrix} - \begin{bmatrix} 6 & 2 \\ 2 & 4 \\ 4 & 3 \end{bmatrix} = \begin{bmatrix} 1 & -1 \\ 1 & 5 \\ -2 & 2 \end{bmatrix} \qquad (12.11)$$

Multiplication can be performed on matrices if the number of columns in the first matrix is equal to the number of rows in the second. Such matrices will be said to *conform* for multiplication. The two matrices $\mathbf{X}'(2 \times 3)$ and $\mathbf{Y}$ (3×2) can be multiplied and the resulting matrix $\mathbf{X}'\mathbf{Y}$ will be of dimension 2×2, as shown in Equation 12.12. Although $ab = ba$ when a and b are both scalars, in general, $\mathbf{X}'\mathbf{Y}$

(2×2) does not equal **YX′** (3×3), and will not have the same dimensions. When the operation **X′Y** is carried out, **Y** may be said to be premultiplied by **X′**. When **YX′** is carried out, **Y** is postmultiplied by **X′**. A particularly useful matrix product is **X′X**, which provides the sum of squares and cross products for **X**.

$$
\begin{array}{ccccc}
\mathbf{X'} & \cdot & \mathbf{Y} & = & \mathbf{X'Y}
\end{array}
$$

$$
\begin{bmatrix} x_{11} & x_{21} & x_{31} \\ x_{12} & x_{22} & x_{32} \end{bmatrix} \cdot \begin{bmatrix} y_{11} & y_{12} \\ y_{21} & y_{22} \\ y_{31} & y_{32} \end{bmatrix} = \begin{bmatrix} x_{11}y_{11} + x_{21}y_{21} + x_{31}y_{31} & x_{11}y_{12} + x_{21}y_{22} + x_{31}y_{32} \\ x_{12}y_{11} + x_{22}y_{21} + x_{31}y_{32} & x_{12}y_{12} + x_{22}y_{22} + x_{32}y_{32} \end{bmatrix};
$$

$$
\text{or} \quad \begin{bmatrix} 7 & 3 & 2 \\ 1 & 9 & 5 \end{bmatrix} \cdot \begin{bmatrix} 6 & 2 \\ 2 & 4 \\ 4 & 3 \end{bmatrix} = \begin{bmatrix} 56 & 32 \\ 44 & 53 \end{bmatrix} \tag{12.12}
$$

Any matrices or vectors that are to be multiplied must conform for multiplication, with one exception: any matrix or vector of any dimension can be pre- or postmultiplied by a scalar, as shown in Equation 12.13.

$$
a \cdot \mathbf{X} = a \cdot \begin{bmatrix} x_{11} & x_{12} \\ x_{21} & x_{22} \\ x_{31} & x_{32} \end{bmatrix} = \begin{bmatrix} ax_{11} & ax_{12} \\ ax_{21} & ax_{22} \\ ax_{31} & ax_{32} \end{bmatrix} = \mathbf{X} \cdot a; \quad \text{or}
$$

$$
5 \cdot \begin{bmatrix} 7 & 1 \\ 3 & 9 \\ 2 & 5 \end{bmatrix} = \begin{bmatrix} 35 & 5 \\ 15 & 45 \\ 10 & 25 \end{bmatrix} \tag{12.13}
$$

Division is, in general, undefined for matrices. With matrices in which rows equal columns and the *determinant* of the matrix does not equal zero, multiplication of a matrix by its *inverse* produces the same result as division. The *determinant* of a matrix is a scalar defined only for matrices in which rows equal columns. For the 2×2 matrix **W**, the determinant of **W** may be written as shown in Equation 12.14.

$$
|\mathbf{W}| = \begin{vmatrix} w_{11} & w_{12} \\ w_{21} & w_{22} \end{vmatrix} = w_{11}w_{22} - w_{21}w_{12}; \quad \text{or}
$$

$$
|\mathbf{W}| = \begin{vmatrix} 6 & 3 \\ 4 & 7 \end{vmatrix} = (6 \cdot 7) - (4 \cdot 3) = 30. \tag{12.14}
$$

If any column of a matrix is a linear transformation of one or more other columns, the determinant will be zero. If, for example, the matrix **V** is as shown in Equation 12.15, the determinant of **V** will be zero and the *inverse* of **V** (written $\mathbf{V}^{-1}$) will not exist.

$$|\mathbf{V}| = \begin{vmatrix} v_{11} & 2v_{11} \\ v_{21} & 2v_{21} \end{vmatrix} = \begin{vmatrix} 6 & 12 \\ 4 & 8 \end{vmatrix}; \quad \text{then} \quad |\mathbf{V}| = (6 \cdot 8) - (4 \cdot 12) = 0. \quad (12.15)$$

In scalar arithmetic, $a/a = a \times 1/a = aa^{-1} = 1$. If the inverse of a matrix **W** exists (see Equation 12.14 and Equation 12.15), then $\mathbf{WW}^{-1} = \mathbf{I}$, where **I** is a matrix with 1 in each entry on the main diagonal and zero everywhere else. For example, suppose **W** is as defined in Equation 12.16 (the matrix whose determinant is shown in Equation 12.14).

$$\mathbf{W} = \begin{bmatrix} w_{11} & w_{12} \\ w_{21} & w_{22} \end{bmatrix} \quad (12.16)$$

Then, $\mathbf{W}^{-1}$ is as defined in Equation 12.17, where $w_{11}w_{22} - w_{12}w_{21}$ is $|\mathbf{W}|$, as defined in Equation 12.14.

$$\mathbf{W}^{-1} = \begin{bmatrix} \dfrac{w_{22}}{w_{11}w_{22} - w_{12}w_{21}} & \dfrac{-w_{12}}{w_{11}w_{22} - w_{12}w_{21}} \\ \dfrac{-w_{21}}{w_{11}w_{22} - w_{12}w_{21}} & \dfrac{w_{11}}{w_{11}w_{22} - w_{12}w_{21}} \end{bmatrix} \quad (12.17)$$

Finally, $\mathbf{WW}^{-1} = \mathbf{I}$, as shown in Equation 12.18.

$$\mathbf{WW}^{-1} = \begin{bmatrix} w_{11} & w_{12} \\ w_{21} & w_{22} \end{bmatrix} \begin{bmatrix} \dfrac{w_{22}}{w_{11}w_{22} - w_{12}w_{21}} & \dfrac{-w_{12}}{w_{11}w_{22} - w_{12}w_{21}} \\ \dfrac{-w_{21}}{w_{11}w_{22} - w_{12}w_{21}} & \dfrac{w_{11}}{w_{11}w_{22} - w_{12}w_{21}} \end{bmatrix}$$

$$= \begin{bmatrix} \dfrac{w_{11}w_{22} - w_{12}w_{21}}{w_{11}w_{22} - w_{12}w_{21}} & \dfrac{-w_{11}w_{12} + w_{12}w_{11}}{w_{11}w_{22} - w_{12}w_{21}} \\ \dfrac{w_{21}w_{22} - w_{22}w_{21}}{w_{11}w_{22} - w_{12}w_{21}} & \dfrac{-w_{12}w_{21} + w_{11}w_{22}}{w_{11}w_{22} - w_{12}w_{21}} \end{bmatrix} = \begin{bmatrix} 1 & 0 \\ 0 & 1 \end{bmatrix} = \mathbf{I}, \quad \text{or}$$

$$\begin{bmatrix} 6 & 3 \\ 4 & 7 \end{bmatrix} \begin{bmatrix} 7/30 & -3/30 \\ -4/30 & 6/30 \end{bmatrix} = \begin{bmatrix} 1 & 0 \\ 0 & 1 \end{bmatrix} \quad (12.18)$$

Whereas it is relatively easy to find the inverse of a 2×2 matrix, finding the inverse of a 3×3 or larger matrix becomes increasingly difficult. One method developed early on in linear algebra is the square root method—described, for example, in Harmon (1960). Today it is easier to rely on computer programs that have the capability to produce the matrix inverse in order to obtain it. Fortunately, Excel is one such computer program. In the next section, we look at this capability of Excel's and how it works to solve the simultaneous equation problem of multiple regression.

Matrix Capabilities of Excel

Excel provides several functions that are specifically matrix functions and are particularly useful in regard to the solution of the multiple regression problem. Interestingly, Excel refers to matrices as *arrays*, and the term array will be used to refer to a matrix during much of this discussion. But it is often confusing to try to stay with one or the other, so if you see matrix and array used interchangeably here, just remember that they are basically the same things. Excel provides four functions that are specifically designed to manipulate arrays (or matrices). These are =MMULT(), =MINVERSE(), =MDETERM(), and =TRANSPOSE(). The first of these functions, =MMULT(), multiplies any two arrays together as long as the two conform for multiplication. The second, =MINVERSE(), finds the inverse of any square array that has a nonzero determinant. If the determinant of the array is 0, Excel will return NUM# in the cells selected. Excel returns the determinant of the array for =MDETERM() and the transpose of the array for =TRANSPOSE(). To see how these operate and the results obtained, let us look again at the data in Figure 12.1. We will also use the Intercept variable (constant), as shown in Figure 12.4, and this is reproduced in Figure 12.6. In Figure 12.6, the area that is highlighted in black will be referred to with matrix notation as $\mathbf{X}$, (matrices other than those that are $m \times 1$ or $1 \times m$ are always designated with bold roman capitals). The cost column (not highlighted) will be

FIGURE 12.6. HOSPITAL DATA.

	A	B	C	D	E
B3		= 225			
1	Y	X1	X2	X0	
2	Cost	Size	Visibility	Intercept	
3	2750	225	6	1	
4	2400	200	37	1	
5	2920	300	14	1	
6	1800	350	33	1	
7	3520	200	11	1	
8	2270	250	21	1	
9	3100	175	21	1	
10	1980	400	22	1	
11	2680	350	20	1	
12	2720	275	16	1	
13					

FIGURE 12.7. ARRAYS Y, X, AND X'.

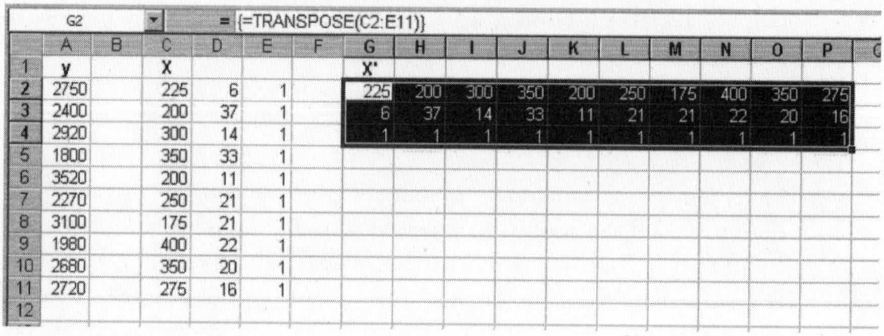

designated with matrix notation as **y** (matrices that are $m \times 1$ or $1 \times m$ are called vectors and are always referred to with bold roman small letters).

Figure 12.7 shows the data given in Figure 12.6, but with several modifications. Now, the independent variable array is designated as simply **y**, the independent variable array is designated as **X**, and a new array, designated as **X'**, is shown in G2:P4. In the formula line in Figure 12.7 is the expression {=TRANSPOSE(C2:E11)}. This is the transpose function, and the resulting array **X'** is the transpose of **X**. It should be noted that the brackets surrounding the =TRANSPOSE() function means that it is one of those functions that enters data into more than one cell and must be invoked by holding down Ctrl/Shift and then hitting enter.

> **IMPORTANT**: In invoking any of the functions that produce results in more than one cell of the spreadsheet, such as the array functions discussed here or the =FREQUENCY() function discussed earlier in the book, it is necessary to highlight the entire area into which the results are to go before typing in the function. In Figure 12.7 the area G2:P4 was highlighted before the =TRANSPOSE() function was typed.

The =MMULT() array function can be used to produce two new arrays, **X'X** and **X'y**, which are shown in Figure 12.8. The array **X'X** is highlighted and the formula for that array is shown in the formula bar. It can be seen there that the array **X'X** is produced with {=MMULT(G2:P4,C2:E11)}. The brackets again indicate that the function was completed with Ctrl/Shift and Enter. The array **X'y** is produced with the array function, {=MMULT(G2:P4,A2:A11)}.

FIGURE 12.8. ARRAYS X′X AND X′y.

G7			= {=MMULT(G2:P4,C2:E11)}												
A	B	C	D	E	F	G	H	I	J	K	L	M	N	O	P
y		x				X′									
2750		225	6	1		225	200	300	350	200	250	175	400	350	275
2400		200	37	1		6	37	14	33	11	21	21	22	20	16
2920		300	14	1		1	1	1	1	1	1	1	1	1	1
1800		350	33	1											
3520		200	11	1		X′X				X′y					
2270		250	21	1		794375	55825	2725		6896750					
3100		175	21	1		55825	4833	201		497750					
1980		400	22	1		2725	201	10		26140					
2680		350	20	1											
2720		275	16	1											

There is something else to note about Figure 12.8 and its comparison with the data in G3:G11 of Figure 12.4. The array $\mathbf{X'X}$ includes all the values in G3 to G8 and the array $\mathbf{X'y}$ includes the values in G9 to G11. The calculation of the $\mathbf{X'X}$ and the $\mathbf{X'y}$ arrays using the matrix capabilities of Excel produces all the values needed for the calculation of the coefficients b_j. It is important to note that the results shown in $\mathbf{X'X}$ (3×3) would not be the same as the results for $\mathbf{XX'}$, which would be 10×10. Moreover, $\mathbf{yX'}$ does not even exist, because the two arrays in that format (10×1) and (3×10) cannot be multiplied.

Using the data in $\mathbf{X'X}$ and $\mathbf{X'y}$ from Figure 12.8, it is possible to rewrite the second three expressions in Equation 12.7, as shown in Equation 12.19. We have already seen that these three equations can be solved for the coefficients b_j with successive elimination. But with our understanding of matrix math, it can also be seen that Equation 12.19 can be rewritten in matrix format, as shown in Equation 12.20.

$$
\begin{aligned}
b_1 794{,}375 + b_2 55{,}825 + b_0 2725 &= 6{,}896{,}750 \\
b_1 55{,}825 \ + b_2 4833 \ + b_0 201_0 &= \ 497{,}750 \\
b_1 2725 \ + b_2 201 \ + b_0 10 \ &= \ 26{,}140
\end{aligned}
\tag{12.19}
$$

$$
\begin{bmatrix} 794{,}375 & 55{,}825 & 2725 \\ 55{,}825 & 4833 & 201 \\ 2725 & 201 & 10 \end{bmatrix}
\begin{bmatrix} b_1 \\ b_2 \\ b_0 \end{bmatrix} =
\begin{bmatrix} 6{,}896{,}750 \\ 497{,}750 \\ 26140 \end{bmatrix}
\tag{12.20}
$$

In matrix notation, the formulation in Equation 12.20 is $\mathbf{X'Xb = X'y}$. Now, how can matrix math be used to solve this equation for b? If we were dealing strictly with scalar arithmetic and we had an equation such as $xb = y$, and x and y

FIGURE 12.9. INVERSE OF X'X.

	M7		▼		= {=MINVERSE(G7:I9)}										
	A	B	C	D	E	F	G	H	I	J	K	L	M	N	O	P
1	y		X				X'									
2	2750		225	6	1		225	200	300	350		200	250	175	400	350	275
3	2400		200	37	1		6	37	14	33		11	21	21	22	20	16
4	2920		300	14	1		1	1	1	1		1	1	1	1	1	1
5	1800		350	33	1											
6	3520		200	11	1		X'X					X'y		X'X⁻¹			
7	2270		250	21	1		794375	55825	2725			6896750		1.98E-05	-2.6E-05	-0.00488	
8	3100		175	21	1		55825	4833	201			497750		-2.6E-05	0.0013	-0.01888	
9	1980		400	22	1		2725	201	10			26140		-0.00488	-0.01888	1.808118	
10	2680		350	20	1											
11	2720		275	16	1											
12																

were known, we could solve for b by $b = y/x$. But this formulation is the same as $1/x \times xb = 1/x \times y$. The expression $1/x$ is the inverse of x, and can also be written as x^{-1}. Similarly, in matrix terms, it turns out that if we can find the inverse of $\mathbf{X'X}$, we can solve the equation $\mathbf{X'Xb = X'y}$ with the equation $\mathbf{X'X^{-1}X'Xb = X'X^{-1}Xy}$, which turns out to be $\mathbf{X'X^{-1}Xy = b}$. Happily, Excel provides the ability to find $\mathbf{X'X^{-1}}$. To see how Excel provides the inverse, we can look at Figure 12.9. In Figure 12.9, the inverse of $\mathbf{X'X}$ is shown in the highlighted area, M7:O9. The {=MINVERSE()} function used to produce the inverse array is shown on the formula bar. Note again that it is enclosed in brackets to denote that it was completed with Ctrl/Shift and Enter. Also, it is important to remember that the entire area M7:O9 was highlighted before the {=MINVERSE()} function was typed in.

A further point that should be made about the inverse array is that the numbers, particularly in M7, N7, and M8, may appear a little strange. The way these numbers are shown is known as scientific notation. In more familiar terms, the number 1.98E-05 is actually the number .0000198. The E-05 means that there are five decimal places before the decimal place in 1.98E-05. It should be recognized that any number that is followed by E with a minus sign and a number is a very small number. Excel uses the E convention to put numbers into cells that otherwise would be two narrow to display the string of decimal places before the actual values begin.

The E convention is also used for very large numbers. For example, a number that would be shown in Excel as 1.98E+11 would actually be 198,000,000,000. This is a relatively economical way for Excel to display very large numbers.

Having found the inverse of $\mathbf{X'X}$, it is now possible to solve for the vector $\mathbf{b}$. This solution is shown in Figure 12.10. As can be seen there, the coefficients b_j (found by the =MMULT() function, as shown in the formula line of Figure 12.10),

FIGURE 12.10. THE *b* COEFFICIENTS.

	G12		▼		=	{=MMULT(M7:O9,K7:K9)}									
	A	B	C	D	E	F	G	H	I	J	K	L	M	N	O	P
1	**y**		**X**				**X'**									
2	2750		225	6	1		225	200	300	350	200	250	175	400	350	275
3	2400		200	37	1		6	37	14	33	11	21	21	22	20	16
4	2920		300	14	1		1	1	1	1	1	1	1	1	1	1
5	1800		350	33	1											
6	3520		200	11	1		**X'X**				**X'y**		**X'X⁻¹**			
7	2270		250	21	1		794375	55825	2725		6896750		1.98E-05	-2.6E-05	-0.00488	
8	3100		175	21	1		55825	4833	201		497750		-2.6E-05	0.0013	-0.01888	
9	1980		400	22	1		2725	201	10		26140		-0.00488	-0.01888	1.808118	
10	2680		350	20	1											
11	2720		275	16	1		**b**									
12							-3.7623									
13							-29.896									
14							4240.13									

are exactly the same (except for order and decimal places) as the b_j values found by using the built-in Excel package under Tools/Data Analysis/Regression, which is shown in Figure 12.3.

In general, the calculation of all the important results relative to multiple regression—the predicted value of $y(\hat{y})$, the total sums of squares (SS_T), regression sums of squares (SS_R) and error sums of squares (SS_E), the value of R^2 and the correlation coefficient (R), the standard error of estimate (Syx), and the F tests—can all be developed, once the b coefficients are available. These follow the same development as that described for simple linear regression in the previous chapter. There is one place in which the remaining calculations diverge from that shown for simple linear regression, in the calculation of the standard errors for the coefficients b_j. The calculation of the standard errors of the coefficients for multiple regression relies on values that appear only in the matrix $\mathbf{X'X^{-1}}$.

Recall that the standard error of estimate, Syx, the standard error of the predicted values of y, is found by dividing the error sums of squares, SS_E, by $n - 2$ and taking the square root of the result. In simple linear regression, the standard error of b_j is found by dividing the Syx by the square root of the sums of squares in x (SS_X). This is essentially the same as multiplying Syx by the square root of $1/SS_X$. In multiple regression, the equivalent result is obtained by multiplying Syx by the square root of each of the main diagonal elements of $\mathbf{X'X^{-1}}$.

To see the calculation of the standard errors for the coefficients b_j consider Figure 12.11. Here the value of Syx has been copied from Figure 12.3. The formula bar shows that the cell highlighted in white is calculated by multiplying the value in cell $M$11 (Syx) by the square root of the value in cell M7 (here 1.98E-05). Because cell $M$11 is fixed, the formula can then be copied

FIGURE 12.11. CALCULATION OF STANDARD ERRORS OF *b*.

	=$M$11*SQRT(M7)		
M	**N**	**O**	**P**
X'X⁻¹			
1.98E-05	-2.6E-05	-0.00488	
-2.6E-05	0.0013	-0.01888	
-0.00488	-0.01888	1.808118	
323.9537			
1.442784	#NUM!	#NUM!	
#NUM!	11.663	#NUM!	
#NUM!	#NUM!	435.6084	

into the other cells in M and in N and O to produce, on the main diagonal, the standard errors for all the values of the coefficients *b*. The expression #NUM! that appears in the off-diagonal cells indicates, in this case, that we tried to take the square root of a negative number. In any case, it is the main diagonal elements that are of interest. It can be seen that except for ordering, they match the values found for the standard errors of the coefficients *b* in Figure 12.3. These standard error values can be used directly to perform the *t* test that determines whether the appropriate coefficients are different from 0 or not.

Calculation of All Multiple Regression Results

Figure 12.12 shows the analysis as given in Figure 12.10 and Figure 12.11, but, in addition, it shows all the other important results of multiple regression, as shown originally in Figure 12.3. The section of column A labeled $\hat{y}$ was calculated using the matrix function =MMULT(C2:E11,G13:G15), which is essentially the formula for the prediction of the *y* values cast in matrix form. The values in column C labeled $y - \bar{y}$ represent the difference between the actual values of *y* and the mean of *y*. The value in C14 was calculated with the formula =A2-AVERAGE ($A$2:$A$11). That formula can be copied all the way to C23 to produce all the $y - \bar{y}$ values. The value for the total sums of squares, SS_T, in cell H18, is calculated using the Excel function =SUMSQ(C14:C23).

The column labeled *yh* (for $\hat{y}$) –*yb* (for $\bar{y}$) was calculated by subtracting the predicted values of *y*, $\hat{y}$, from the average values for *y*. The formula for the cell D14 is =A14-AVERAGE($A$2:$A$11). That formula can be copied to all the cells from D14 to D23 to create all the values of *yh* – *yb*. The value of the sums of squares

FIGURE 12.12. CALCULATION OF ALL RESULTS FROM FIGURE 12.3.

#	A	B	C	D	E	F	G	H	I	J	K	L	M	N	O	P
1	y	x					x'									
2	2750	225	6	1			225	200	300	350	200	250	175	400	350	275
3	2400	200	37	1			6	37	14	33	11	21	21	22	20	16
4	2920	300	14	1			1	1	1	1	1	1	1	1	1	1
5	1800	350	33	1												
6	3520	200	11	1		X'X	794375	55825	2725	X'y	6896750	X'X-1	1.98E-05	-2.6E-05	-0.00488	
7	2270	250	21	1			55825	4833	201		497750		-2.6E-05	0.0013	-0.01888	
8	3100	175	21	1			2725	201	10		26140		-0.00488	-0.01888	1.808118	
9	1980	400	22	1												
10	2680	350	20	1												
11	2720	275	16	1												
12							b	S.E.b	t	p			1.442784	#NUM!	#NUM!	
13	yhat	y-ybar		yh-yb	y-yh		-3.7623	1.44278	-2.61	0.03503			#NUM!	11.66298	#NUM!	
14	3214	136		600.2	-464		-29.896	11.663	-2.56	0.03737			#NUM!	#NUM!	435.6084	
15	2382	-214		-232.5	18.47		4240.13	435.608	9.734	2.6E-05						
16	2693	306		78.9	227.1											
17	1937	-814		-677.2	-137			SS	d.f.	MS	F	p				
18	3159	906		544.8	361.2		SST	2413440	9							
19	2672	-344		57.75	-402		SSR	1678818	2	839409	7.99849	0.016				
20	2954	486		339.9	146.1		SSE	734622	7	104946						
21	2078	-634		-536.5	-97.5											
22	2325	66		-288.6	354.6		R^2	0.69561								
23	2727	106		113.2	-7.17		S.E.	323.954								

due to regression, SS_R, in cell H19 is calculated using =SUMSQ (D14:D23). The column labeled $y - yh$ (for $\hat{y}$) was calculated by subtracting each value of $\hat{y}$ from y. The formula for cell E14 is =A2-A14. The sums of squares error, SS_E, in cell H20 was calculated using =SUMSQ(E14:E23).

Degrees of freedom in any multiple regression will always be $n - 1$ for SS_T, equal to m (the number of predictor variables) for SS_R, and $n - m - 1$ for SS_E. In the case of this analysis, these values are shown in Cells I18:I20 as 9, 2, and 7, respectively. The mean square values in cells J19 and J20 are the sums of squares values divided by their degrees of freedom. The overall F test for the independence of y from the two variables x is calculated by dividing the mean square due to regression by the mean square error. The probability of the F value, p, is given by the Excel function =FDIST(K19,2,7).

The R^2 value in cell H22 is calculated by dividing SS_R by SS_T. The value of S.E. (standard error of estimate) in cell H23 is obtained by dividing SS_E by its degrees of freedom and taking the square root of the result. This value was used to multiply by the square root of the values in M12, N13, and O14 to produce the standard error of each value of b_j in cells H13:H15. The t values for each of the b_j is calculated by dividing each value of b by its standard error. The probabilities of the t values are given by =TDIST(t,d.f.,2). The degrees of freedom for any value of b_j is equal to the degrees of freedom for SS_E. Since two of the b_j values are negative, however, the =TDIST() function will produce only the result #NUM!. In order to produce the actual probability of the coefficients, it is necessary to include the Excel =ABS( ) function to get the absolute value of t before getting the probability of the t value. So, for example, the probability in cell J13 was obtained with =TDIST(ABS(I13),7,2).

Exercises for Section 12.2

1. Use the data on the Hospitals worksheet of Chpt 12–1.xls and replicate the analysis shown in Figure 12.12.

   a. Set up the data from the Hospitals worksheet, as shown in Figure 12.12, with the variables X_1 and X_2 in cells C2:C11 and D2:D11, respectively, and supply a third independent variable, the constant, as shown in cells E2:E11.

   b. Generate the transpose of the matrix **X** in cells G2:P4 by using the =TRANSPOSE(C2:E11) function. Remember that the entire area into which the transpose matrix will go must be highlighted prior to invoking the function and that the function must be invoked with Ctrl/Shift and Enter.

   c. Calculate the values of **X′X** in cells G7:I9 by using the =MMULT (G2:P4,C2:E11) function. This function, too, requires highlighting of the entire three-by-three cell area and Ctrl/Shift and Enter.

   d. Use =MMULT(G2:P4,A2:A11) to calculate the values of **X′y** in cells K7:K9.

   e. Use =MINVERSE(G7:I9) to obtain the inverse of the matrix **X′X** in cells M7:O9.

   f. Calculate the values of b in cells G13:G15, using the =MMULT (M7:O9,K7:K9) function.

   g. Using the values of b and the original matrix **X**, generate the values of $\hat{y}$ in cells A14:A23 with =MMULT(C2:D11,G13:G15).

   h. Generate the values of $y - \bar{y}$ in cells C14:C23, using y-AVERAGE ($A$2:$A$11) and calculate the total sums of squares (SS_T) in cell H18, using the =SUMSQ(C14:C23) function.

   i. Generate the values of $yh - yb$ in cells D14:D23, using yhat-AVERAGE ($A$2:$A$11) and calculate the regression sums of squares (SS_R) in cell H19, using the =SUMSQ(D14:D23) function.

   j. Generate the values of $y - yh$ in cells E14:E23 and calculate the error sums of squares (SS_E) with the =SUMSQ(E14:E23) function.

   k. Calculate the value of R^2 in cell H22 by dividing the regression sums of squares by the total sums of squares.

   l. Calculate the value of *S.E.* in cell H23 by taking the square root of $[SS_E/(n - m - 1)]$.

m. Determine the degrees of freedom for SS_T $(n - 1)$, SS_R (m), and SS_E $(n - m - 1)$ and put these into cells H13:H15. Calculate the values of MS_R and MS_E in cells J19 and J20 and calculate the value of F in cell K19 to determine its probability in cell K19.

n. Calculate the values of the *S.E. b* by multiplying the value of *S.E.* by the square root of each value in M7:O9 and by putting the answer in cells M12:O14. Copy the main diagonal cells (the standard error of the coefficients) to cells H13:H15.

o. Calculate the values of t in cells I13:I15 and determine the probability of these values of t in cells J13:J15.

2. Give an interpretation of this analysis by briefly stating in words the following:

a. The meaning of the three *b* coefficients in cells G13:G15

b. The meaning of the three t tests and their probabilities

c. The meaning of the values of SS_T, SS_R, and SS_E

d. The meaning of the F test and its probability

e. The meaning of R^2

f. The meaning of *S.E.*

3. Use the data on the SWC worksheet of Chpt 12–1.xls and carry out an analysis, as shown in Figure 12.12

a. Supply a third independent variable—the constant.

b. Generate the transpose of the matrix **X**, using the =TRANSPOSE() function. Remember that the entire area into which the transpose matrix will go must be highlighted prior to invoking the function, and that the function must be invoked with Ctrl/Shift and Enter.

c. Calculate the values of **X′X**, using the =MMULT() function. This function, too, requires highlighting the entire three-by-three cell area and Ctrl/Shift and Enter.

d. Use =MMULT() to calculate the values of **X′y**.

e. Use =MINVERSE() to obtain the inverse of the matrix **X′X**.

f. Calculate the values of *b*, using the =MMULT() function.

g. Using the values of *b* and the original matrix **X**, generate the values of $\hat{y}$ with =MMULT().

h. Generate the values of $y - \bar{y}$, using y-AVERAGE() and calculate the total sums of squares (SS_T), using the =SUMSQ() function.

i. Generate the values of $yh - yb$, using yhat-AVERAGE() and calculate the regression sums of squares (SS_R), using the =SUMSQ() function.

j. Generate the values of $y - yh$ and calculate the error sums of squares (SS_E) with the =SUMSQ() function.

k. Calculate the value of R^2 by dividing the regression sums of squares by the total sums of squares.

l. Calculate the value of *S.E.* by taking the square root of $[SS_E/(n - m - 1)]$.

m. Determine the degrees of freedom for SS_T $(n - 1)$, SS_R (m) and SS_E $(n - m - 1)$. Calculate the values of MS_R and MS_E the value of F and determine its probability.

n. Calculate the values of the *S.E. b* by multiplying the value of *S.E.* by the square root of each value in $\mathbf{X'X^{-1}}$.

p. Calculate the values of t and determine the probability of these values of t.

4. Give an interpretation of this analysis by briefly stating in words the following:
   a. The meaning of the three b coefficients in cells G13:G15
   b. The meaning of the three t tests and their probabilities
   c. The meaning of the values of SS_T, SS_R, and SS_E
   d. The meaning of the F test and its probability
   e. The meaning of R^2
   g. The meaning of *S.E.*

References

Harmon, H. H. *Modern Factor Analysis.* Chicago: University of Chicago Press, 1960.

The State of the World's Children 2001, UNICEF, New York, Dec. 2000. [http://www.unicef.org/sowc01/tables/#].

CHAPTER THIRTEEN

EXTENSIONS OF MULTIPLE REGRESSION

Chapter 12 provided an introduction to multiple regression. This chapter continues the discussion of multiple regression. In particular, this chapter considers the use and effect of dummy variables in multiple regression, the selection of best models in multiple regression, correlation among independent variables and the effect of this correlation, and assessing non-linear relationships.

Section 13.1 Dummy Variables in Multiple Regression

Chapter Eleven discussed the correspondence between regression and the *t* test and showed that the results of both analyses were essentially the same when a dummy variable alone was employed as the predictor variable in regression. This section examines the inclusion of a dummy variable, along with other continuous variables in multiple regression analysis, to produce what is sometimes called analysis of covariance.

A Dummy Variable with No Interaction

Suppose we examine again the data shown in Figure 11.3, which shows twenty hospital stays and the total charge for each. But this time we will include a second variable: sex of the patient. It should be pointed out that whereas the length of stay and charges data were taken from actual hospital discharge records, the

FIGURE 13.1. DATA FOR TWENTY HOSPITAL DAYS WITH SEX AS A DUMMY VARIABLE.

	A	B	C	D
1	Stay	LOS (x1)	Sex (x2)	TC (y)
2	1	3	0	$2,613.91
3	2	10	0	$8,769.03
4	3	2	1	$2,448.60
5	4	3	0	$2,568.70
6	5	3	0	$1,936.19
7	6	5	1	$7,230.71
8	7	5	1	$5,342.61
9	8	3	1	$4,108.13
10	9	1	0	$1,596.91
11	10	2	1	$4,061.28
12	11	2	0	$1,761.53
13	12	5	0	$4,779.19
14	13	1	1	$2,078.30
15	14	3	1	$4,713.61
16	15	4	0	$3,946.68
17	16	2	1	$2,902.74
18	17	1	0	$1,438.85
19	18	1	0	$820.21
20	19	1	1	$3,309.41
21	20	6	0	$5,476.33
22				

FIGURE 13.2. RESULTS OF REGRESSION FOR TWENTY HOSPITALS.

	H	I	J	K	L	
16		Coefficients	Standard Error	t Stat	P-value	Low
17	Intercept	143.6974749	285.4721068	0.503368	0.621165	-4
18	LOS (x1)	875.0476353	62.5665606	13.98587	9.35E-11	74
19	Sex (x2)	1544.552164	273.445291	5.648487	2.89E-05	96
20						

included sex variable was made up to fit the example we will look at. The new data set for the twenty discharges is shown in Figure 13.1. This figure shows the length of stay as x1 and sex as x2. It should be clear that sex is a categorical variable that has been labeled 1 and 0 (1 = female). This allows the categorical variable sex to be treated as a numeric variable in regression (as shown in Chapter Eleven).

Now, if the regression coefficients for the two independent variables and the intercept are calculated for these data, the results are as shown in Figure 13.2. It can be seen in the figure that the coefficients for both length of stay and sex are different from 0, according to the t tests and probabilities of t (cells K18 and 19 and L18 and 19, respectively).

With the results shown in Figure 13.2, the equation for the predicted values of total charges (TC), given the length of stay and the sex of the patient, is as shown in Equation 13.1. But since sex takes on only the two values 1 and 0, the predicted values of total charges actually form two lines—one when the categorical variable sex is coded 0 (male) and one when sex is coded 1 (female). The equation of these two lines is as shown in Equation 13.2. The part within the parentheses in Equation 13.2 is read TC_{pred}, *given that* sex equals 0 (male), and TC_{pred}, *given that* sex equals 1 (female).

$$TC_{pred} = 875.05 \text{ LOS} + 1544.55 \text{ sex} + 143.70 \tag{13.1}$$

$$
\begin{aligned}
(TC_{pred} \,|\, \text{sex} = 0) &= 875.05 \text{ LOS} + 143.70, \quad \text{and} \\
(TC_{pred} \,|\, \text{sex} = 1) &= 875.05 \text{ LOS} + 1{,}688.25
\end{aligned}
\tag{13.2}
$$

It should be clear that these two lines are exactly parallel to one another (they have the same slope of \$875.05) and are exactly \$1,544.55 apart (1688.25–143.70). The predicted lines for male and female patients among the twenty in the data set are shown in Figure 13.3. Also shown in the figure are the actual observations. The observations for women are shown as black diamonds and, for men, as gray squares. As the two parallel predictor lines show, the cost goes up by \$875.05 per day, but for every day, the cost is higher for women than for men by \$1,544.55. It might also be noted that the two regression lines defined by the equations in Equation 13.1 and Equation 13.2 account for 92 percent of the variance in total charges ($R^2 = .92$)

Having looked at the effect of a single dummy variable added to a regression analysis, it is useful to provide a general formula for the effect of a dummy variable alone in a multiple regression model. This is shown in Equation 13.3.

$$
\begin{aligned}
\text{if} \quad \hat{y} &= b_1 x + b_D D + b_0, \quad \text{then} \\
(\hat{y} \,|\, D = 0) &= b_1 x + b_0, \quad \text{and} \\
(\hat{y} \,|\, D = 1) &= b_1 x + (b_D + b_0)
\end{aligned}
\tag{13.3}
$$

where D is the dummy, and b_D is the coefficient of the dummy.

When a dummy variable is included in regression, the effect of the dummy could be more complex than simply to define two parallel regression lines. It is possible that the two lines (or planes, or hyperspaces) defined by the dummy

FIGURE 13.3. GRAPH OF COST DATA BY LENGTH OF STAY.

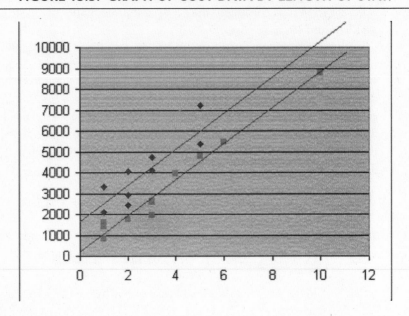

may not be parallel. But for this to occur, the regression analysis would have to include not only the dummy but also an interaction term between the dummy and at least one continuous variable. Consider again the data for hospital charges shown in Figure 13.1 but now including an interaction between the continuous variable length of stay and the dummy variable sex, as shown in Figure 13.4. In that figure, it can be seen that the interaction is simply the multiplication of the continuous variable by the dummy variable. When the dummy variable is 0, the interaction term (x1*x2) is 0. When the dummy variable is 1, the interaction term is equal to the continuous variable.

If we now carry out regression analysis with charges as the dependent variable and the three independent variables as shown in Figure 13.4, the resulting regression coefficients, their standard errors, and the appropriate t tests are shown in Figure 13.5. These regression coefficients also account for 92 percent of variance. The fact that the interaction term adds nothing to the regression equation in terms of the variance accounted for is confirmed by the t statistic for the interaction term, shown in L40. The t statistic is .55, which has a 59 percent probability of occurrence under the null hypothesis that charges are independent of the interaction between the length of stay and sex. In essence, we conclude that the coefficient on the interaction term is 0.

FIGURE 13.4. HOSPITAL CHARGES WITH DUMMY AND INTERACTION.

	A	B	C	D	E	
	Stay	**LOS (x1)**	**Sex (x2)**	**x1*x2**	**TC (y)**	
1						
2	1	3	0	0	$2,613.91	
3	2	10	0	0	$8,769.03	
4	3	2	1	2	$2,448.60	
5	4	3	0	0	$2,568.70	
6	5	3	0	0	$1,936.19	
7	6	5	1	5	$7,230.71	
8	7	5	1	5	$5,342.61	
9	8	3	1	3	$4,108.13	
10	9	1	0	0	$1,596.91	
11	10	2	1	2	$4,061.28	
12	11	2	0	0	$1,761.53	
13	12	5	0	0	$4,779.19	
14	13	1	1	1	$2,078.30	
15	14	3	1	3	$4,713.61	
16	15	4	0	0	$3,946.68	
17	16	2	1	2	$2,902.74	
18	17	1	0	0	$1,438.85	
19	18	1	0	0	$820.21	
20	19	1	1	1	$3,309.41	
21	20	6	0	0	$5,476.33	
22						

FIGURE 13.5. REGRESSION COEFFICIENTS WITH DUMMY AND INTERACTIONS.

	I	J	K	L	M	
36		Coefficients	Standard Error	t Stat	P-value	Low
37	Intercept	205.7500125	312.5326393	0.658331	0.519687	-4!
38	LOS (x1)	857.5456375	71.35928576	12.0173	2.01E-09	70(
39	Sex (x2)	1293.925913	533.9772408	2.423186	0.027613	1(
40	x1*x2	88.21714028	160.2076205	0.550643	0.589485	-2!

A Dummy Variable with an Interaction

But now let us consider an example in which the interaction term is statistically significant—that is, in which we would conclude that the coefficient on the interaction term is different from 0. Such an example is shown in Figure 13.6. This figure shows the same charges and the same length of stay as that shown in

FIGURE 13.6. HOSPITAL CHARGES WITH DUMMY AND INTERACTION: II.

	A Stay	B LOS (x1)	C Sex (x2)	D x1*x2	E TC (y)
1	Stay	LOS (x1)	Sex (x2)	x1*x2	TC (y)
2	1	3	0	0	$2,613.91
3	2	10	0	0	$8,769.03
4	3	2	1	2	$2,448.60
5	4	3	1	3	$2,568.70
6	5	3	1	3	$1,936.19
7	6	5	1	5	$7,230.71
8	7	5	0	0	$5,342.61
9	8	3	1	3	$4,108.13
10	9	1	1	1	$1,596.91
11	10	2	0	0	$4,061.28
12	11	2	1	2	$1,761.53
13	12	5	0	0	$4,779.19
14	13	1	0	0	$2,078.30
15	14	3	0	0	$4,713.61
16	15	4	0	0	$3,946.68
17	16	2	1	2	$2,902.74
18	17	1	1	1	$1,438.85
19	18	1	1	1	$820.21
20	19	1	0	0	$3,309.41
21	20	6	0	0	$5,476.33
22					

FIGURE 13.7. REGRESSION COEFFICIENTS WITH DUMMY ONLY: II.

	I	J Coefficients	K Standard Error	L t Stat	M P-value	Low
37		Coefficients	Standard Error	t Stat	P-value	Lov
38	Intercept	1488.76838	533.051131	2.792919	0.01249	3€
39	LOS (x1)	755.066654	108.7859451	6.940847	2.38E-06	5₂
40	Sex (x2)	-544.16469	473.0625337	-1.1503	0.265944	-1
41						

Figure 13.1 and Figure 13.4, but the sex designations have changed to present a different picture of the data. Now if regression is carried out using only the dummy variable with no interaction term, the results are shown in Figure 13.7.

For the regression coefficients shown in Figure 13.7, only the coefficients for length of stay and the intercept are different from 0. Sex is no longer a statistically significant predictor of charges. In this case, it would be a reasonable practice to simply drop sex from the analysis and predict charges with the length of stay only—except for one thing. It may be that the interaction between the length of

FIGURE 13.8. REGRESSION COEFFICIENTS WITH DUMMY AND INTERACTION: II.

	I	J	K	L	M
16		Coefficients	Standard Error	t Stat	P-value	Low
17	Intercept	1959.00894	483.7201956	4.04988	0.000929	93
18	LOS (x1)	637.506515	101.7513079	6.26534	1.13E-05	42
19	Sex (x2)	-2280.0527	747.4511603	-3.05044	0.007632	-3
20	x1*x2	667.841641	242.5195211	2.753764	0.014124	15

stay and sex could have a statistically significant relationship to charges. To answer that question, it would be necessary to analyze all three variables, the length of stay, sex, and the length of stay*sex interaction simultaneously. The coefficients that result from this analysis are shown in Figure 13.8. In that figure it is possible to see that not only is the coefficient for sex statistically different from 0, but so, too, is the interaction coefficient, while the coefficient on the length of stay remains statistically significant. What does this mean in terms of the prediction of charges? It means not only will charges be predicted by two lines with different intercepts for males and females, but the slopes of those lines will be different also. This can be seen in the equations for the two lines, as shown in Equation 13.4. For men (sex = 0), the charge increases by \$637.51 for each additional day of stay, with a fixed cost of \$1,959.01 for a stay of zero days. For women, the cost increases by \$1,305.35 per day of stay from a fixed cost of −\$221.04 for a stay of zero days. Of course, since no hospital admission will be a zero-day stay, the intercept terms only represent the y axis anchor for the respective lines.

$$(TC_{pred}) = 637.51 \text{ LOS} + -2,280.05 \text{ sex} + 667.84 \text{ LOS} \cdot \text{sex} + 1,959.01, \quad \text{or}$$
$$(TC_{pred}| \text{sex} = 0) = 637.51 \text{ LOS} + 1,959.01, \quad \text{and}$$
$$(TC_{pred}| \text{sex} = 1) = 1,305.35 \text{ LOS} + -221.04 \tag{13.4}$$

Having now seen that the regression lines are different, it may be useful to see how these are pictured in a two-dimensional graphic presentation. Figure 13.9 shows the graph of the charges data with the two regression lines as defined by Equation 13.4, included in the graph. The more steeply sloped graph with the intercept below 0 is the line for women. The actual observations for women are shown as gray diamonds. The less steeply sloped graph with the regression line crossing the y axis at about \$2,000 is the slope for men. The actual observations for men are shown as black squares.

It should be remembered that these examples, although based on actual charge and length of stay data, have fabricated data for sex. The sex variable has been manipulated in each case just presented, to produce the outcomes that

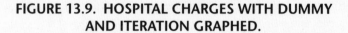

FIGURE 13.9. HOSPITAL CHARGES WITH DUMMY AND ITERATION GRAPHED.

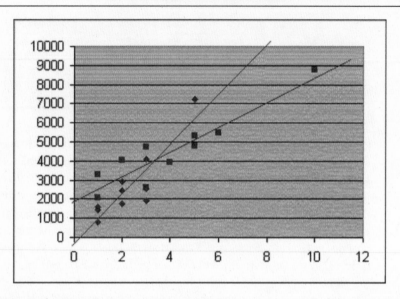

have been found. It is highly unlikely that over a large sample of data any difference would be found for men and women in hospital charges, and the result of an interaction effect would be even more unlikely. Nevertheless, there are many situations in which dummy variables and interaction terms could have realistic meaning. With that in mind, it is useful to present a general formula for determining the slope and intercept of lines when dummy variables and interactions are present. Such a formula is given in Equation 13.5.

$$\text{if} \quad \hat{y} = b_1 x + b_D D + b_2 x D + b_0, \quad \text{then}$$
$$(\hat{y} \mid D = 0) = b_1 x + b_0, \quad \text{and} \qquad (13.5)$$
$$(\hat{y} \mid D = 1) = (b_1 + b_2)\, x + (b_D + b_0)$$

where D is the dummy, and b_D is the coefficient of the dummy.

If there is more than one continuous independent variable, the slope of the line defined by the continuous variable will change only for those variables for which there are dummy—continuous variable interaction terms.

General Comments on Dummy and Interaction Terms

In general, if an interaction is expected and an interaction term is included in an analysis with a continuous variable and a 1/0 dummy, the full regression model, including the interaction term, should be run. If the interaction term is not different from 0 (that is, if the absolute *t* value is less than 2), the interaction term can be dropped and the analysis rerun with only the continuous variable and the dummy variable included. This simpler model will describe the data as adequately as the more complex model, including the interaction. If, in this further analysis, the coefficient for the dummy is not different from 0, it is possible to drop the dummy as well and simply predict the dependent variable on the basis of the continuous variable (or continuous variables).

If an interaction term is included in an analysis and the coefficient for the interaction term is different from 0 but the coefficients for the continuous variable and the dummy variables are not different from 0, a similar decision may be made. It is sometimes possible to drop the continuous variable and the dummy variable and predict the dependent variable solely on the strength of the interaction variable itself. The results of the analysis may produce slightly different coefficients, but the predicted values of the dependent variable will be very much the same. To see an example of this, consider the imaginary hospital charge data shown in Figure 13.10. In this data set, Inpatient = 1 means that the patient was actually in the hospital during the length of stay indicated, whereas

FIGURE 13.10. CHARGE DATA SHOWING AN INTERACTION EFFECT.

	A	B	C	D	E
1	**Obs**	**LOS**	**Inpatient**	**Inter**	**Charges**
2	1	7	0	0	2900
3	2	5	0	0	2539
4	3	7	0	0	2427
5	4	7	0	0	2202
6	5	9	0	0	2682
7	6	8	0	0	2581
8	7	3	0	0	2862
9	8	5	0	0	2857
10	9	4	0	0	2257
11	10	11	0	0	3190
12	11	3	1	3	3317
13	12	2	1	2	2970
14	13	9	1	9	5443
15	14	9	1	9	5011
16	15	8	1	8	4717
17	16	10	1	10	5214
18	17	3	1	3	3955
19	18	9	1	9	4906
20	19	2	1	2	2544
21	20	3	1	3	3987
22					

Inpatient = 0 means that the patient was being treated during the time period indicated as LOS on an outpatient basis. The question is whether there is an interaction effect of LOS and Inpatient. Using the Tools/Data Analysis/ Regression add-in produces the coefficients shown in Figure 13.11. In that figure it can be seen by the t tests on the three coefficients representing the independent variables and the probabilities of those t tests (cells M18:M20 and N18:N20, respectively) that only the coefficient for the interaction is different from 0. This essentially means that neither the continuous variable LOS nor the dummy variable Inpatient contributes in a statistically significant way to the prediction of charges. The total proportion of the variance in charges accounted for by all three variables (R^2) is .91.

Because neither the coefficient on LOS nor that on Inpatient is statistically different from 0 in the analysis of the data in Figure 13.10, it is not unreasonable to consider dropping those from the analysis in order to predict charges. Conceptually, this amounts to imputing a fixed fee to outpatient contacts with the hospital, regardless of the amount of time over which they extend, and predicting inpatient stays on the basis of the time in the institution. The result of this analysis is shown in Figure 13.12. Here, the coefficient for the interaction has changed from 230.39 (Figure 13.11) to 270.61, but the total proportion of the variation accounted for remains essentially at .91. In essence, either model is equally good at predicting hospital charges as represented by the data in Figure 13.10. Graphing the actual data points and both predicted values for the data, those using

FIGURE 13.11. COEFFICIENTS FOR CHARGE DATA SHOWING AN INTERACTION EFFECT.

	J	K	L	M	N	
16		Coefficients	Standard Error	t Stat	P-value	Low
17	Intercept	2360.91221	338.1670817	6.981496	3.09E-06	1
18	LOS	43.7557252	48.40847693	0.903886	0.379464	-5
19	Inpatient	255.441953	407.1281721	0.627424	0.539233	-6
20	Inter	230.390108	59.2131279	3.890862	0.001299	10

FIGURE 13.12. COEFFICIENTS FOR CHARGE DATA SHOWING ONLY THE INTERACTION EFFORT.

	J	K	L	M	N	
39		Coefficients	Standard Error	t Stat	P-value	Low
40	Intercept	2643.26954	96.27864552	27.45437	3.83E-16	2
41	Inter	270.613952	20.4801831	13.21345	1.05E-10	2

FIGURE 13.13. GRAPH OF CHARGE DATA WITH PREDICTED LINES.

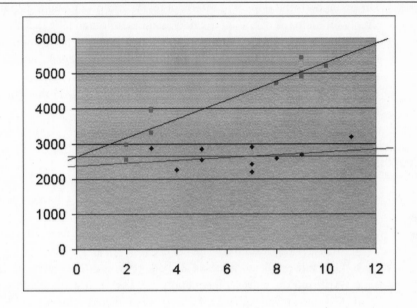

the coefficients in Figure 13.11 and those using the coefficients in Figure 13.12 will show this. The result is shown in Figure 13.13.

In Figure 13.13, the gray squares represent charges for actual hospital stays and the black diamonds represent charges for outpatient contacts with the hospital over the numbers of days indicated on the horizontal axis. The sloping line from about 2360 when days of contact with the hospital are zero, to about 2800 when days of contact with the hospital are twelve represents the predicted charges for those who were treated on an outpatient basis when the predicted values are calculated using all three coefficients, as given in Figure 13.11. The horizontal line at 2643 represents the predicted charges for those people who were treated on an outpatient basis, using only the coefficients given in Figure 13.12. Because there is no separate term to represent the length of contact with the hospital for the outpatient group in generating this line, it is essentially nothing more than the mean of the outpatient charges. The diagonal line sloping from about 2600 when length of stay is zero days, to about 5700 when length of stay is twelve days represents the predicted value of charges for those people who actually had hospital stays, using either set of coefficients. The lines are so close together that they cannot be shown separately on the graph. (The predicted line given the coefficients in Figure 13.11 is Charges = 274.05 LOS + 2,616.35, whereas for the coefficients in Figure 13.12, it is Charges = 270.61 LOS + 2,643.27.)

In considering the preceding discussion, an important point should be noted. Dropping both the slope and intercept terms and predicting the charges values simply on the basis of the interaction assumes automatically that the outpatient contacts (given as 0 in the dummy variable) actually have no relationship to number of days of contact with the hospital. If they did, the coefficients for days and the intercept would have had to be included in the analysis, even if they were not statistically different from zero. Otherwise, the predicted values for charges for outpatients would always be a flat line.

Exercises for Section 13.1

1. Use the data shown in Figure 13.1 (available on the Charges1 worksheet in Chpt 13–1.xls).
   a. Replicate the analysis given in Figure 13.2 by using the Tools/Data Analysis/Regression add-in.
   b. Generate predicted values of TC on the basis of the regression coefficients.
   c. Write out the regression equations for TC when sex = 0 and sex = 1.
   d. Develop an *xy* graph with TC and the predicted values of TC as the *y* variable and LOS as the *x* variable and confirm that the predicted values of TC form two parallel lines.

2. The data file on the Costs worksheet of Chpt 13–1.xls is the same data file as that given on the Costs worksheet of Chpt 10–1.xls, and it is discussed in Section 10.1 of Chapter Ten. The only difference is that the variable length of stay (LOS) has been added to the worksheet in Chpt 13–1.xls. Use these data to do the following:
   a. Insert a new column at column C and create a variable called Catawba— that is, 1 for Catawba and 0 for the other three hospitals.
   b. Develop the multiple regression analysis by using the Tools/Data Analysis/Regression add-in with both the variables Catawba and LOS as the independent variables and Costs as the dependent variable.
   c. Interpret the *t* values and probabilities for the coefficients to determine whether either or both independent variables are statistically significant (different from 0).
   d. Write out the regression equations for costs when Catawba = 0 (for any other hospital) and Catawba = 1.
   e. Generate predicted values of costs on the basis of the regression coefficients.
   f. Develop an *xy* graph with costs and the predicted values of costs as the *y* variable and LOS as the *x* variable and decide if the predicted values of costs form two parallel lines.

3. Use the data shown in Figure 13.6 (or use the data given on the Charges2 worksheet, insert a column, and add an interaction term).

   a. Replicate the analysis given in Figure 13.8 by using the Tools/Data Analysis/Regression add-in.

   b. Generate predicted values of TC on the basis of the regression coefficients.

   c. Write out the regression equations for TC when sex = 0 and sex = 1.

   d. Develop an *xy* graph with TC and the predicted values of TC as the *y* variable and LOS as the *x* variable and confirm that the predicted values of TC form two parallel lines.

4. Use the data file on the Costs worksheet of Chpt 13–1.xls with the addition of the variable for Catawba.

   a. Insert a column next to the Catawba variable and label it Inter (interaction), and then create a new variable that is the multiplication of the variable Catawba by the LOS.

   b. Carry out a regression analysis with Costs as the dependent variable and the three independent variables—Catawba, Inter, and LOS—as the independent variables.

   c. On the basis of the results, decide whether Inter is a statistically significant predictor of costs.

   d. On the basis of this analysis and that in Exercise 2, decide on which of the two analyses seem best for costs.

Section 13.2 The Best Regression Model

In Section 13.1, the discussion focused on dummy variables and their treatment in regression. In that discussion there arose the question of whether to include a dummy variable or an interaction term in a general regression model if either was not statistically significant (that is, different from 0). The conclusion of the discussion was that it did not make much difference either way in the prediction of the dependent variable, and, in general, that result holds. However, the question of whether it is appropriate or not appropriate to drop variables from a regression model if they are not statistically significant is one that is widely debated, and there is no generally accepted agreement on which is correct.

Theory or Dust Bowl Empiricism?

The argument for dropping statistically nonsignificant variables from a regression model is based on two points. First, including statistically nonsignificant variables in a model will not improve the prediction of the dependent variable in any statistically significant way. Second, including statistically nonsignificant variables unnecessarily complicates the understanding of the dependent variable with extraneous independent variables that have no predictive value.

The argument for not dropping statistically nonsignificant variables from a regression model is based primarily on a single point—but it is an important one. This point is that a regression equation implies a causal relationship in which the values of the dependent variable are actually caused by the values of the independent variable set. This causal relationship in turn implies some underlying theoretical model that says a certain set of independent variables should be included in a regression model. The fact that in a particular instance under analysis this may not have been found to be true does not necessarily invalidate the theory, and neither does it allow the analyst to drop a variable from the predictor model. To do so is not only to abandon the theory but, as we have seen in regard to dummy variables, also to change the values of the coefficients.

The argument that a regression model represents a theory is further supported by the empirical evidence that one set of predictor variables may be as useful as another completely different set of predictor variables in predicting a dependent variable. In such a situation, only a theory—and not simply the regression analysis alone—can determine which variables to include in the regression equation.

To explore some of these issues, we will use data taken from *The State of the World's Children 1996* (1996). These data are for seventy-five countries in the world for which all the data to be examined were available. (It should be noted that UNICEF publishes these data every year, so that more recent data are available. It happens that the data from 1996 demonstrate several points that are to be made in this section, whereas data from later years do not necessarily demonstrate the same points. This is one of the difficult things about regression analysis. The data do not always behave in the same ways from one sample to another.)

A sample of the data under consideration is shown in Figure 13.14. The data represent eight independent variables and one dependent variable. The dependent variable is U5Mort in column K, the under-five mortality for each country for 1994. The eight independent variables include five variables related to the public health system. The variable SafeW is the proportion of households with access to safe water. The variable Sanit is the proportion of households with access to sanitary facilities. The variable HealthS is the proportion of households within a specified travel distance of a health facility. The variable DPT is the proportion of children immunized for diphtheria, pertussis, and tetanus by age one. The variable CPR is the contraceptive prevalence rate. Also included as independent variables are three that are not dimensions of the health care system. The variable LogGNP is the log of the gross national product per capita (the log is used because the actual value of GNP is not linearly related to under-five mortality, whereas the log is).

FIGURE 13.14. DATA FROM *THE STATE OF THE WORLD'S CHILDREN, 1996.*

	B	C	D	E	F	G	H	I	J	K
1		SafeW	Sanit	HealthS	DPT	CPR	LogGNP	FemLit	TFR	U5Mort
2	Niger	54	15	32	20	4	2.4314	5	7.3	320
3	Angola	32	16	30	27	1	2.8451	29	7	292
4	Sierra Leone	34	11	38	43	4	2.1761	14	6.4	284
5	Mozambique	33	20	39	55	4	1.9542	19	6.4	277
6	Guinea-Bissau	53	21	40	74	1	2.3802	37	5.7	231
7	Guinea	55	21	80	70	1	2.6990	18	6.9	223
8	Malawi	47	53	80	98	13	2.3010	37	7	221
9	Liberia	46	30	39	43	6	2.6532	18	6.7	217
10	Mali	37	31	30	39	5	2.4314	17	7	214
11	Somalia	37	18	27	23	1	2.0792	14	6.9	211
12	Zambia	50	37	75	85	15	2.5798	65	5.8	203
13	Ethiopia	25	19	46	37	2	2.0000	21	6.9	200
14	Nigeria	40	35	66	41	6	2.4771	39	6.3	191
15	Zaire	27	23	26	29	1	2.3424	61	6.6	186
16	Uganda	34	57	49	79	5	2.2553	44	7.1	185
17	Burundi	70	51	80	48	9	2.2553	19	6.6	176
18	Central African Rep.	18	45	45	31	15	2.6021	41	5.6	175
19	Burkina Faso	78	18	90	41	8	2.4771	7	6.4	169
20	Madagascar	29	3	65	66	17	2.3424	73	6	164
21	Tanzania, U. Rep. of	50	64	80	79	18	1.9542	50	5.8	159
22	Lesotho	52	28	80	58	23	2.8129	57	5.1	156

The variable FemLit is the female literacy rate for the country. The variable TFR is the average number of births per woman.

Each one of the independent variables in Figure 13.14 is approximately linear in its relation to U5Mort, and each is a statistically significant predictor of U5Mort. Figure 13.15 is a composite of eight separate regression analyses, one for each of the independent variables predicting U5Mort on its own. As the t statistics and their probabilities indicate (columns AJ and AK respectively), each of the independent variables, taken separately, is a statistically significant predictor of under-five mortality. Furthermore, the R^2 value, shown in column AM, indicates that the independent variables, taken alone, account for between 43.7 percent (for HealthS) and 71.6 percent (for CPR) of the variance in under-five mortality across the seventy-five countries for which all the data are available.

Consider first the question of what to do about statistically nonsignificant variables in a multiple regression model. To do this, we will look at all eight of the independent variables shown in Figure 13.14 and Figure 13.15, analyzed *simultaneously*. The result of this analysis is shown in Figure 13.16.

As Figure 13.16 shows, when all seven independent variables are included in the regression model, only one coefficient, that for Sanit, is different from 0 (that is, a probability of less than 0.05). This is despite the fact that when each variable is examined separately in regard to under-five mortality, each of the eight has

FIGURE 13.15. COEFFICIENTS FOR EACH OF THE PREDICTOR VARIABLES FOR U5Mort INDEPENDENTLY.

AG	AH	AI	AJ	AK	AL	AM
1	Coefficients	Standard Error	t Stat	P-value	Intercept	R Square
2 SafeW	-2.364	0.312	-7.567	9.14E-11	255.452	0.440
3 Sanit	-2.308	0.239	-9.640	1.19E-14	227.016	0.560
4 HealthS	-2.271	0.302	-7.532	1.06E-10	265.128	.0.437
5 DPT	-2.479	0.291	-8.534	1.4E-12	284.451	0.499
6 CPR	-2.665	0.197	-13.557	1.26E-21	196.177	0.716
7 FemLit	-2.177	0.223	-9.764	6.97E-15	225.211	0.499
8 TFR	37.340	3.079	12.126	3.66E-19	-70.733	0.668
9 LogGNP	-116.564	12.628	-9.231	6.88E-14	438.092	0.539

FIGURE 13.16. MULTIPLE REGRESSION COEFFICIENTS OF PREDICTORS FOR U5Mort.

M	N	O	P	Q	L
16	Coefficients	Standard Error	t Stat	P-value	L(
17 Intercept	264.8972296	71.10592989	3.725389	0.000406	1
18 SafeW	0.030147374	0.332918971	0.090555	0.928121	·
19 Sanit	-0.733757198	0.279558794	-2.6247	0.010765	·
20 HealthS	-0.318333165	0.259903869	-1.22481	0.225	·
21 DPT	-0.523582754	0.286016159	-1.83061	0.071675	·
22 CPR	-0.605704804	0.494921411	-1.22384	0.225364	·
23 LogGNP	-21.91231273	14.69602134	-1.49104	0.140716	·
24 FemLit	-0.289953578	0.292665598	-0.99073	0.325434	·
25 TFR	7.640583579	6.954863453	1.098596	0.275936	·

a nonzero coefficient. The total variance accounted for (R^2) by all eight variables in the regression model (even though only one is statistically different from 0) is .815.

Within the context of the view that holds that a theory must be the basis of the regression model analyzed, it would have been assumed that some theory specified that all eight variables should be included in the multiple regression model. Within this perspective, the fact that only one variable (Sanit) actually shows a statistically significant coefficient would not be sufficient cause to eliminate any of the variables used as a way to simplify the regression model. Within the context of the alternative view, which seeks the simplest regression model for predicting the dependent variable, it is clear that some variables in the model are not useful and should be dropped. One approach to this would be simply to fall back to the use of Sanit alone to predict U5Mort. But we already know that Sanit alone is not the best predictor of U5Mort, that distinction being held by CPR (see Figure 13.15). So how should we proceed?

A common approach to seeking the best multiple regression model is what is often called *stepwise regression*. Stepwise regression is a term that denotes a number of different methods of varying levels of complexity for seeking the best set of independent variables for simultaneously predicting the dependent variable of interest. In general, the various stepwise regression approaches can be characterized as either *backward stepwise elimination* or *forward stepwise inclusion*.

The simplest example of backward stepwise elimination begins with the complete model, as shown in Figure 13.16, and it successively eliminates in a stepwise manner the predictor with the least significant coefficient. This process continues until only variables with statistically significant coefficients remain. If the backward elimination approach to stepwise regression is employed, the first variable to be eliminated is SafeW, with a *P*-value of .928. Although the result of that analysis with six independent variables is not shown, the next variable to be eliminated would be TFR. The stepwise process would continue until only variables with statistically significant coefficients remain.

Figure 13.17 shows the results of the backward elimination process beginning with all variables shown in Figure 13.16. As Figure 13.17 shows, four variables— LogGNP, Sanit, DPT, and CPR—have coefficients that are statistically different from 0 when the other four variables are eliminated in a stepwise fashion. The resulting *R* square is .798.

Forward stepwise inclusion begins with the single variable that accounts for the largest proportion of the variance and proceeds at each step by adding a next variable that accounts for as much of the unexplained variance as possible. This essentially means selecting the next variable which, with the two variables taken together, accounts for the largest proportion of variance (has the largest *R* square).

FIGURE 13.17. MULTIPLE REGRESSION COEFFICIENTS OF BEST PREDICTORS FOR U5Mort: BACKWARD ELIMINATION.

	M	N	O	P	Q
114		Coefficients	Standard Error	t Stat	P-value	L
115	Intercept	321.9082	34.59634683	9.3047	7.3E-14
116	LogGNP	-29.967464	13.39720112	-2.237	0.02848
117	Sanit	-0.7018368	0.25167603	-2.789	0.00681
118	DPT	-0.6947679	0.275624748	-2.521	0.01399
119	CPR	-1.2991115	0.317337595	-4.094	0.00011

From the forward inclusion approach, the first variable into the model would be CPR, because it accounts for the largest proportion of variance in under-five mortality when each variable is taken singly (R^2 = .716 in Figure 13.15). With CPR included, the next best predictor is Sanit. Together, CPR and Sanit account for .768 percent of the variance in U5Mort. With CPR and Sanit included, the next best predictor turns out to be TFR, which, when included with CPR and Sanit, account for .789 percent of the variance in U5Mort.

But now a problem arises in the analysis. When TFR is included with CPR and Sanit, the coefficient for CPR is no longer different from 0 (that is, the probability for the t statistic is greater than .05—actually, .068). This requires a decision that, in general, does not usually arise with backward elimination. Should we continue with CPR, Sanit, and TFR, even though CPR is no longer statistically different from 0, or should we drop CPR and replace it with TFR and continue to develop the model on the basis of TFR and Sanit? In this case, we will elect the latter approach.

The results of the forward inclusion method (substituting TFR for CPR because when TFR, CPR, and Sanit are included in the same model, CPR no longer has a coefficient different from zero) are shown in Figure 13.18. Three variables—TFR, Sanit, and DPT—have coefficients different from zero. Adding any other variable to this set of three results in a probability greater than .05 for the coefficient of the added variable, but all three included variables retain statistically significant coefficients. This model, with three predictor variables, accounts for 79.6 percent of the variance in U5Mort.

It is possible that with a more sophisticated approach to backward elimination, both approaches would have reached the same result, which is that shown in Figure 13.18. But a more sophisticated approach to forward inclusion—for example, selecting the best three predictors simultaneously, regardless of how good any single one was—might have also resulted in a different set of predictor variables. The bottom line, then, is this. In general, stepwise regression, though it may

**FIGURE 13.18. MULTIPLE REGRESSION COEFFICIENTS OF BEST
PREDICTORS FOR U5Mort: FORWARD INCLUSION.**

	BA	BB	BC	BD	BE	
16		*Coefficients*	*Standard Error*	*t Stat*	*P-value*	L
17	Intercept	109.91	34.18740328	3.2149	0.00196	
18	TFR	21.65734	3.580406439	6.0488	6.2E-08	
19	Sanit	-1.1491147	0.209352248	-5.4889	5.9E-07	
20	DPT	-0.6447902	0.264066091	-2.4418	0.01711	

result in a simplified model, is probably less desirable as an approach to regression analysis than analysis based on a clear understanding of which independent variables should be included in a given model. This can only be determined from a clear understanding of the process that actually produces the results in the dependent variable of interest. The best place to obtain this understanding is a good theory.

Doing Stepwise Regression with Excel

Dedicated statistics packages often have a few commands that will allow the user to perform a host of forward, backward, and sideways regression analyses (the sideways is apocryphal), producing vast reams of printout. Excel, though an outstanding statistical tool, does not produce stepwise regression results quite so easily—or perhaps quite so promiscuously. It is necessary with Excel to do each regression separately. So if one is to replicate the discussion in the previous (first) subsection of this section (13.2), as is suggested in Exercise 1 of this section, a little direction is probably useful.

To replicate the results in the previous discussion, begin with the data on the U5Mort1 Worksheet of Chpt 13–1.xls. The first task is to reproduce the single variable regression results shown in Figure 13.15. Begin with the data on the U5Mort1 worksheet, which are the data given in Figure 13.14. Using Tools/Data Analysis/Regression, specify U5Mort as the dependent variable and SafeW as the independent variable. Specify the output cell as M1. This will produce the regression that will allow you to replicate line 2 in Figure 13.15. Now recall the Tools/Data Analysis/Regression window and change the independent variable to Sanit and the output cell to M21. This will produce the result to replicate line 3 in Figure 13.15. Proceed this way with the remaining six variables, putting the results in M41, M61, M81, and so on. This allows you to produce all of the results shown in Figure 13.15.

To replicate the results in Figure 13.16, the entire independent variable set from SafeW to TFR should be included in a single regression model. Because this is the first step to the backward elimination process, insert a new worksheet, label it U5Mort1-b for backward elimination, and copy the data in cells A1:K76 to the new worksheet. Now invoke Tools/Data Analysis/Regression and specify all the variables from SafeW to TFR as the independent variables. Put this result in cell M1. This replicates Figure 13.16 and also provides the starting point for backward elimination.

As the analysis in Figure 13.16 shows, SafeW has the smallest p value in the complete model. This is the first variable to be eliminated in the next step. Copy all the data from D1 to J1 (that is, all the independent variables except for

SafeW) and paste the copy in cell W1. This now leaves seven independent variables in columns W through AC. Invoke Tools/Data Analysis/Regression again and change the variable fields to reflect the moved data set. (It is necessary only to change the reference for the independent variables, because the dependent variable remains in column K.) Put the result into cell AE. In this analysis you will discover that TFR has the largest p value (.273) and is the next to be eliminated.

Copy the six independent variables (columns W to AB) and paste them in cell AO1. This eliminates TFR. Now invoke Tools/Data Analysis/Regression and specify the new set of six independent variables and specify the output cell as AV1. In this analysis you will discover that HealthS has the largest p value (.137) and will be the next variable eliminated. The easiest way to do this is to copy all the columns—AO through AT—and paste them into BF1. Then click on the BG at the top of the HealthS column and eliminate the entire column. This will now put the five remaining independent variables into columns AO:BJ. Analysis proceeds in this fashion until all variables in the model have p values of .05 or less, at which time the regression analysis result should look exactly like that in Figure 13.17 (it will take two more steps, and the variables will not appear in the same order, but the coefficients, t tests, and p values will be the same).

Replicating forward stepwise inclusion to produce the result shown in Figure 13.18 is a similar, but somewhat more complicated, process. To begin the process, return to the U5Mort1 worksheet on which the regressions with each independent variable as a predictor of U5Mort was carried out, and select the variable with the largest R^2 value. This happens to be CPR (shown in Figure 13.15).

Copy the variable CPR to column W, beginning in W1. Now select the first of the other independent variables, SafeW, and copy it to column X, beginning in X1. Now invoke Tools/Data Analysis/Regression and specify the two variables CPR and SafeW in columns W and X as the independent variables. Put the results into cell Z1. Now it is time to pair CPR with Sanit. Recall that it is necessary for the entire independent variable set in regression to be in contiguous columns. So Sanit must be contiguous with CPR. The easiest way to do this is to click on the X that heads the column containing SafeW and insert a new column at this point. This moves the variable SafeW to column Y and the output from the most recent regression to column AA. Now copy the data for Sanit and put it into column X, beginning in X1. Using the variables CPR and Sanit, replicate the previous regression and put the output into cell AA21. In doing this, it will be necessary to change only the destination cell.

To continue with the two variable regression, continue to add a new column at X for each new variable to be paired with CPR until all the other six variables have been analyzed this way. It should not be necessary ever to change the data references, but it will be necessary to change the output reference each time to ensure that all the output is in the same column. The cell into which the last regression output will go for this sequence (which will be the pairing of CPR with TFR if you are following this example) will be cell AF121.

After completing this sequence of two variables, it will be seen that CPR and Sanit, taken together, have the largest R^2 at .768. So these two variables will be those included at the next step. This next step will proceed just as the last, except that now the two variables—CPR and Sanit—will be copied to the columns AP and AQ, beginning in the first cell in those columns. Now the first of the remaining variables, SafeW will be copied to column AR and a new regression analysis will be performed with these three variables as the predictors. It will be necessary to change the x input range to reflect the three variables being analyzed, and also the output range, which should be specified as cell AT1.

Just as in the last sequence, we now insert a column at AR and copy the next variable, HealthS, to that column. Having done this, regression is again performed, changing only the output destination to AU22. Now another column is inserted at AR and the process continues. The destination of the last regression analysis will be cell AY106. Having completed this stage of the analysis, we will see that the largest R^2 (.789) is associated with regression that includes CPR, Sanit, and TFR. But as noted previously, CPR no longer has a statistically significant coefficient ($p = .068$). So we will drop CPR in favor of TFR and replicate the two variable analysis with Sanit and TFR.

In the repeat of the two variable analysis with Sanit and TFR, it turns out that only one of the other six variables, DPT, has a coefficient different from 0, and that is the last variable to be included. This set of three variables accounts for 79.6 percent of the variance ($R^2 = .796$), and the analysis is complete.

An Alternative Look at the Importance of Theory

This concern with a theoretical approach to regression is also supported with a somewhat different analysis of these same data. Suppose we have one group of analysts who believe that the important determinant of under-five mortality is the health and health services environment of a country. With that in mind, they might reasonably decide to predict under-five mortality by using those available variables that are health-related, which, in this case, could include the variables SafeW, Sanit, HServe, DPT, and CPR. Another group of analysts might believe that the important determinant of under-five mortality is not the health environment of the country but, rather, the general cultural environment, and they might determine that they should predict under-five mortality by using the cultural variables, FemLit, LogGNP, and Fert.

FIGURE 13.19. MULTIPLE REGRESSION COEFFICIENTS OF BEST PREDICTORS FOR U5Mort: HEALTH PREDICTORS.

	I	J	K	L	M	
		Coefficients	Standard Error	t Stat	P-value	L
61						
62	Intercept	253.64387	16.74887038	15.1439	6.3E-24	
63	Sanit	-0.9348755	0.235470915	-3.9702	0.00017	
64	DPT	-0.6163626	0.280988904	-2.1935	0.03154	
65	CPR	-1.6090868	0.293419628	-5.4839	6E-07	
66						

FIGURE 13.20. MULTIPLE REGRESSION COEFFICIENTS OF BEST PREDICTORS FOR U5Mort: CULTURAL PREDICTORS.

	G	H	I	J	K	
		Coefficients	Standard Error	t Stat	P-value	
16						
17	Intercept	183.29635	61.75869844	2.9679	0.00408	
18	LogGNP	-44.275924	14.03687157	-3.154	0.00236	
19	FemLit	-0.7447152	0.286887575	-2.596	0.01146	
20	TFR	18.90089	5.19210462	3.6403	0.00051	
21						

Taking the health approach, and using backward elimination of nonsignificant coefficients, the results of the analysis are shown in Figure 13.19. The three variables—Sanit, DPT, and CPR—together account for 78.3 percent of the variance in under-five mortality. If the general cultural environment approach is taken, the results of the analysis are shown in Figure 13.20. Here, all three variables had statistically significant coefficients on the first analysis. The three variables—LogGNP, FemLit, and Fert—taken together account for 73.6 percent of the variance in under-five mortality. It is possible to account for similar proportions of the variation in under-five mortality, approaching it as strictly a health issue, or as a cultural issue. The bottom line is that the statistical analysis alone is a weak tool for deciding which variables should or should not be included in the analysis.

Despite the problems of determining the correct regression model on the basis of the statistical analysis alone, there will continue to be those who use the stepwise method—either forward or backward, or both—to uncover the "best" regression models. There will also continue to be many who say that the regression model can only be determined by a theoretical framework and confirmed or not confirmed by the analysis. Perhaps the best that can be said about the two approaches is that the former is largely exploratory, whereas the latter is an attempt at the confirmation of theory. Short of that, the controversy is not likely to be resolved.

Exercises for Section 13.2

1. The data on the U5Mort1 worksheet of Chpt 13–1.xls show the entire data set shown in Figure 13.14. Use this data set to replicate the analysis discussed in this section.

   a. Use the Tools/Data Analysis/Regression add-in to perform the eight single variable regressions needed to replicate Figure 13.15 and replicate the figure.

   b. Use the Tools/Data Analysis/Regression add-in to perform the multiple regression needed to replicate Figure 13.16 and replicate the figure.

   c. Beginning with the lowest probability value in the result of b, proceed with backward stepwise elimination of the least important variable to replicate the result shown in Figure 13.17. *Remember that to use the Tools/Data Analysis/ Regression add-in, all independent variables must be in contiguous columns.*

   d. Beginning with the highest probability value in the result in a, carry out forward stepwise inclusion to arrive at the results shown in Figure 13.18.

   e. Use stepwise backward elimination to replicate the analysis shown in Figure 13.19 for the health predictor set: SafeW, Sanit, HealthS, DPT, and CPR.

   f. Use stepwise backward elimination to replicate the analysis shown in Figure 13.20 for the cultural variables: LogGNP, FemLit, and TFR.

2. The data on the U5Mort2 worksheet in Chpt 13–1.xls show the same data as those shown in Section 13.2, except that it is for the year 2001 (http://www.unicef.org/sowc01/tables/#). Use the data and replicate the analyses carried out in Section 13.2. (The variable HealthS was not available for 2001.)

   a. Use the Tools/Data Analysis/Regression add-in to perform the seven single variable regressions needed to replicate Figure 13.15 and replicate the figure for these data.

   b. Use the Tools/Data Analysis/Regression add-in to perform the multiple regression needed to replicate Figure 13.16 and replicate the figure for these data.

   c. Beginning with the lowest probability value in the result of b, proceed with backward stepwise elimination of the least important variable to replicate the result shown in Figure 13.17 for these data.

   d. Beginning with the highest probability value in the result in a, carry out forward stepwise inclusion to replicate the result shown in Figure 13.18 for these data.

   e. Use stepwise backward elimination to replicate the analysis shown in Figure 13.19 for the health predictor set: Sanit, HealthS, DPT, and CPR.

f. Use stepwise backward elimination to replicate the analysis shown in Figure 13.20 for the cultural variables: LogGNP, FemLit, and TFR.

g. Decide what the consequences of these results are for understanding the relationship between the seven independent variables and U5Mort.

Section 13.3 Correlation and Multicolinearity

How is it that different independent variables can produce similar results in predicting a dependent variable? Or how is it that two variables can each separately predict 50 percent or more of the variance in an independent variable but, together, cannot predict more than 70 percent. The answer is that the predictor variables themselves are related. This is frequently called *multicolinearity*. Multicolinearity has two effects in multiple regression analysis—one of little consequence and the other of some significant consequence. The first result is what we have already seen, which is that different variables can produce similar results as predictors of a dependent variable and that the proportion of variance attributable to two variables taken together will not generally be the sum of the variance attributable independently by each. The second result—that of some consequence—is that as colinearity increases, the standard errors of the coefficients that are multicolinear will increase. This can result, for example, in two variables that are both statistically significant predictors of a third variable when taken independently, being neither statistically significant when taken together.

To examine multicolinearity, consider first the relationship between the independent variables examined in Section 13.2, the eight variables taken from *The State of the World's Children, 1996* (1996). Figure 13.21 shows the correlation between the eight predictors of U5Mort. This was generated using the Excel

FIGURE 13.21. CORRELATION AMONG THE PREDICTORS FOR U5Mort.

	L	M	N	O	P	Q	R	S	T
2		SafeW	Sanit	HealthS	DPT	CPR	LogGNP	FemLit	TFR
3	SafeW	1							
4	Sanit	0.66827	1						
5	HealthS	0.58598	0.53536	1					
6	DPT	0.5708	0.53551	0.57861	1				
7	CPR	0.69504	0.68752	0.64122	0.72175	1			
8	LogGNP	0.66665	0.69559	0.50875	0.47242	0.71137	1		
9	FemLit	0.41646	0.60439	0.57115	0.63066	0.77748	0.6083	1	
10	TFR	-0.63155	-0.58507	-0.6523	-0.68206	-0.91374	-0.72151	-0.78688	1

add-in for correlation in Tools/Data Analysis/Correlation. A correlation is exactly the same as the value of Multiple R in regression analysis that would be generated if only one independent variable was considered at a time. You will recall that the Multiple R is just the square root of R square. So the correlations shown in Figure 13.21 are essentially the square roots of the amount of variance shared between each of the variables shown. For example, the correlation between SafeW and Sanit (cell M4) is .668. This means that SafeW and Sanit share about 44.7 percent of their variance ($.668^2 = .447$).

Thus far, the correlation between two variables has been computed either by using the correlation add-in in Tools/Data Analysis or as the Multiple R in regression. The correlation coefficient can be calculated directly by using the formula given in Equation 13.6, where x refers to one of the two variables and y refers to the other.

$$r = \frac{\sum (x_i - \bar{x})(y_i - \bar{y})}{\sqrt{\sum (x_i - \bar{x})^2 \times \sum (y_i - \bar{y})^2}} \tag{13.6}$$

If the correlation table in Figure 13.21 is examined closely, it is possible to see that the highest correlation is between CPR (contraceptive prevalence rate) and TFR (total fertility rate) (.914 in cell Q10). There is every reason to expect that these two variables would be highly correlated because there is reason to believe that higher contraceptive prevalence rates will actually produce lower total fertility rates. If these two variables are examined independently with regard to U5Mort, CPR accounts for 71.6 percent of the variance in U5Mort and TFR accounts for 66.8 percent (Figure 13.15), and both variables have statistically significant coefficients ($p = 1.26E-21$ for CPR and $3.66E-19$ for TFR). Now consider what happens if the two variables are considered simultaneously. The result of the simultaneous analysis of CPR and TFR produces the coefficients and t tests shown in Figure 13.22. Now, the two variables together account for 72.8 percent

FIGURE 13.22. CPR AND TFR TOGETHER AS PREDICTORS FOR U5Mort.

	K	L	M	N	O
21		Coefficient	Standard E	t Stat	P-value	L
22	Intercept	111.753	48.17262	2.319845	0.023188
23	TFR	12.29324	6.914236	1.777961	0.079633
24	CPR	-1.89031	0.476815	-3.96445	0.000172

FIGURE 13.23. CPR AND TFR TOGETHER AS PREDICTORS FOR U5Mort: REDUCED SAMPLE.

	K	L	M	N	O	
20		Coefficient	Standard Er	t Stat	P-value	
21	Intercept	59.73911	99.59955	0.599793	0.551945	
22	TFR	20.36392	14.20315	1.433761	0.159223	
23	CPR	-1.30266	0.987915	-1.3186	0.194621	

of the variance in U5Mort, but TFR is no longer statistically different from 0 (p = .079). Furthermore, the probability for CPR now reaches only .0002. But this could be a function only of the variance shared between the two variables canceling out each other, so to speak. Is there a better demonstration of the effect of multicolinearity as an inflator of standard errors? To find one, it is necessary to modify the data a little.

CPR and TFR are highly correlated—that is, .914, which means they share about 83 percent of their variance ($.914^2$ = .83). But the effects of extreme multicolinearity do not arise at that level. To see the effects, it is necessary to increase the relationship between CPR and TFR. To do that, thirty-one countries that had the lowest correlations between CPR and TFR were removed from the data set, resulting in forty-four countries for which CPR and TFR were correlated .962. At that level of correlation, they share about 92 percent of their variance. When each of the variables is separately related to U5Mort, the results are quite like those in Figure 13.15. The probability of the coefficient for CPR is 2.76E−12 and the probability of the coefficient for TFR is 2.36E−12. Each of the variables independently accounts for about 69 percent of the variance in U5Mort. But when they are examined simultaneously, the results are as those shown in Figure 13.23. It can be seen there that neither coefficient (CPR or TFR) has a statistically significant probability. This is the consequence of extreme multicolinearity. It inflates the standard errors to the extent that variables no longer show statistical significance. But it is important to note that this happened at a correlation between CPR and TFR of .962. In general, multicolinearity is not a problem to be concerned about unless the correlation between variables exceeds about .90.

Exercises for Section 13.3

1. Use the data on the U5Mort1 worksheet and the formula in Equation 13.6 to calculate the correlation between FemLit and CPR, between TFR and CPR.
2. Use the data on the U5Mort2 worksheet and the formula in Equation 13.6 to calculate the correlation between FemLit and CPR and between TFR and CPR.

Section 13.4 Nonlinear Relationships

Up to this point, we have considered regression analysis in its classical context, which is as a way to examine linear relationships between independent and dependent variables. But regression analysis can also be used in certain cases to analyze nonlinear relationships. This section discusses some of the ways in which Excel can be used to perform nonlinear regression analysis.

Estimating a Nonlinear Relationship

In examining the relationship between the independent variables taken from the State of *The State of the World's Children, 1996* (1996) and U5Mort, LogGNP, rather than GNP itself, was used as a predictor, because it was indicated that GNP is not linearly related to U5Mort, whereas LogGNP is. This decision deserves somewhat more discussion and, along with that discussion, some observations on the analysis of nonlinear relationships. To begin the discussion it is useful actually to look at the relationship in an *xy* graph.

A graph of the relationship between GNP and U5Mort is shown in Figure 13.24. It is possible to see there that the relationship is highly nonlinear. Below a GNP of about $5,000 per year, U5Mort falls precipitously from over three hundred to below fifty. For the four countries above $5,000 per year, the differences in U5Mort are comparatively small. Although a straight line might fit the data either

FIGURE 13.24. RELATIONSHIP BETWEEN GNP AND U5Mort.

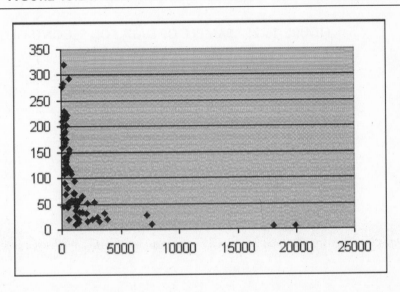

below or above $5,000, a straight line does not fit both segments of the data simultaneously.

There are a number of different ways in which an attempt to fit the data represented by the relation between GNP and U5Mort might be approached. Consider first the possibility of fitting the line with a *second-degree curve*. In general, a second-degree curve is any relationship between a dependent and an independent variable that is defined by the independent variable and a power of the independent variable. But, typically, a second-degree curve is defined by the original independent variable and its square. A major characteristic of a second-degree curve is that it produces a graphed line that has one change of direction. In the data shown in Figure 13.24, the data essentially change direction one time, at about twenty-five deaths per thousand live births or at about $1,500 in GNP per capita. A third degree curve would have two changes of direction, a fourth degree three, and so on. In general, data that are encountered in health-related applications will rarely benefit from going beyond a second degree curve.

A sample of the data (for the first ten countries) for analyzing the relationship in Figure 13.24 is shown in Figure 13.25. Column A is the actual value of GNP per capita and column B is the square of GNP per capita. Column C is the actual value of U5Mort and column D is the best fitting second-degree curve through the data. The actual regression equation that predicts that curve (which was found by using Tools/Data Analysis/Regression) is shown in Equation 13.7. This equation accounts for 39.6 percent of the variance in U5Mort ($R^2 = .396$), compared with only 17.5 percent of the variance accounted for when GNP alone (not the log of GNP) is used as a predictor. Clearly, from the point of view of the R square, the second degree curve is a better fit for the data than the straight line (a first-degree curve).

FIGURE 13.25. SAMPLE OF DATA FOR SECOND-DEGREE CURVEY ANALYSIS OF U5Mort.

	A	B	C	D	E
1		GNP	GNP^2	U5Mort	U5MortP
2	Niger	270	72900	320	141.94
3	Angola	700	490000	292	122.26
4	Sierra Leone	150	22500	284	147.57
5	Mozambique	90	8100	277	150.41
6	Guinea-Bissau	240	57600	231	143.34
7	Guinea	500	250000	223	131.31
8	Malawi	200	40000	221	145.21
9	Liberia	450	202500	217	133.60
10	Mali	270	72900	214	141.94
11	Somalia	120	14400	211	148.99
12	Zambia	380	144400	203	136.83

FIGURE 13.26. RELATIONSHIP BETWEEN GNP AND U5Mort WITH U5Mort PREDICTED: SECOND-DEGREE CURVE.

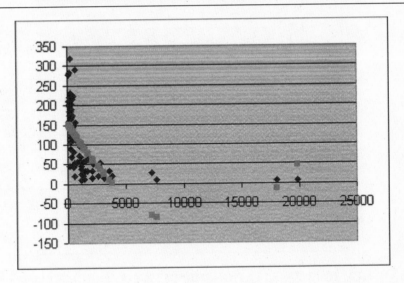

But let us see how well the second-degree curve, based on the square of GNP, actually fits the data. To see that, we will look at the predicted values of U5Mort, along with the actual values as graphed in Figure 13.26.

$$U5Mort = -.048 \, GNP + .00000214 \, GNP^2 + 154.697 \qquad (13.7)$$

As Figure 13.26 shows, the predicted values of U5Mort (shown as the gray squares) do not lie along a straight line. But at the same time, they do not fit the actual values of U5Mort as well as would be hoped. In particular, the predicted values of under-five mortality for three countries with GNP per capita above $5,000 are actually negative. Since this is clearly an impossibility, and since we already know that the log of GNP is a better predictor of U5Mort (R square = .539 from Figure 13.15), it is useful to look at that relationship more closely.

Figure 13.27 shows the actual values of U5Mort and the predicted values, based on LogGNP on the LogGNP scale. By using the log of GNP as the predictor, the distribution has become much more linear than when GNP itself is used. But the relationship is still not truly linear, as the figure shows, and furthermore, the predicted values of U5Mort are again below zero for some of the countries, particularly for those with LogGNP per capita in excess of about 3.8. You will recall that the coefficient for the log of GNP and the constant for this model were both given in Figure 13.15.

FIGURE 13.27. RELATIONSHIP BETWEEN LogGNP AND U5Mort.

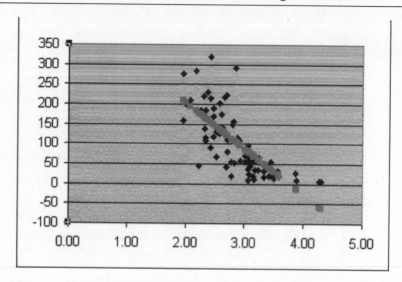

FIGURE 13.28. RELATIONSHIP BETWEEN LogGNP AND LogU5Mort.

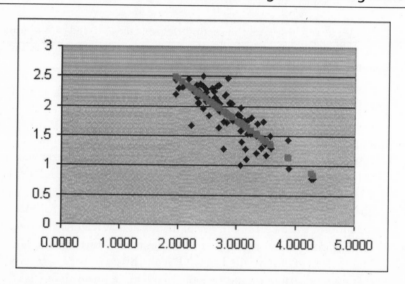

In an effort to come closer to a linear relationship, consider the possibility of taking the log of both GNP and of U5Mort. Figure 13.28 shows the relationship between LogGNP and LogU5Mort. As is evident in that figure, the relationship between the logs of these two variables is a very good approximation of a linear relationship. The figure also shows the predicted values for LogU5Mort.

These are based on the regression equation in Equation 13.8, which was calculated by using Tools/Data Analysis/Regression. Furthermore, LogGNP accounts for about 68 percent of the variance in LogU5Mort, which is right up in the range of the best predictors of U5Mort itself: CPR and TFR.

$$\text{LogU5Mort} = -.706 \ \text{LogGNP} + 3.874 \tag{13.8}$$

There is one last way that we will consider for assessing the nonlinear relationship between GNP and U5Mort, which is based on the use of a dummy variable. In this case, the dummy variable will simply be assigned as a 1 to countries with GNP greater than \$1,500 and 0 to other countries. So the regression equation that will be used to describe the relationship between GNP and U5Mort will contain GNP and a variable we will call HiGNP, along with an interaction term—GNP*HiGNP, as predictors.

Figure 13.29 shows the result of this analysis. As can be seen in the figure, the inclusion of a dummy representing high-income countries and an interaction produces predicted values along two separate regression lines—one representing those countries with GNP per capita less than \$1,500 and one representing countries with GNP per capita greater than \$1,500. The regression equation for this analysis is given in Equation 13.9.

$$\begin{aligned} \text{U5Mort} = -.126 \ \text{GNP} + -163.833 \ \text{HiGNP} \\ + .124 \ \text{GNP} \times \text{HiGNP} + 200.976 \end{aligned} \tag{13.9}$$

FIGURE 13.29. RELATIONSHIP BETWEEN GNP AND U5Mort WITH HiGNP DUMMY.

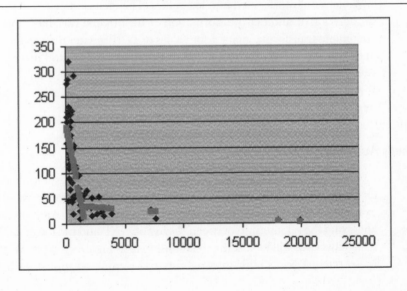

This model accounts for 59 percent of the variance in U5Mort—not as much as that accounted for when the log transformation of each variable was chosen, but more than that accounted for by any of the other models examined here. A question arises from this analysis, however, and that question is, why decide to use a dummy and why chose $1,500 as the cutoff point? The answer is simple: by looking at the scatterplot (for example, Figure 13.24) of the relationship between GNP and U5Mort. It just looks from that graph that there is a discontinuity in the relationship between these two at about $1,500 (or $1,300, or $1,800). If we are seeking the best linear regression model to describe the relationship between GNP and U5Mort, it is a good idea not only to look at the data plots but also to benefit from them when specifying a model.

But is this not simply mining the data for anything we can find? Yes, but so is any other approach to regression analysis—in particular, stepwise regression, whether forward or backward, that does not begin with some type of theory. If all we hope to do is to get the best description that we can of the relationship, all of these tools are appropriate. However, if we wished to test the hypothesis that there is a discontinuity in the relationship between GNP and U5Mort at $1,500, based on prior information available to us, then that is also a legitimate reason to include the dummy variable.

To conclude this section, there are a number of ways that nonlinear relationships might be examined using regression. They all involve some modification of the original data. When the second-degree equation was examined, the square of the original predictor, GNP, was employed, along with GNP. When the log values were examined, both the independent variable and the dependent variable were transformed into log values. The inclusion of a dummy variable is the addition of another transformation of the original variable—this time, a discontinuous transformation of 1 for values of GNP greater than some cutoff point, and 0 otherwise. All are reasonable strategies to employ (and there are others as well) if the purpose is to try to find the best-fitting line for a nonlinear relationship. Excel provides a shortcut for some of this activity, which is discussed in the next section.

Excel's Automatic Curve Fitter

Excel has the built-in capability to examine some of the possible alternative ways for fitting regression lines with data. To look at this capability, we will stay with the example of the relationship between GNP and U5Mort. And since we already know that the relationship between the log of GNP and the log of U5Mort is virtually linear, we will look at that relationship first. Figure 13.30 shows the first step in accessing Excel's built-in capability to examine relationships between two

FIGURE 13.30. FORMAT DATA SERIES WINDOW.

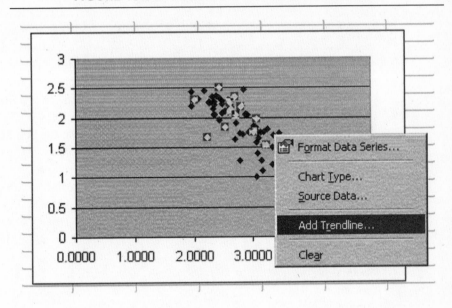

variables. If the cursor is placed over a point in the data series and right-clicked, the window Format Data Series comes up. There are several options with this window, but we will concentrate on only one: Add Trendline.

If we select the Add Trendline option in the Format Data Series window, the Add Trendline window, shown in Figure 13.31, comes up. In that window it is possible to select from six different options: linear, logarithmic, polynomial, power, exponential, and moving average.

The linear option, which we will examine first, is essentially a simple linear regression model that relates a single independent variable (the variable that defines the horizontal access) to the dependent variable (the variable that defines the vertical axis). Having selected the linear option, we can ask Excel to calculate the regression equation and the R square and display both on the graph. The selection of the regression equation and the R square are done on the window produced by selecting the Options tab in the Add Trendline window, as shown in Figure 13.32. Notice in that figure that there are check marks in both the boxes that precede Display equation on chart and Display R-squared value on chart.

With the linear model selected and both the equation and R square values checked, the result is the best-fitting straight line shown on the chart with the original data, along with the regression equation and the R square value, as seen in Figure 13.33. (It may be necessary to grab the regression formula and the R square with the cursor and drag these to a spot on the chart where they will be fully visible,

FIGURE 13.31. ADD TRENDLINE WINDOW.

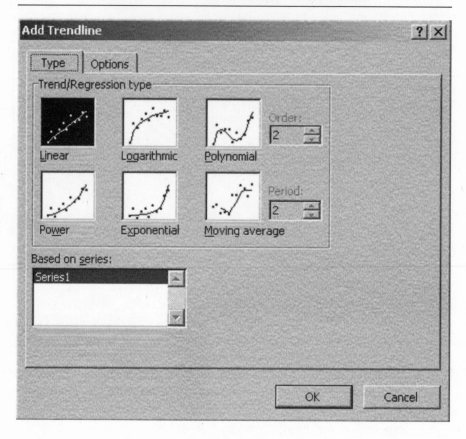

as they tend to pop up right in the midst of the data.) Now it should be clear that the results shown in Figure 13.33 are exactly the same as the results shown in Figure 13.28, and the regression formula and R square are the same as those produced for the latter figure. So, essentially, the charting capability of Excel has reproduced exactly what is produced by the regression add-in (albeit, with not nearly as much information; there are no significance tests, for example).

Having introduced the capabilities of the Add Trendline window, it is necessary to say a little about each of the other trendline options. The Logarithmic option produces a curve that is based on conversion of the x axis variable (GNP, in this case) to its natural logarithm. Ordinary least squares are then performed to generate the regression coefficients and R square, and then the resulting predicted values are graphed on the chart with the actual values of GNP. This produces the curve, the regression equation, and the R square shown in Figure 13.34. It is useful to note that the regression constant of 438.09 and the

FIGURE 13.32. ADD TRENDLINE WINDOW: OPTIONS TAB.

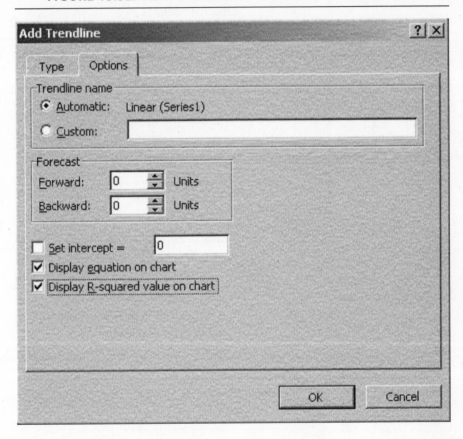

R square of .5386 are the same, as they were generated for the relationship shown in Figure 13.27 and detailed in row 9 of Figure 13.15. The only difference between the equation shown in Figure 13.34, and that indicated in row 9 of Figure 13.15, is the value of the coefficient on LogGNP, which is −116.56 rather than −50.52. The reason for this difference is that the data used to generate the values in Figure 13.15 were the log of GNP to the base 10, whereas Excel uses the natural logarithm (base 2.71828) for the regression equation shown in Figure 13.34. Since there is a constant relationship between the log to the base ten and the natural log, the coefficient of logGNP in Figure 13.15 can be generated from the coefficient in Figure 13.34 by multiplying by the constant value 2.30585. Thus, the logarithmic model in the Add Trendline window is simply the model generated by taking the log of the independent variable and relating it—using ordinary least squares regression—to the actual value of the dependent variable.

FIGURE 13.33. BEST-FITTING LINE FOR LogGNP AND LogU5Mort: LINEAR MODEL.

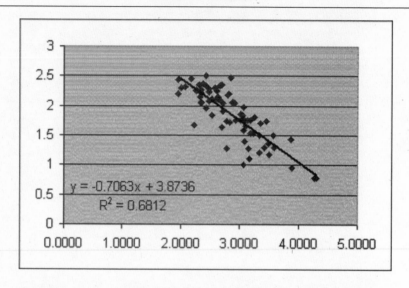

$y = -0.7063x + 3.8736$

$R^2 = 0.6812$

FIGURE 13.34. BEST-FITTING LINE FOR GNP AND U5Mort: LOGARITHMIC MODEL.

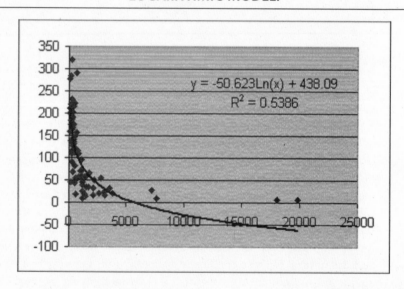

$y = -50.623\mathrm{Ln}(x) + 438.09$

$R^2 = 0.5386$

The third option in the Add Trendline window is the Polynomial option. If the Polynomial option is selected, it is possible to select 2 through 6 from the up and down arrows beside the Polynomial option. If you select 2, you produce a second degree curve with one change of direction. Selection of 3 produces a third degree curve with two changes of direction, and so on. Selection of 2 produces exactly the same result in terms of predicted values and the same regression equation and R square as were produced for Figure 13.26 and given in Equation 13.7. If the Polynomial option is selected, it is important to realize that there will be as many predictors in the model as the number selected plus a constant. In other words, if 2 is selected, the model will contain the x axis variable plus its square and a constant. If 3 is selected, the model will contain the x axis variable plus its square, its cube, and a constant, and so on.

The fourth option available in the Add Trendline window is the Power option. The Power option is shown in Figure 13.35. The equation for the power option, given in the figure, is the most complex yet encountered. But look at the R square for the power option. At .6812, it looks suspiciously like the R square for the model in which both GNP and U5Mort are converted to their log values (Figure 13.33). Furthermore, the $-.7063$ power to which x is raised in Figure 13.35 looks very much like the $-.7063$, by which x is multiplied in Figure 13.33. Moreover, if we take the 3.8736 in Figure 13.33 and raise 10 to that power, we get 7,475.5, which is the multiplier of x in Figure 13.35. Thus, the formula for the Power model can be found by using ordinary least squares, converting both the independent and dependent variables to their log values (base 10) and calculating the regression coefficients. The next step is to set up an equation in which the actual value of the dependent variable is predicted by using the actual value of the independent variable, raised to the power of the coefficient on the log of the

FIGURE 13.35. BEST FITTING LINE FOR GNP AND U5Mort: POWER MODEL.

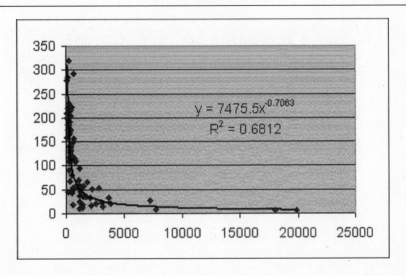

dependent variable and multiplied by 10, raised to the power of the intercept. The result is the Power model.

The fifth option in the Add Trendline window is the Exponential model. The line, equation, and R square for the exponential model are shown in Figure 13.36. The coefficients of the exponential model can be found, using ordinary least squares by first converting the dependent variable to its natural logarithm. The next step is to calculate the ordinary least square coefficients, using the actual value of the independent variable and the natural log of the dependent variable. In the case of the GNP and U5Mort data, this produces the result shown in Equation 13.10. To get the values of U5Mort as expressed in the formula given in Figure 13.36, then, it is necessary to raise e (2.718282) to the power of the coefficient of GNP shown in Equation 13.10 times the actual value of GNP, and then multiply that result by e raised to the power of the intercept term in Equation 13.10. This produces the result shown in Figure 13.36.

$$\text{LnU5Mort} = -.0002\,\text{GNP} + 4.603 \qquad (13.10)$$

The last model shown in the Add Trendline window is a Moving Average model. The moving average model applies specifically to time-related data—data where there is one measure for each of a string of time intervals. Since this book does not deal with time-related data, the moving average model will not be discussed.

FIGURE 13.36. BEST-FITTING LINE FOR GNP AND U5Mort: EXPONENTIAL MODEL.

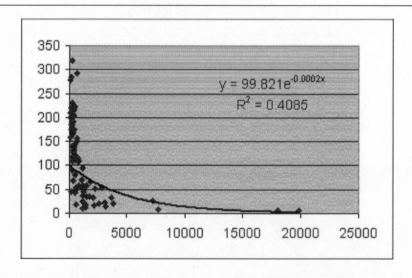

Exercises for Section 13.4

1. The worksheet GNP1 in Chpt 13–1.xls contains the GNP per capita, the log of GNP per capita, and U5Mort for seventy-five countries of the world from *The State of the World's Children, 1996* (1996).
   a. Use the GNP data along with GNP squared as independent variables to generate a regression analysis to predict U5Mort.
   b. Generate the predicted values of U5Mort, based on this analysis.
   c. Graph the actual and predicted values of U5Mort against GNP to replicate Figure 13.26.
   d. Use the Add Trendline window and the options tab to add a second degree polynomial to the graph for the values of GNP and U5Mort, along with the regression equation and the R square and compare this with the predicted values generated in b (preceding).

2. Use the worksheet GNP1 in Chpt 13–1.xls.
   a. Use the log of GNP to generate a regression analysis to predict U5Mort.
   b. Generate the predicted values of U5Mort, based on this analysis.
   c. Graph the actual and predicted values of U5Mort against logGNP to replicate Figure 13.27.
   d. Graph the actual values of U5Mort against GNP and use the Add Trendline window and the options tab to add the Logarithmic model with the regression equation and the R square to the graph.
   e. Confirm that the proportion of variance accounted for and the intercept are the same in both a and d and that the regression coefficient for LogGNP in a is 2.302585 times larger than the coefficient in d (the ratio of the natural log to the log base ten).

3. Use the worksheet GNP1 in Chpt 13–1.xls.
   a. Generate a new variable LogU5Mort by using the =LOG() function.
   b. Use the log of GNP to generate a regression analysis to predict LogU5Mort.
   c. Generate the predicted values of LogU5Mort, based on this analysis.
   d. Graph the actual and predicted values of LogU5Mort against logGNP to replicate Figure 13.28.
   e. Graph the actual values of U5Mort against GNP and use the Add Trendline window and the options tab to add the Power model with the regression equation and the R square to the graph.
   f. Confirm that the proportion of variance accounted for are the same in both b and e. Also, confirm that the power regression equation as given in e can

be replicated by raising the actual value of GNP to the power of the regression coefficient on LogGNP ($-.70633$) and multiplying by 10 raised to the power of the intercept term (3.8736).

4. The data on worksheet BirthW in Chpt 13–1.xls represent constructed data for the mother's age and the child's birth weight for a sample of two hundred mothers and children. Use the graphing capability of Excel and alternative curvilinear models to find the best-fitting nonstraight line for these data.

5. The data on worksheet Wait in Chpt 13–1.xls represent constructed data for length of time in quarter of hours and time from scheduled appointment to admission to the physicians office in a clinic for a sample of 220 people selected randomly from clinic records. Use the graphing capability of Excel and alternative curvilinear models to find the best-fitting nonstraight line for these data.

6. The data on worksheet Size in Chpt 13–1.xls represents constructed data for hospital size measured in the number of beds and the hospital occupancy rate. Use the graphing capability of Excel and alternative curvilinear models to find the best-fitting nonstraight line for these data.

Reference

The State of the World's Children, 1996, UNICEF, New York, 1996. [http://www.unicef.org/sowc96/stats.htm].

CHAPTER FOURTEEN

ANALYSIS WITH A DICHOTOMOUS CATEGORICAL DEPENDENT VARIABLE

The chi-square statistic deals with categorical data in both the independent and the dependent variables, but with the general limitation that only two variables—one independent and one dependent, or, occasionally, two independent and one independent—can be analyzed at one time. Furthermore, the chi-square is limited by the need to retain relatively large values (at least five or more) in all the cells of the tables in the analysis. The *t* test and ANOVA deal with categorical data in the independent variable but require a numerical variable in the dependent variable. Again, though, *t* tests are limited to a single independent variable that can take on only two values, whereas ANOVA is usually limited to no more than one or two independent variables. Regression analysis, the topic of the last three chapters, is more flexible than any of the other three analysis methods, in that it can deal simultaneously with a large number of independent variables and these can be either numerical or categorical. And regression has no particular cell size requirements. But like *t* tests and ANOVA, regression as discussed thus far is limited to numerical data in the dependent variable. But, frequently, there may arise a need to deal with categorical data in the dependent variable, and the desire may be to examine several (or many) independent variables simultaneously. This chapter addresses some alternative approaches to this problem—when the dependent variable is a dichotomous categorical variable.

Section 14.1 Introduction to the Dichotomous Dependent Variable

As has been discussed, a dichotomous categorical variable is one that takes on only two values. Sex is a dichotomous categorical variable. Emergency or not emergency is a dichotomous categorical variable. Medicare patient or non-Medicare patient is a dichotomous categorical variable. These variables are also frequently referred to as dummy variables, especially when used as predictor or independent variables in regression. They are universally coded 1 and 0, 1 designating one of the two alternatives and 0 designating the other. But it is also possible to consider a dichotomous categorical variable as a dependent variable. When this is done, the variable is again universally coded 1 or 0 to designate the two levels of the variable.

In early treatments of dichotomous dependent variables, it was common to use ordinary least squares regression, which is essentially what has been presented in the last three chapters. In this form, regression has commonly been referred to as a linear probability model. This is because the predicted value of the dependent variable, based on the analysis, was considered the probability that an observation would be a 1 or a 0, not whether it actually was a 1 or a 0. As with any other regression model, there is a direct mathematical solution to the problem of finding regression coefficients with dichotomous categorical dependent variables—dummy variables, as it were. But there are also some clear problems to using regression with dummy variables. These problems are discussed in somewhat more detail as we proceed.

In more recent years, two things have led to the virtual abandonment of ordinary least squares regression to analyze dummy dependent variables. The first has been the recognition of the problems in using ordinary least squares regression to deal with dummy dependent variables. The second has been the increasing availability of computers to carry out complex and time-consuming calculations. Especially because of the latter, there has been a universal shift to what is called *maximum likelihood estimators,* to derive the relationship between one or more independent variables and a dichotomous dependent variable. Two maximum likelihood estimators have gained the most favor in dealing with dichotomous categorical dependent variables. One of these is called Logit and the other is called Probit. These two estimation procedures produce nearly identical results in practice. Because the Logit approach is substantially less complex, Logit is discussed in this chapter. But before turning to Logit, we will examine the ways in which dichotomous dependent variables have been analyzed in the past as a way of demonstrating the problems attendant with these treatments.

Section 14.2 An Example with a Dichotomous Dependent Variable: Traditional Treatments

The staff at a well-baby clinic is concerned about the immunization levels of children being treated at the clinic. The clinic staff hopes to achieve full immunization levels for all children seen at the clinic. The staff also knows that some mothers are more likely than others to seek full immunization for their children and thus need little or no push from the clinic. What clinic staff would like to know is whether it is possible to predict which mothers are likely not to seek full immunization for their children so that they can concentrate their effort on those women in promoting full immunization.

Clinic staff also perceive from observation that younger mothers, mothers with less education, and low-parity women are less likely to have their children fully immunized. They are hopeful that knowing this will allow them to better concentrate their effort in education and the promotion of immunization. They have also observed that if a child is a second, third, or higher birth-order child, it is more likely that the mother will seek full immunization on her own. The clinic has collected data on thirty-two mothers who are coming to the clinic. Each of these mothers has a child between one and two years of age. The data available to the health department include the mother's age, her years of formal education, the birth order of the child, and whether the child is fully immunized for one year of age. The data (which are wholly fabricated for this example) are shown in Figure 14.1. As Figure 14.1 shows, the mothers range in age from seventeen to twenty-eight years. They have between five and fifteen years of formal education and they have one to six children (remember that these are fabricated data). Of the children, twenty-one are fully immunized (those coded 1 in the column labeled Immun); the other eleven children are not fully immunized. The question is whether the clinic can gain any information from these data to help them better target their education efforts about immunization.

A Chi-Square Analysis

One way to approach the problem of deciding where to put education efforts is to use contingency table analysis and the chi-square statistic, since this approach can deal with categorical dependent variables. However, since the contingency table and chi-square statistic approach basically requires some observations in every cell, it would not be feasible to use this approach without collapsing the independent variable data—age, education, and parity—into some smaller set of categories. One way to collapse the independent variable data would be simply to

Statistics for Health Policy and Administration Using Microsoft Excel

FIGURE 14.1. DATA FOR THIRTY-TWO MOTHERS.

	A	B	C	D	E	F	G	H	I	J	K
1	Mother	Age	Educ	Order	Immun		Mother	Age	Educ	Order	Immun
2	1	21	7	3	0		17	21	12	1	1
3	2	19	12	2	1		18	21	8	4	0
4	3	23	10	3	0		19	22	6	3	0
5	4	25	8	2	1		20	21	8	3	0
6	5	25	7	2	1		21	21	10	3	1
7	6	26	15	4	1		22	21	10	1	1
8	7	17	6	1	0		23	25	10	3	1
9	8	21	6	3	0		24	22	10	3	1
10	9	25	13	6	1		25	22	7	3	0
11	10	19	11	3	1		26	21	8	3	0
12	11	20	13	4	1		27	27	7	2	1
13	12	18	10	1	1		28	24	12	3	1
14	13	17	6	2	0		29	28	14	5	1
15	14	20	12	4	1		30	20	7	2	1
16	15	21	7	1	1		31	26	13	2	1
17	16	17	5	3	0		32	18	10	1	1

FIGURE 14.2. ONE-ZERO CONVERSION OF DATA FOR THIRTY-TWO MOTHERS.

	A	B	C	D	E	F	G	H	I	J	K
20	Mother	Age	Educ	Order	Immun		Mother	Age	Educ	Order	Immun
21	1	0	0	1	0		17	0	1	0	1
22	2	0	1	0	1		18	0	0	1	0
23	3	1	1	1	0		19	1	0	1	0
24	4	1	0	0	1		20	0	0	1	0
25	5	1	0	0	1		21	0	1	1	1
26	6	1	1	1	1		22	0	1	0	1
27	7	0	0	0	0		23	1	1	1	1
28	8	0	0	1	0		24	1	1	1	1
29	9	1	1	1	1		25	1	0	1	0
30	10	0	1	1	1		26	0	0	1	0
31	11	0	1	1	1		27	1	0	0	1
32	12	0	1	0	1		28	1	1	1	1
33	13	0	0	0	0		29	1	1	1	1
34	14	0	1	1	1		30	0	0	0	1
35	15	0	0	0	1		31	1	1	0	1
36	16	0	0	1	0		32	0	1	0	1

split them into high and low at the mean. If we do that, the resulting data for the thirty-two mothers would be as those shown in Figure 14.2, where a 1 designates a value of the original variable that is greater than the mean and 0 represents a value of the original variable less than the mean.

The data in Figure 14.2 can be used to generate two-by-two contingency tables and chi-square values to determine whether immunization status of the

FIGURE 14.3. CHI-SQUARE ANALYSIS OF IMMUNIZATION BY AGE OF MOTHER.

	O17	▼	=	=((ABS(O11-O5)-0.5)^2)/O11	
	N	O	P	Q	R
3	Count of Immun	Age ▼			
4	Immun ▼	0	1	Grand Total	
5	0	8	3	11	
6	1	11	10	21	
7	Grand Total	19	13	32	
8					
9	Count of Immun	Age	0	0	
10	Immun	0	1	Grand Total	
11	0	6.531	4.469	11	
12	1	12.47	8.531	21	
13	Grand Total	19	13	32	
14					
15	Count of Immun	Age	0	0	
16	Immun	0	1	Grand Total	
17	0	0.144	0.21	11	
18	1	0.075	0.11	21	
19	Grand Total	19	13	32	
20					
21			chi sq	0.5389698	
22			p	0.46286	

child is dependent on any of the three variables—age, education, or parity. One such analysis—that for age—is shown in Figure 14.3. That figure shows the pivot table results of crossing immunization with age in cells N3:Q7. In cells N9:Q13, the expected values for the cells in the original pivot table are given. One problem with using chi-square analysis for these data is immediately obvious from either the original data table or the expected value table. That problem is the small cell sizes, especially for the older age-no immunization category. In consequence, the chi-square is computed by using the Yates's correction that was discussed in Chapter Ten. The formula for the contribution to the chi-square of cell O17 is shown in the formula bar. Note that the absolute value of the difference between the observed and expected values and the −.5 of the Yates's correction is shown there.

With or without the Yates's correction, the chi-square value produced by the analysis of full immunization by the mother's age suggests that the two variables are statistically independent. The chi-square is given in cell Q21 and its probability is given in cell Q22. Given that the probability of finding a chi-square value as large as .539 (if a mother's age and immunization status are independent of one another) is .46, we will conclude that they are in fact independent. The bottom line is, you can't predict a child's immunization status from the age of its mother.

We can carry out a similar analysis for both a mother's education and the birth order of the child. If we do so, the results are a chi-square of 10.49, with a probability of .001 for the mother's education, and a chi-square of 2.24, with a probability of .136 for the birth order of the child. The conclusion that we would draw, based on these data (remember, they are constructed data), is that of the three things about which the clinic has information, it is only the mother's education that is related to the child's immunization status. Consequently, it would not be unreasonable for clinic staff to conclude that if they hope to have an effect with a targeted information program, they should target women with lower education.

There are a couple problems with these analyses, though. First, since we have collapsed the data regarding the mother's education and the birth order of the child from multiple levels to just two, we have lost information. It is generally better, if possible, to select an analysis that uses all the available data. Second, we have looked only at one variable at a time. It is also generally better, if possible, to select an analysis that treats all variables of interest simultaneously. Although contingency tables and chi-square analysis can, in certain circumstances, be used to examine more than one independent variable at a time, in this case, the cell sizes would be too small to make it practical.

We have seen in Chapters Twelve and Thirteen that multiple regression uses the full range of data available in the analysis. Multiple regression can also deal simultaneously with a number of independent variables (sixteen for the Excel add-in, but, theoretically, the number of independent variables is limited to one fewer than the number of observations). So can we use multiple regression—in this case, ordinary least squares, or OLS—to analyze these data? The answer turns out to be yes—and no. To help us see why, the next section discusses the use of OLS with the data on immunization.

Ordinary Least Squares with a Dichotomous Dependent Variable

Let us consider the data on children's immunization status, using OLS. Figure 14.4 shows the results of the regression analysis for the data shown in Figure 14.1. The data have been rearranged to carry out the analysis and only the data for the first twenty women and their children are shown. The results of the analysis, using the Excel regression add-in, are given in cells G1:L20. The analysis indicates that 58 percent of the variance in immunization rates has been accounted for (cell H5). It also indicates a significant overall F test (cells K12 and L12). Furthermore, it confirms the conclusions about the age and education of the mother. Even with the additional data, the age of the mother is not a statistically significant predictor of immunization status (cells H18:K18). The additional data confirm also that a mother's education is a statistically significant predictor of immunization status

FIGURE 14.4. RESULTS OF OLS FOR IMMUNIZATION DATA.

	A	B	C	D	E	F	G	H	I	J	K	L	
1	Mother	Age	Educ	Order	Immun		SUMMARY OUTPUT						
2	1	21	7	3	0								
3	2	19	12	2	1		Regression Statistics						
4	3	23	10	3	0		Multiple R	0.759847					
5	4	25	8	2	1		R Square	0.577368					
6	5	25	7	2	1		Adjusted R Squ	0.532085					
7	6	26	15	4	1		Standard Error	0.330091					
8	7	17	6	1	0		Observations	32					
9	8	21	6	3	0								
10	9	25	13	6	1		ANOVA						
11	10	19	11	3	1			df	SS	MS	F	ignificance F	
12	11	20	13	4	1		Regression	3	4.167872	1.389291	12.75047	1.96E-05	
13	12	18	10	1	1		Residual	28	3.050878	0.10896			
14	13	17	6	2	0		Total	31	7.21875				
15	14	20	12	4	1								
16	15	21	7	1	1			Coefficient	andard Err	t Stat	P-value	Lower 95%	Uppe
17	16	17	5	3	0		Intercept	-0.90395	0.439026	-2.05899	0.048905	-1.80326	-0.0
18	17	21	12	1	1		Age	0.039752	0.022498	1.766921	0.088142	-0.00633	0.08
19	18	21	8	4	0		Educ	0.125969	0.024454	5.151268	1.83E-05	0.075878	0.17
20	19	22	6	3	0		Order	-0.17968	0.055634	-3.22959	0.003159	-0.29364	-0.0
21	20	21	8	3	0								

(cells H19:K19). With the additional data provided by the OLS analysis for birth order of the child, that variable too appears to be a statistically significant predictor of immunization status. So the use of OLS instead of contingency tables and chi-square would lead clinic personnel to conclude that they might effectively concentrate their education effort not only on low-education women but also on low parity women.

But there are also problems with this analysis. The problems have to do with the restriction of the dependent variable to two values: 1 and 0. In this situation the predicted regression values will not be actually 1 or 0 but, rather, some number that must be interpreted as the probability that the true value will be 1 or 0. For this reason, OLS used in this manner is called a linear probability model (LPM). The fact that the actual values of the dependent variable take on only the values of 1 and 0 is not a problem for the regression coefficients themselves. They remain unbiased. The problem lies with the error terms, and thus with statistical tests based on the error terms. A basic assumption of the statistical tests (F test and t tests) in regression is that the error terms are uncorrelated with the independent variables and have a constant variance and an expected value of 0. Aldrich and Nelson (1984) have provided a clear discussion of why these assumptions cannot be maintained when the dependent variable is restricted to 1 and 0. The basic problem is that the variance of the error terms turns out to be correlated systematically with the independent variables. In this situation the statistical tests based on OLS regression are invalid, even in large samples.

But there is a relatively simple fix for this situation in regard to the statistical test, which was originally proposed by Goldberger (1964) and clearly laid out by Aldrich and Nelson (1984). This is a weighted least squares (WLS) procedure for estimating the linear probability model.

WLS for Estimating Linear Probability Models

The weighted least squares procedure for the linear probability model is carried out in two steps. The first step is to estimate the regression model by using OLS. The second step is to use the results of OLS to create weights by which the original variables—both the independent variables x_i and the dependent variable y—are transformed, and then to estimate the regression model a second time, on the basis of the transformed variables.

The weights for the transformation are as those given in Equation 14.1. Equation 14.1 says that a weight for each observation is created by first calculating the predicted values of the dependent variable, using the OLS estimates of the coefficients. Then the predicted value of the dependent variable is multiplied by 1 minus the predicted value, and the square root of that number is taken. Finally, 1 is divided by the resulting value to obtain the appropriate weight. As Aldrich and Nelson (1984) point out, this is just the reciprocal of the estimated standard errors of the error term.

$$w_i = 1/[\hat{y}_i(1 - \hat{y}_i)]^{1/2} \qquad (14.1)$$

There is, however, a basic problem with this procedure for generating weights. Even though the predicted values of the dependent variable are appropriately interpreted as the probability that the dependent variable will be 1 or 0, it is likely that at least some of the predicted values will be either greater than 1 or less than 0. When a number greater than 1 or less than 0 is multiplied by 1 minus itself, it produces a negative result. The square root of a negative number is an imaginary number, and Excel will generate a #NUM! result in the cell that includes the square root of a negative number. Aldrich and Nelson (1984) suggest a relatively simple solution to this problem, which is to use some large number less than 1, such as .999, in place of the true predicted value when it is greater than 1 and some small number greater than 0, such as .001, when the predicted value is less than 0.

Figure 14.5 shows the original OLS data for the thirty-two mothers (only the first twenty are shown), along with the calculation of the weights for WLS. As it is possible to see, the actual OLS regression analysis has been moved to the right and three new columns have been inserted. The first of the new columns (column F) is the predicted value of the dependent variable Immun (which is $\hat{y}$ in Equation 14.1) and is called Ipred for Immun predicted. The values of Ipred

FIGURE 14.5. CALCULATION OF WEIGHTS FOR WLS.

| H2 | | $=1/(G2*(1-G2))^{0.5}$ | | | | | | | | |

	A	B	C	D	E	F	G	H	I	J	K
1	Mother	Age	Educ	Order	Immun	Ipred	Ipredadj	w		SUMMARY OUTPUT	
2	1	21	7	3	0	0.27359	0.27359	2.24314			
3	2	19	12	2	1	1.00361	0.999	31.6386		*Regression Statistics*	
4	3	23	10	3	0	0.73101	0.73101	2.25511		Multiple R	0.759847
5	4	25	8	2	1	0.73825	0.73825	2.27485		R Square	0.577368
6	5	25	7	2	1	0.61228	0.61228	2.05242		Adjusted R Squ	0.532085
7	6	26	15	4	1	1.30043	0.999	31.6386		Standard Error	0.330091
8	7	17	6	1	0	0.34797	0.34797	2.0994		Observations	32
9	8	21	6	3	0	0.14763	0.14763	2.81906			
10	9	25	13	6	1	0.64939	0.64939	2.09573		ANOVA	
11	10	19	11	3	1	0.69797	0.69797	2.17799			*df*
12	11	20	13	4	1	0.80998	0.80998	2.54898		Regression	3 4.1
13	12	18	10	1	1	0.8916	0.8916	3.2166		Residual	28 3.0
14	13	17	6	2	0	0.16829	0.16829	2.67289		Total	31 7.
15	14	20	12	4	1	0.68402	0.68402	2.15097			
16	15	21	7	1	1	0.63295	0.63295	2.07468			*Coefficients and*
17	16	17	5	3	0	-0.13735	0.001	31.6386		Intercept	-0.90395 0.4
18	17	21	12	1	1	1.26279	0.999	31.6386		Age	0.039752 0.0
19	18	21	8	4	0	0.21989	0.21989	2.41446		Educ	0.125969 0.0
20	19	22	6	3	0	0.18738	0.18738	2.5627		Order	-0.17968 0.0
21	20	21	8	3	0	0.39956	0.39956	2.04161			
22	21	21	10	3	1	0.5545	0.5545	2.0986			

were calculated using the regression formula with the original independent data in columns B, C, and D and the coefficients in cells K17:K21. By inspection of column F, it is possible to see that three of the first twenty predicted values of immunization are outside the range 0 to 1. Cells F3, F7 and F18 have values greater than 1 and cell F17 has a value less than 0. To accommodate that problem in the calculation of weights, a new column, Ipredadj—or Immun predicted adjusted, was included as column G. In column G, the Excel =IF() function is used to adjust the predicted values to ensure that they are all in the range 0 to 1. The =IF() statement as it appears in cell G2, for example, is =IF(F2>1, .999, IF(F2<0, .001, F2). That =IF() statement is then copied to each cell in column G.

The final new column in Figure 14.5 is the actual weight calculated from the adjusted predicted value of Immun. The formula for the calculation of the weights is given, for cell H2, in the formula bar above the spreadsheet. These are the values by which the independent variable set is modified for WLS.

The regression analysis based on the weighted values of the variables is shown in Figure 14.6. Figure 14.6 again shows the first twenty mothers in the data set in column A. Column B, labeled Const for constant, is simply the weight calculated in Figure 14.5, but it can be thought of as the constant term in regression (1) multiplied by the weight. Each column—C, D, E, and F—is the original value of each variable—Age, Educ, Order, and Immun—multiplied by the weight from Figure 14.5.

FIGURE 14.6. WEIGHTED LEAST SQUARES RESULTS.

	A	B	C	D	E	F	G	H	I	J	K	L	M
	G37	▼	=	=$J$53+B2*$J$54+C2*$J$55+D2*$J$56									
36	Mother	Const	Age	Educ	Order	Immun	Ipred		SUMMARY OUTPUT				
37	1	2.243	47.11	15.7	6.729	0	0.32768						
38	2	31.64	601.1	379.7	63.28	31.6386	0.94838		*Regression Statistics*				
39	3	2.255	51.87	22.55	6.765	0	0.66463		Multiple R	0.990383			
40	4	2.275	56.87	18.2	4.55	2.27485	0.5817		R Square	0.980859			
41	5	2.052	51.31	14.37	4.105	2.05242	0.47573		Adjusted R Sqr	0.943094			
42	6	31.64	822.6	474.6	126.6	31.6386	1.11311		Standard Error	1.860843			
43	7	2.099	35.69	12.6	2.099	0	0.40346		Observations	32			
44	8	2.819	59.2	16.91	8.457	0	0.22171						
45	9	2.096	52.39	27.24	12.57	2.09573	0.67177		ANOVA				
46	10	2.178	41.38	23.96	6.534	2.17799	0.73247			df	SS	MS	F	igni.
47	11	2.549	50.98	33.14	10.2	2.54898	0.844		Regression	4	4968.374	1242.094	358.7027	5.
48	12	3.217	57.9	32.17	3.217	3.2166	0.83685		Residual	28	96.95666	3.462738	
49	13	2.673	45.44	16.04	5.346	0	0.29353		Total	32	5065.331		
50	14	2.151	43.02	25.81	8.604	2.15097	0.73803						
51	15	2.075	43.57	14.52	2.075	2.07468	0.54755			Coefficient	andard Err	t Stat	P-value	Low
52	16	31.64	537.9	158.2	94.92	0	0.07762		Intercept	0	#N/A	#N/A	#N/A	
53	17	31.64	664.4	379.7	31.64	31.6386	1.07737		Const	-0.2844	0.147475	-1.92849	0.063989	-C
54	18	2.414	50.7	19.32	9.658	0	0.3237		Age	0.00953	0.011832	0.80545	0.427347	-C
55	19	2.563	56.38	15.38	7.688	0	0.23124		Educ	0.105965	0.012779	8.291955	5.05E-09	0.I
56	20	2.042	42.87	16.33	6.125	0	0.43364		Order	-0.10994	0.019975	-5.50364	7.01E-06	-C
57	21	2.099	44.07	20.99	6.296	2.09866	0.64557						

The WLS analysis can be carried out on these data by using the regression package in Excel. But it must be employed somewhat differently from most regression situations. The WLS procedure requires that each variable, including the dependent variable and the constant term—(the value that will determine the intercept),—be multiplied by the weight before proceeding with the regression analysis. This means that the variable Const (column B) becomes the set of values that will determine the intercept. In order to carry out the regression analysis with the variable Const as the determinant of the intercept, it is necessary to specify that the intercept is 0 in the regression window.

Recall the regression analysis window that is shown again in Figure 14.7. The Input X range now includes columns B through E. Column B, which represents the intercept term, is now part of the analysis, unlike the previous situations in which Excel was simply assumed to provide the constant for the calculation of the intercept term. At the same time, the box Constant is Zero, is now checked. This means that Excel will calculate the regression results without including the column of ones for the intercept. Everything else in the regression window remains the same.

The results of the WLS analysis are shown beginning in column I in Figure 14.6. A major difference between the regression results using OLS (Figure 14.4) and those using WLS are that the place in the regression output where the intercept usually appears (J52) is simply a zero, indicating that, in fact, the intercept is being considered 0 by the analysis. It is the value in cell J53 that now represents the intercept term and has the same sign and is of the same order of magnitude

FIGURE 14.7. REGRESSION SETUP FOR WEIGHTED LEAST SQUARES ANALYSIS.

	A	B	C	D	E	F	G	H	I	J
36	Mother	Const	Age	Educ	Order	Immun	Ipred		SUMMARY OUTPUT	
37	1	2.243	47.11	15.7	6.729	0	0.32768			
38	2	31.64	601.1	379.7	63.28	31.6386	0.94838		Regression Statistics	
39	3	2.255								
40	4	2.275								
41	5	2.052								
42	6	31.64								
43	7	2.099								
44	8	2.819								
45	9	2.096								
46	10	2.178								
47	11	2.549								4
48	12	3.217								9
49	13	2.673								5
50	14	2.151								
51	15	2.075								an
52	16	31.64								
53	17	31.64								0
54	18	2.414								0
55	19	2.563								0
56	20	2.042								0
57	21	2.099								
58	22	31.64								
59	23	2.552								

Regression dialog box:
- Input Y Range: $F$36:$F$68
- Input X Range: $B$36:$E$68
- ☑ Labels ☑ Constant is Zero
- ☐ Confidence Level 95 %
- Output options:
  - ☉ Output Range: $I$36
  - ☐ New Worksheet Ply:
  - ☐ New Workbook
- Residuals:
  - ☐ Residuals ☐ Residual Plots
  - ☐ Standardized Residuals ☐ Line Fit Plots
- Normal Probability:
  - ☐ Normal Probability Plots
- OK, Cancel, Help

as the intercept term in the OLS analysis. Similarly, whereas the other regression coefficients have changed somewhat, these have the same sign and are of the same order of magnitude as the coefficients calculated by using OLS.

The statistical tests (F and t tests) are now unbiased, but they essentially confirm what was determined by using OLS, which is that both a mother's education level and the birth order of her child, but not the mother's age—influence immunization. On the basis of these results, the clinic might appropriately decide that it should focus education efforts to improve full immunization on women with low education and whose child was low in the birth order.

One thing that might seem somewhat anomalous in the regression output is the magnitude of the R square. In fact, the R square is not meaningful in this case, as it generally is when regression is carried out with a continuous dependent variable. In this case, it represents the proportion of variance in the weighted dependent variable that can be accounted for by the weighted independent variables. But the R square of interest is that which represents the proportion of variance in the original 1, 0 dependent variable that is accounted for by the original independent variables, using the WLS coefficients.

There is some argument about whether an R square with a 1, 0 variable is even meaningful, but assuming that it is desirable to have some measure comparable to the R square for the WLS analysis, it is possible to construct a pseudo R square by the formula in Equation 14.2. Equation 14.2 is probably the least conservative (that is, it will create the largest R square value) of several possible ways in which a pseudo R square might be calculated. The initial step in generating this R square value is to calculate predicted values based on the regression weights given by the WLS analysis, but using the original unweighted data. These predicted values are shown, for the first twenty women, in column G of Figure 14.6. The Excel formula used to create the predicted values is given in the formula bar. The cells B2, C2, and D2 contain the original variables as shown in Figure 14.5. (It should be noted that the original data is in rows 2 through 33). Having calculated the predicted values based on the original data and the WLS coefficients, it is then possible to calculate error terms for each variable, as shown in Figure 14.8.

$$\text{pseudo } R^2 = (SS_{\text{T}} - SS_{\text{E}})/SS_{\text{T}} \tag{14.2}$$

where SS_{T} is the familiar $\sum_{i=1}^{n}(y_i - \bar{y})^2$ and SS_{E} is $\sum_{i=1}^{n}(y_i - \sum_{j=1}^{m}\tilde{b}_j x_{ij})^2$ with the values of y_i and x_{ij} being from the original data and $\tilde{b}_j$ being the coefficients from the WLS analysis.

FIGURE 14.8. CALCULATION OF PSEUDO R SQUARE FOR WLS.

	G	H	I	J	K
	H37		= =E2-G37		
36	lpred	Error	SSerror		
37	0.32768	-0.3277	0.10737	SSE	3.482462
38	0.94838	0.05162	0.00267	SST	7.21875
39	0.66463	-0.6646	0.44173	R^2	0.517581
40	0.5817	0.4183	0.17498		
41	0.47573	0.52427	0.27485		
42	1.11311	-0.1131	0.01279		
43	0.40346	-0.4035	0.16278		
44	0.22171	-0.2217	0.04916		
45	0.67177	0.32823	0.10773		
46	0.73247	0.26753	0.07157		
47	0.844	0.156	0.02434		
48	0.83685	0.16315	0.02662		
49	0.29353	-0.2935	0.08616		
50	0.73803	0.26197	0.06863		
51	0.54755	0.45245	0.20471		
52	0.07762	-0.0776	0.00603		
53	1.07737	-0.0774	0.00599		
54	0.3237	-0.3237	0.10478		
55	0.23124	-0.2312	0.05347		
56	0.43364	-0.4336	0.18804		

Figure 14.8 shows the predicted values of Immun based on the WLS coefficients, as given originally in Figure 14.6, for the first twenty women (column G). Column H shows the error as calculated from the predicted values in column G and the original values of Immun. The equation in the formula bar shows that the first error term is based on the value of Immun in E2, as shown in Figure 14.5. Column I is the square of column H, and the sum of the squared errors (SS_E) is given in K37. The total sums of squares (SS_T) is taken from cell I14 in Figure 14.4 but could be calculated as given in Equation 14.2. The pseudo R square, calculated as $(SS_T - SS_E)/SS_T$, is given in cell K39 as .518. In general, the pseudo R square calculated this way (or in any other manner) will always be less than the original R square from the OLS analysis.

Up to this point the WLS results provide a statistically acceptable analysis of the data. The coefficients are unbiased and the statistical tests are appropriate. But the predicted values of y remain problematic for most serious statisticians. It was mentioned earlier that OLS or WLS employed with a dichotomous dependent variable is referred to as a linear probability model because the predicted values of the dependent variable are essentially equivalent to the probability that the dependent variable will be 1 or 0, depending on the values of the independent variable. All probabilities must be in the range 0 to 1; either a negative probability (one less than 0) or a probability greater than 1 is meaningless. But, as can be seen in Figure 14.5 and Figure 14.6, some of the predicted values using either OLS or WLS are greater than 1 or less than 0. The desire on the part of statisticians to remedy this situation in predicting values of dichotomous categorical dependent variables has led to the ascendance of Logit analysis.

Exercises for Section 14.2

1. Use the data on the Immun worksheet of Chpt 14–1.xls.
    a. Convert each of the variables Age, Educ, and Order to 1, 0 variables at their mean and carry out the three chi-square analyses that relate these three variables to FI (full immunization).
    b. Generate the OLS regression analysis of FI, with Age, Educ, and Order as independent variables, and confirm that the results are as shown in Figure 14.4.
    c. Calculate the appropriate weights for weighted least squares (WLS) analysis of the Immun data and carry out the weighted least squares analysis, following the discussion in the third subsection of Section 14.2, including Figure 14.5 and Figure 14.7, to replicate the results given in Figure 14.6.
    d. Calculate a pseudo R square, using the approach given by the formula in Equation 14.2.

2. The data on the ChildF (child-friendly) worksheet of Chpt 14–1.xls was taken from *The State of the World's Children, 2001* (2000). Use these data to relate safe water (SafeW), the log of GNP per capita (LogGNP), and female literacy (FemLit) to child friendliness (ChildF) for the ninety-five countries of the world. (*Child-friendly* are countries with under-five mortality of forty-five per thousand live births or less.)

   a. Convert each of the variables SafeW, LogGNP, and FemLit to 1, 0 variables at their mean and carry out the three chi-square analyses that relate these three variables to U5Mort. What would you conclude from these analyses?

   b. Generate the OLS regression analysis of U5Mort with SafeW, LogGNP, and FemLit as independent variables. What would you conclude from this analysis?

   c. Calculate the appropriate weights for weighted least squares (WLS) analysis of the U5Mort data and carry out the weighted least squares analysis, following the discussion in the third subsection of Section 14.2. What would you conclude from this analysis?

   d. Calculate a pseudo R square, using the approach given by the formula in Equation 14.2.

Section 14.3 Logit for Estimating Dichotomous Dependent Variables

The previous sections of this chapter have considered chi-square and both ordinary least squares and weighted least squares as ways of dealing with dichotomous dependent variables. This section now takes up the discussion of Logit as a means of analyzing dichotomous dependent variables.

Setting up the Logit Model

The coefficients from a linear probability model, whether calculated using OLS or WLS, will produce a linear relationship between the independent and the dependent variables. If there is only one independent variable x, as well as a dichotomous dependent variable y, the predicted values of the dependent variable (the probabilities of the dependent variable being 0 or 1) will lie along a straight line—for example, as shown by the black diagonal line in Figure 14.9. The diagonal line in Figure 14.9 is actually generated by the linear equation $y = .09x + -.04$. The diagonal line could be interpreted as a true probability as long as the value of the independent variable x is between about 5 and 15. If x is less than 5, y is less than 0 and thus cannot be interpreted as a probability. If

FIGURE 14.9. GRAPH OF TWO RELATIONSHIPS BETWEEN INDEPENDENT AND DEPENDENT VARIABLES.

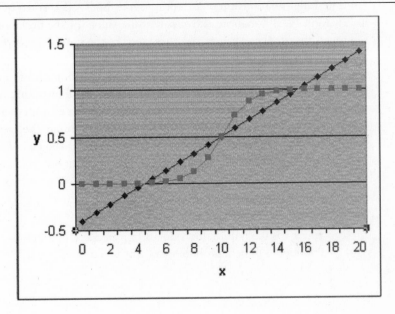

x is greater than 15, y is greater than 1 and similarly cannot be interpreted as a probability. Since, in general, there is nothing to constrain x to a range from 5 to 15, it would be desirable to be able to specify a relationship—clearly a nonlinear one—that would constrain y to the range 0 to 1 for any values of x.

A number of nonlinear relationships allow the x to vary across any range while confining y to the range 0 to 1. Aldrich and Nelson (1984) describe several of these. Of these several alternatives, two have found favor among statisticians— what have come to be called the Logit relationship and the Probit relationship. As the Logit relationship is the simpler of the two, and as they produce almost identical results in the dichotomous dependent variable case, the remainder of this chapter focuses on the Logit relationship.

The Logit relationship can be characterized by the gray curved line in Figure 14.9. It might also be called an S curve because it takes on that shape. For the particular Logit relationship pictured, the value of y when x is 10 is .5, exactly the same as it is for the linear relationship pictured by the black line. But the Logit relationship approaches both 1 and 0 much more rapidly than does the linear relationship, right to the point where the linear relationship crosses the 1, 0 boundary. When x is 14, for example, the value of y in the linear relationship is .86, but for the Logit relationship it is .98. But the Logit relationship never allows the value of y to exceed 1. In fact, it never actually reaches 1 but only approaches it from below. Similarly, the Logit relationship never reaches 0 but only approaches it from above.

The Logit relationship pictured in Figure 14.9 is described by the formula in Equation 14.3. Equation 14.3 says that the values of the probability p_i (which represents the predicted values of y_i) are given by the value 1 divided by the quantity 1 plus e (approximately 2.718), raised to the power of the regression equation as characterized in OLS or WLS. But the coefficients of the regression equation in Logit are not simply the coefficients derived from OLS or WLS and substituted into the Logit equation. It is necessary to find a whole new set of coefficients to describe the Logit relationship. For example, the actual equation that produced the graph shown in Figure 14.9 was as that shown in Equation 14.4. This can be compared with the equation for the straight line given earlier.

$$p_i = \frac{1}{1 + e^{-b_j x_{ij}}} \tag{14.3}$$

where e is the natural log value of approx. 2.718. and p_i is considered to be a probability of any value of y_i.

$$p_i = \frac{1}{1 + e^{-10 + 1x}} \tag{14.4}$$

The graph in Figure 14.9 was actually created in Excel. The formula for the Logit relationship as expressed in Excel was =1/(1+EXP(–(–10+1*x))), where x refers to each value of the independent variable.

If the coefficients for the Logit relationship are not found simply by substituting OLS or WLS coefficients, how then are they found? With OLS and WLS, there is a set of linear equations, derived through calculus, that can be solved to find the regression coefficients directly. With the Logit relationship, there is no such set of equations. The Logit relationship is found by a process known as *maximum likelihood*. Whereas least squares, the process in both OLS and WLS, is an attempt to minimize the sum of squared error terms through the best selection of coefficients, maximum likelihood is an attempt to maximize the fit between the observed data and a specified model of the data through the best selection of coefficients. The fit is based on the *product* of all values in the data set times the probability that the values will or will not occur. But since products are mathematically difficult to deal with, the common solution is to convert the probabilities to logarithms and maximize the fit between the observed data and the log of the specified model. Because of this, the actual value to be maximized in maximum likelihood is referred to as the *log-likelihood*.

How will this work in the case of Logit and in the specific case of the data on immunization of children? The first step is to set up the relationship for the log-likelihood to be maximized. The log-likelihood function to be maximized is as that

FIGURE 14.10. FIRST STEP IN FINDING logL.

	F3	▾		=	=1/(1+EXP(-($A$1+$B$1*B3+$C$1*C3+$D$1*D3)))			
	A	B	C	D	E	F	G	H	I
1	1	0	0	0					
2	Mother	Age	Educ	Order	Immun	p	(1-p)		
3	1	21	7	3	0	0.7311	0.2689		
4	2	19	12	2	1	0.7311	0.2689		
5	3	23	10	3	0	0.7311	0.2689		
6	4	25	8	2	1	0.7311	0.2689		
7	5	25	7	2	1	0.7311	0.2689		
8	6	26	15	4	1	0.7311	0.2689		
9	7	17	6	1	0	0.7311	0.2689		
10	8	21	6	3	0	0.7311	0.2689		
11	9	25	13	6	1	0.7311	0.2689		
12	10	19	11	3	1	0.7311	0.2689		
13	11	20	13	4	1	0.7311	0.2689		
14	12	18	10	1	1	0.7311	0.2689		
15	13	17	6	2	0	0.7311	0.2689		
16	14	20	12	4	1	0.7311	0.2689		
17	15	21	7	1	1	0.7311	0.2689		
18	16	17	5	3	0	0.7311	0.2689		
19	17	21	12	1	1	0.7311	0.2689		
20	18	21	8	4	0	0.7311	0.2689		
21	19	22	6	3	0	0.7311	0.2689		
22	20	21	8	3	0	0.7311	0.2689		
23	21	21	10	3	1	0.7311	0.2689		

given in Equation 14.5. Equation 14.5 is somewhat intimidating, so we will look at the construction of the log-likelihood function to be maximized using Excel.

$$\text{logL} = \sum_{i=1}^{n} [\log p_i y_i + \log(1 - p_i)(1 - y_i)] \tag{14.5}$$

where p_i is as given in Equation 14.3.

Figure 14.10 shows the initial step in constructing the log-likelihood function to be maximized. This step is to set up the Logit relationship that defines the probability in Equation 14.3. In column A of Figure 14.10 is shown the identifier for each mother in the study, up to mother 20. Columns B, C, D, and E show the three independent variables—Age, Educ, and Order—and the dependent variable Immun for the first twenty mothers as well. Column F contains the initial calculation of the probability as given in Equation 14.3, and as expressed in Excel. The actual formula for cell F3 is given in the formula bar. In examining the formula for F3 in the formula bar, it is clear that the probability in cell F3 includes the values in cells A1, B1, C1, and D1. These values, 1, 0, 0, and 0, respectively, are initial values of the true coefficients to be found by maximizing the log-likelihood. The first of these, 1, represents the coefficient of the constant. Each of the 0 values represent the coefficient of the variable in the column in which they are

FIGURE 14.11. COMPLETE LAYOUT FOR MAXIMIZING logL.

	J3		▼		=	=LN(F3)*H3					
	A	B	C	D	E	F	G	H	I	J	K	L
1	1	0	0	0	-21						log(1-p)	
2	Mother	Age	Educ	Order	Immun	p	(1-p)	y	(1-y)	logp*y	*(1-y)	logL
3	1	21	7	3	0	0.7311	0.2689	0	1	0	-1.3133	-1.3133
4	2	19	12	2	1	0.7311	0.2689	1	0	-0.3133	0	-0.3133
5	3	23	10	3	0	0.7311	0.2689	0	1	0	-1.3133	-1.3133
6	4	25	8	2	1	0.7311	0.2689	1	0	-0.3133	0	-0.3133
7	5	25	7	2	1	0.7311	0.2689	1	0	-0.3133	0	-0.3133
8	6	26	15	4	1	0.7311	0.2689	1	0	-0.3133	0	-0.3133
9	7	17	6	1	0	0.7311	0.2689	0	1	0	-1.3133	-1.3133
10	8	21	6	3	0	0.7311	0.2689	0	1	0	-1.3133	-1.3133
11	9	25	13	6	1	0.7311	0.2689	1	0	-0.3133	0	-0.3133
12	10	19	11	3	1	0.7311	0.2689	1	0	-0.3133	0	-0.3133
13	11	20	13	4	1	0.7311	0.2689	1	0	-0.3133	0	-0.3133
14	12	18	10	1	1	0.7311	0.2689	1	0	-0.3133	0	-0.3133
15	13	17	6	2	0	0.7311	0.2689	0	1	0	-1.3133	-1.3133
16	14	20	12	4	1	0.7311	0.2689	1	0	-0.3133	0	-0.3133
17	15	21	7	1	1	0.7311	0.2689	1	0	-0.3133	0	-0.3133
18	16	17	5	3	0	0.7311	0.2689	0	1	0	-1.3133	-1.3133
19	17	21	12	1	1	0.7311	0.2689	1	0	-0.3133	0	-0.3133
20	18	21	8	4	0	0.7311	0.2689	0	1	0	-1.3133	-1.3133
21	19	22	6	3	0	0.7311	0.2689	0	1	0	-1.3133	-1.3133
22	20	21	8	3	0	0.7311	0.2689	0	1	0	-1.3133	-1.3133
23	21	21	10	3	1	0.7311	0.2689	1	0	0.3133	0	0.3133

located. When the maximization process is finished, these values will have changed to those that maximize logL, as is given in Equation 14.5. It can also be seen that column G contains the value $(1 - p)$, which also enters into the calculation of logL. The Excel formula for cell G3, for example, is simply =1–F3.

The complete layout for maximizing logL is given in Figure 14.11. Columns A through G remain the same as in Figure 14.10. Column H simply repeats the data in column E but is now designated y to conform to Equation 14.5. Column I is 1 minus column H. Columns J and K represent the calculation of log $p_i y_i$ and log$(1 - p_i)(1 - y_i)$, respectively. The Excel formula for cell J3 is given in the formula bar. =LN() is the Excel function for the natural logarithm. Column L is the sum of columns J and K. It should be clear that when y is 1, column L will be log $p_i y_i$. When y is 0, column L will be log$(1 - p_i)(1 - y_i)$. There is also a new number, -21, in cell E1. This is the sum of the numbers in column L. It is the log-likelihood, the number to be maximized. There is no accident that the number in E1 is -21. When the coefficient of the constant (cell A1) is 1 and all other coefficients are 0, the log-likelihood for the Logit will always be the negative of the number of ones in the dependent variable.

We have now laid out the spreadsheet for the maximization of the log-likelihood function. Now how do we find the maximum value of the cell E1?

Unfortunately, there is no single set of equations (as with least squares) that can be solved for the answer. Basically, the maximization of the log-likelihood function is a trial and error process. But there are better and worse methods of going about the process of trial and error to find the set of coefficients that maximize the log-likelihood function. Madalla (1997) provides a detailed description of the best process for finding the maximum of the log-likelihood function for the Logit model. However, that discussion is complex enough that for our purposes here, it is bypassed, and we will rely on an add-in capability of Excel to maximize the log-likelihood function.

The Solver Add-In

Excel includes an add-in called *Solver*. It is accessed in the same way as the data analysis add-in, under Tools/Solver on the Menu bar. Solver is a general maximization routine that works on a wide variety of applications. In this chapter it is discussed only as it applies to the maximization of the log-likelihood function in Logit.

The Solver window is shown in Figure 14.12. The value to be maximized, in this case, cell E1, is shown in the box next to 'Set Target Cell:'. Solver provides

FIGURE 14.12. SOLVER WINDOW FOR MAXIMIZING logL.

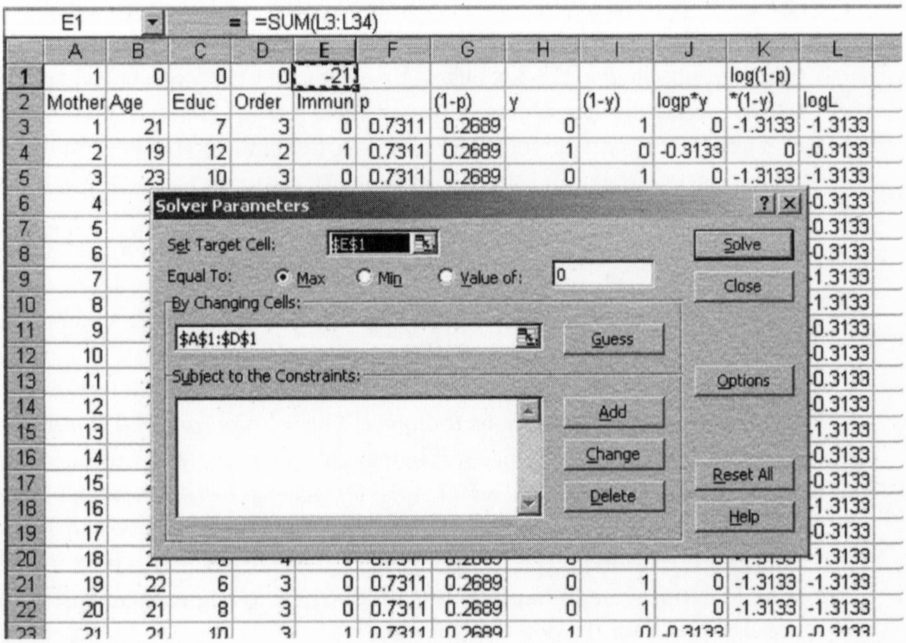

FIGURE 14.13. SOLVER SOLUTION FOR LOGIT MODEL.

	E1	▼		=	=SUM(L3:L34)							
	A	B	C	D	E	F	G	H	I	J	K	L
1	-17.7	0.52	1.655	-2.61	-6.24						log(1-p)	
2	Mother	Age	Educ	Order	Immun	p	(1-p)	y	(1-y)	logp*y	*(1-y)	logL
3	1	21	7	3	0	0.0472	0.9528	0	1	0	-0.0484	-0.0484
4	2	19	12	2	1	0.9989	0.0011	1	0	-0.0011	0	-0.0011
5	3	23	10	3	0	0.9526	0.0474	0	1	0	-3.0494	-3.0494
6	4	25	8	2	1	0.9656	0.0344	1	0	-0.035	0	-0.035
7	5	25	7	2	1	0.843	0.157	1	0	-0.1708	0	-0.1708
8	6	26									0	-4E-05
9	7	17									5	-0.1965
10	8	21									4	-0.0094
11	9	25									0	-0.2661
12	10	19									0	-0.0733
13	11	20									0	-0.0221
14	12	18									0	-0.0036
15	13	17									9	-0.0159
16	14	20									0	-0.1106
17	15	21									0	-0.1043
18	16	17	5	3	0	0.0002	0.9998	0	1	0	-0.0002	-0.0002
19	17	21	12	1	1	1	3E-05	1	0	-3E-05	0	-3E-05
20	18	21	8	4	0	0.0188	0.9812	0	1	0	-0.019	-0.019
21	19	22	6	3	0	0.0157	0.9843	0	1	0	-0.0158	-0.0158
22	20	21	8	3	0	0.2059	0.7941	0	1	0	-0.2306	-0.2306
23	21	21	10	3	1	0.8767	0.1233	1	0	-0.1316	0	-0.1316

Solver Results dialog: "Solver has converged to the current solution. All constraints are satisfied." Options: ● Keep Solver Solution ○ Restore Original Values. Reports: Answer, Sensitivity, Limits. Buttons: OK, Cancel, Save Scenario..., Help.

several options for what to do with the value in E1. It can be maximized, minimized, or set equal to some specified value as determined by the 'Equal To:' row. The cells that are to be changed to seek the solution desired (in this case, a maximum) are specified in the box below 'By Changing Cells:'. Solver will guess which cells to modify if you wish, and it usually gets it right. Finally, a number of constraints can be set on the solution Solver reaches in the box below 'Subject to the Constraints:'. In general, no constraints are required to reach a solution for the Logit model. Solver is invoked by clicking Solve.

The solution to the Logit model arrived at by Solver is given in Figure 14.13. The value of logL produced by Solver is −6.24 (cell E1). The coefficients of the model that produce this value are given in cells A1:D1. Cell A1 represents the intercept or constant value, and B1:D1 represent the coefficients of the three independent variables. Clicking on OK will keep the solution reached by Solver.

There are clear limitations to Solver. The solution reached can depend on the initial values of the coefficients. In general, beginning with the value 1 for the constant and 0 for the independent variables will lead to a solution that represents the best fit between the model and the data. But beginning with other initial values can result in logL blowing up, so that the result would be a #NUM! in cell E1. If this were to happen, it would be best to begin again with 1 for the intercept and 0 for the other coefficients.

Overall Significance Test with Logit

Having found the coefficients developed by solver, what is the next step? In least squares regression, one next step would be an overall *F* test to determine if any of the coefficients of the independent variables are different from 0. With Logit, there is no *F* test as such, but there is a chi-square test that accomplishes essentially the same thing. The formula for the appropriate chi-square is shown in Equation 14.6. The value of $\log L_1$ is given in cell E1 in Figure 14.13. The value of $\log L_0$ can be found by recalculating the Solver solution but restricting the cells to be changed (By Changing Cells box) to A1 (the intercept term) only. However, the value of $\log L_0$ can also be found, as is given in Equation 14.7.

$$X^2 = -2(\log L_0 - \log L_1) \tag{14.6}$$

where $\log L_0$ is the value of logL when all coefficients except the intercept are 0 and $\log L_1$ is the value of logL for the best model.

$$\log L_0 = n_0(\log(n_0/n)) + n_1(\log(n_1/n)) \tag{14.7}$$

where n is the total sample size, n_0 is the number of observations where y equals 0, and n_1 is the number of observations where y equals 1.

Figure 14.14 shows the calculation of the chi-square value for the Logit solution shown in Figure 14.13. The value of n, given in B1, is 32. The values of n_0 and n_1, in cells B2 and B3, respectively, are 11 and 21. The value -1.06784 in cell C2 was calculated with the Excel function =LN(B2/B1). Similarly, the value -0.4212 in cell C3 was calculated with the Excel function =LN(B3/B1). L_1 in cell B5 was taken from cell E1 in Figure 14.13. Cell B6 was calculated by the Excel statement =B2*C2+B3*C3. The formula for the chi-square value in cell B8 is given in the formula bar. The degrees of freedom for this chi-square are equal

FIGURE 14.14. CALCULATION OF CHI-SQUARE FOR LOGIT.

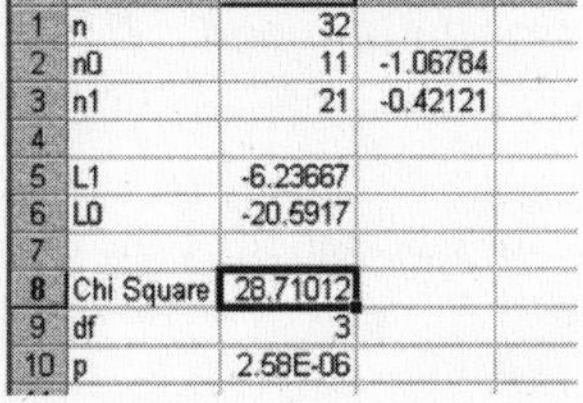

B8 = =-2*(B6-B5)

	A	B	C	D
1	n	32		
2	n0	11	-1.06784	
3	n1	21	-0.42121	
4				
5	L1	-6.23667		
6	L0	-20.5917		
7				
8	Chi Square	28.71012		
9	df	3		
10	p	2.58E-06		

to the number of regressors, not counting the intercept, or, in this case, three. The probability of the chi-square value was found with the Excel function, =CHIDIST(B8,B9). The conclusion of this chi-square test, as with the OLS and WLS F tests, is that at least one of the regression coefficients other than the intercept coefficient is statistically different from 0.

Significance of Individual Coefficients

Of course, this now leads to the question of how to determine which of the coefficients can be considered different from 0. The test of this is the same as that with OLS or WLS; that is, it is the coefficient divided by its standard error. Unfortunately, though Solver can give us the coefficients, it cannot directly give us the standard errors of those coefficients. To find the standard errors, we must use the coefficients to produce something called the *information matrix*. The information matrix can most easily be produced using the matrix multiplication capabilities of Excel. To demonstrate the calculation of the information matrix, we must begin with the predicted values of the dependent variable Immun.

Maddala (1997) calls the information matrix, based on the best-fit coefficients for the Logit model, $I(\hat{\beta})$. The standard errors of the coefficients will be the square root of the main diagonal elements in $[I(\hat{\beta})]^{-1}$, the inverse of the information matrix. To find the information matrix and, hence, its inverse, we need first to find q_i for each value of the dependent variable. The value q_i can be found as shown in Equation 14.8. The calculation of q_i for the data on immunization is shown in Figure 14.15.

$$q_i = \frac{e_i^{bx_j}}{[1 + e_i^{bx_j}]^2} \tag{14.8}$$

where x_j includes all regressors and the intercept term.

Figure 14.15 shows again the data for the first twenty mothers and the coefficients (in row 1) that were generated by Solver in Figure 14.13. A new column has been added as column B, into which has been inserted a column of ones to represent the intercept or constant term. We will use this later in the calculations. All other variables have been shifted one column to the right. Column G is the calculation for the numerator of q_i and column H is the calculation of the denominator. The formula bar shows the way that cell G3 was calculated. The value q_i is shown in column I.

The next step in the calculation of the information matrix is to calculate $q_i \times x_{ij}$ for each x_j, including the intercept term. In the Immunization example, there are three independent variables—Age, Educ, and Order, in addition to the intercept. The construction of the $q_i \times x_{ij}$ for the intercept and the three independent

FIGURE 14.15. FIRST STEP IN THE CALCULATION OF THE INFORMATION MATRIX.

G3		=	=EXP($B$1+$C$1*C3+$D$1*D3+$E$1*E3)					
	A	B	C	D	E	F	G	H	I
1		-17.691	0.520	1.655	-2.606	-6.237			
2	Mother	Const	Age	Educ	Order	Immun	exp(bxj)	(1+exp(bxj))^2	qi
3	1	1	21	7	3	0	0.050	1.102	0.045
4	2	1	19	12	2	1	932.977	872313.770	0.001
5	3	1	23	10	3	0	20.103	445.317	0.045
6	4	1	25	8	2	1	28.111	847.444	0.033
7	5	1	25	7	2	1	5.370	40.574	0.132
8	6	1	26	15	4	1	27749.932	770114252.750	0.000
9	7	1	17	6	1	0	0.217	1.481	0.147
10	8	1	21	6	3	0	0.009	1.019	0.009
11	9	1	25	13	6	1	3.280	18.317	0.179
12	10	1	19	11	3	0	13.154	200.334	0.066
13	11	1	20	13	4	1	44.747	2092.796	0.021
14	12	1	18	10	1	1	274.260	75767.916	0.004
15	13	1	17	6	2	0	0.016	1.032	0.016
16	14	1	20	12	4	1	8.548	91.159	0.094
17	15	1	21	7	1	1	9.094	101.886	0.089
18	16	1	17	5	3	0	0.000	1.000	0.000
19	17	1	21	12	1	1	35754.134	1278429621.959	0.000
20	18	1	21	8	4	0	0.019	1.039	0.018
21	19	1	22	6	3	0	0.016	1.032	0.015
22	20	1	21	8	3	0	0.259	1.586	0.164
23	21	1	21	10	3	1	7.107	65.726	0.108

variables is shown in Figure 14.16. The first five columns in Figure 14.16 are, again, the data for the first twenty mothers. The two columns—G and H—that appear in Figure 14.15 have been hidden in Figure 14.16, simply to provide additional room to display the rest of the columns. Column I is q_i, as calculated in Figure 14.15. Column J, K, L, and M represent the values of $q_i \times x_{ij}$, column J being the intercept, which simply repeats the value of q_i.

The next step in the formation of the information matrix is to prepare to use =MMULT to multiply the matrix represented by the original data by the transpose of the values in columns J, K, L, and M. To generate the transpose, the best approach is to use the Excel function =TRANSPOSE() and put the result somewhere on the spreadsheet where it will not interfere with other data.

Figure 14.17 shows the first eight columns of the transpose matrix that will be used as the premultiplier for the information matrix. The formula bar shows the =TRANSPOSE() function that was used to create the transpose matrix. The labels were copied from the first row of columns K, J, L, and M to V2:V5. If you remember the use of Excel functions that put values into more than one cell (=FREQUENCY(), for example), you remember that the entire area in which the result is to appear must be highlighted before pressing Ctrl/Shift and Enter. The easiest way to know exactly what to highlight as the set of target cells

FIGURE 14.16. CALCULATION OF $q_i \times x_{ij}$.

	K3		=	=$I3*C3						
	A	B	C	D	E	F	I	J	K	L	M
1		-17.691	0.520	1.655	-2.606	-6.237					
2	Mother	Const	Age	Educ	Order	Immun	qi	qi*Const	qi*Age	qi*Educ	qi*Immun
3	1	1	21	7	3	0	0.045	0.045	0.9444	0.3148	0.1349
4	2	1	19	12	2	1	0.001	0.001	0.0203	0.0128	0.0021
5	3	1	23	10	3	0	0.045	0.045	1.0383	0.4514	0.1354
6	4	1	25	8	2	1	0.033	0.033	0.8293	0.2654	0.0663
7	5	1	25	7	2	1	0.132	0.132	3.3086	0.9264	0.2647
8	6	1	26	15	4	1	0.000	0.000	0.0009	0.0005	0.0001
9	7	1	17	6	1	0	0.147	0.147	2.4917	0.8794	0.1466
10	8	1	21	6	3	0	0.009	0.009	0.1950	0.0557	0.0279
11	9	1	25	13	6	1	0.179	0.179	4.4765	2.3278	1.0744
12	10	1	19	11	3	1	0.066	0.066	1.2475	0.7223	0.1970
13	11	1	20	13	4	1	0.021	0.021	0.4276	0.2780	0.0855
14	12	1	18	10	1	1	0.004	0.004	0.0652	0.0362	0.0036
15	13	1	17	6	2	0	0.016	0.016	0.2639	0.0931	0.0310
16	14	1	20	12	4	1	0.094	0.094	1.8753	1.1252	0.3751
17	15	1	21	7	1	1	0.089	0.089	1.8744	0.6248	0.0893
18	16	1	17	5	3	0	0.000	0.000	0.0038	0.0011	0.0007
19	17	1	21	12	1	1	0.000	0.000	0.0006	0.0003	0.0000
20	18	1	21	8	4	0	0.018	0.018	0.3870	0.1474	0.0737
21	19	1	22	6	3	0	0.015	0.015	0.3392	0.0925	0.0463
22	20	1	21	8	3	0	0.164	0.164	3.4340	1.3082	0.4906
23	21	1	21	10	3	1	0.108	0.108	2.2708	1.0813	0.3244

FIGURE 14.17. FORMATION OF THE TRANSPOSE MATRIX.

	W2		=	{=TRANSPOSE(J3:M34)}					
	V	W	X	Y	Z	AA	AB	AC	AD
1									
2	qi*Const	0.045	0.001	0.045	0.033	0.132	0.000	0.147	0.009
3	qi*Age	0.9444	0.0203	1.0383	0.8293	3.3086	0.0009	2.4917	0.1950
4	qi*Educ	0.3148	0.0128	0.4514	0.2654	0.9264	0.0005	0.8794	0.0557
5	qi*Immun	0.1349	0.0021	0.1354	0.0663	0.2647	0.0001	0.1466	0.0279

for the =TRANSPOSE() function is to use Edit/Copy to copy the entire original matrix (in this case, cells J3:M34) and then, in the place where you wish to put the transpose matrix, use Edit/Paste Special/Transpose. This will put values into the cells in which you wish the results of =TRANSPOSE() to go, so that you can then highlight that entire area and invoke the =TRANSPOSE() function.

The information matrix $I(\hat{\beta})$ can now be found by premultiplying the original data matrix (cells B3:E34) by the transpose matrix. Since the transpose is 4×32 and the original data matrix is 32×4, the resulting information matrix will be 4×4. The information matrix, as calculated using the Excel function =MMULT(), is shown, beginning in cell O3 of Figure 14.18. Now the reason for adding the column of ones representing the intercept should be clear. It is necessary to include this column in the calculation of the information matrix.

FIGURE 14.18. INFORMATION MATRIX AND *t* TESTS.

	O3	▼	= {=MMULT(W2:BB5,B3:E34)}		
	N	O	P	Q	R
1					
2		I(betahat)			
3		1.777573	38.25721	15.33456	5.073644
4		38.25721	834.406	333.1399	111.8517
5		15.33456	333.1399	141.1063	48.26349
6		5.073644	111.8517	48.26349	17.61185
7					
8		I(betahat)-1			
9		60.67729	-2.38825	-2.62688	4.886309
10		-2.38825	0.116771	0.034863	-0.14913
11		-2.62688	0.034863	0.433041	-0.65136
12		4.886309	-0.14913	-0.65136	1.381241
13					
14	bj	-17.691	0.520	1.655	-2.606
15	SEbj	7.790	0.342	0.658	1.175
16	t	-2.271	1.521	2.516	-2.218
17	p	0.031	0.139	0.018	0.035

Figure 14.18 also shows the inverse of the information matrix that is calculated using the =MINVERSE() function, which begins in cell O9. The standard errors of the Logit coefficients are found by taking the square root of the values on the main diagonal of the inverse of the information matrix. The Logit coefficients themselves are shown in cells O14:R14. The standard errors for each coefficient are shown below them in O15:R15. The value in O15 (the standard error of the intercept) is the square root of the main diagonal element in the inverse of the information matrix at cell O9. The standard error of the coefficient on Age (cell P15) is the square root of the main diagonal element at cell P10. The standard error of the coefficient on Educ (cell Q15) is the square root of the value in cell Q11. Finally, the standard error of the coefficient for Order (cell R15) is the square root of the value in cell R12.

The *t* tests are shown in O16:R16, and their probabilities are shown in O17:R17. The conclusion reached with Logit is exactly the same as that reached with WLS. Both a mother's education level and the birth order of her child influence whether the child is fully immunized or not, while Age does not. So, based on this analysis, if the clinic wishes to increase the proportion of children fully immunized, the staff should concentrate on children whose birth order is low and whose mother's level of education is low.

As a final topic in the solution of the Logit problem, it seems reasonable to consider a pseudo *R* square that can be calculated for the Logit. Aldrich and Nelson (1984) suggest as a pseudo *R* square the value shown in Equation 14.9. Using the formula in Equation 14.9 and the chi-square value from Figure 14.14, the pseudo R square for the Logit analysis is .4729. This contrasts with .5774 for the OLS analysis and .5176 for the WLS analysis.

$$\text{pseudo } R^2 = X^2/(n + X^2) \qquad (14.9)$$

where X^2 is taken from Equation 14.6.

Exercises for Section 14.3

1. Use the data on the Immun worksheet of Chpt 14–1.xls.
   a. Set up the spreadsheet for maximizing LogL for these data, following the example in Figure 14.10 and Figure 14.11.
   b. Use the Solver add-in to find the values of the coefficients of Age, Educ, and Order to replicate Figure 14.13.
   c. Calculate the overall chi-square value for this analysis, using Equation 14.6 and Equation 14.7 to replicate Figure 14.14.
   d. Set up the worksheet for calculating the information matrix $I(\hat{\beta})$ as given in Figure 14.15, Figure 14.16, and Figure 14.17 and complete the t tests of the individual coefficients, as shown in Figure 14.18.
   e. Confirm that all your results are the same as those given in the figures.

2. Use the data on the ChildF (child friendly) worksheet of Chpt 14–1.xls.
   a. Set up the spreadsheet for maximizing LogL for these data, following the example in Figure 14.10 and Figure 14.11.
   b. Use the Solver add-in to find the values of the coefficients of SafeW LogGNP and FemLit to replicate Figure 14.13.
   c. Calculate the overall chi-square value for this analysis, using Equation 14.6 and Equation 14.7 to replicate Figure 14.14.
   d. Set up the worksheet for calculating the information matrix $I(\hat{\beta})$, as given in Figure 14.15, Figure 14.16, and Figure 14.17, and complete the t tests of the individual coefficients, as shown in Figure 14.18.
   e. Decide if your conclude that the same thing reaches different conclusions, based on this analysis, as compared with ordinary or weighted least squares.

Section 14.4 A Comparison of OLS, WLS, and Logit

Perhaps the last thing to do in this chapter should be to compare the OLS, WLS, and Logit results, in terms of the prediction of whether a child will be fully immunized or not. How well do these three analyses actually predict which children will be immunized, and how do they compare with one another? Since the predicted value of the dependent variable Immun is a probability that the true value

FIGURE 14.19. COMPARISON OF OLS, WLS, AND LOGIT-PREDICTED VALUES.

C2		=	=IF('14-4,5,6'!F2>0.5,1,0)						
	A	B	C	D	E	F	G	H	I	J
1	Mother	Immun	Pols	Pwls	Plog		Count of Pols	Immun ▼		
2	1	0	0	0	0		Pols ▼	0	1	Grand Total
3	2	1	1	1	1		0	10	1	11
4	3	0	1	1	1		1	1	20	21
5	4	1	1	1	1		Grand Total	11	21	32
6	5	1	1	0	1					
7	6	1	1	1	1		Count of Pwls	Immun ▼		
8	7	0	0	0	0		Pwls ▼	0	1	Grand Total
9	8	0	0	0	0		0	10	3	13
10	9	1	1	1	1		1	1	18	19
11	10	1	1	1	1		Grand Total	11	21	32
12	11	1	1	1	1					
13	12	1	1	1	1		Count of Plog	Immun ▼		
14	13	0	0	0	0		Plog ▼	0	1	Grand Total
15	14	1	1	1	1		0	10	1	11
16	15	1	1	1	1		1	1	20	21
17	16	0	0	0	0		Grand Total	11	21	32
18	17	1	1	1	1					
19	18	0	0	0	0					
20	19	0	0	0	0					
21	20	0	0	0	0					
22	21	1	1	1	1					

of Immun will be either 1 or 0, it seems reasonable to assign a 1 to those observations in which the predicted value of Immun is greater than .5 and a 0 to those observations where the predicted value is less than .5. (Since none of the predicted values is exactly .5, we do not have to worry about what we would do in that case.)

Figure 14.19 shows a comparison of the three estimates of the dependent variable Immun. The first column in Figure 14.19 represents the mothers in the sample, again, through mother number twenty. Column B is the actual value of Immun. Column C is a 1 or 0 value of Immun as predicted by OLS. The =IF() statement (as shown in the formula bar) was used to create this as well as columns D and E. Column D is a 1 or 0 value of Immun as predicted by WLS and column D is a 1 or 0 value as predicted by Logit. Simply looking at the three columns C, D, and E reveals that they are very similar.

Beginning in column G are three pivot tables created from the data in columns B to E. The first pivot table compares the actual values of Immun with the predictions based on OLS. The second compares the actual values with the predictions based on WLS. The third compares actual values with Logit. For both OLS and Logit, there are two errors. One true 0 is predicted to be a 1 and one true 1 is predicted to be a 0 by both methods. For WLS there are four errors. One true 0 is predicted to be a 1 and three true ones are predicted to be 0. Though Figure 14.9 does not show this, the match between OLS and Logit predictions is perfect, whereas WLS predicts two observations to be 0, which are predicted to be 1 by OLS and Logit.

Although this is only one example in a number of comparisons between OLS, WLS, and Logit, results on the same data OLS and Logit seem to perform about equally in predicting the actual values of a dichotomous dependent variable, and WLS performs slightly less well. In consequence, if the desire is only to predict which observations will be 1 and which will be 0, it seems that OLS, which is relatively simple, compared with Logit, might be satisfactory. However, in this case, OLS did not reveal that birth order was a statistically significant predictor of Immun, whereas both WLS and Logit did. But, in general, if the dependent variable is dichotomous, you cannot go far wrong assuming the Logit relationship and using the techniques described in the Logit section of this chapter.

Exercises for Section 14.4

1. Use the previous analyses of the data on the Immun worksheet of Chpt 14–1.xls.
   a. Convert the predicted values of Immun to a 1, 0 variable at .05 for each of the prediction methods—OLS, WLS, and Logit.
   b. Generate the comparison table as shown in Figure 14.19.

2. Use the previous analyses of the data on the ChildF worksheet of Chpt 14–1.xls.
   a. Convert the predicted values of ChildF to a 1, 0 variable at .05 for each of the prediction methods—OLS, WLS, and Logit.
   b. Generate the comparison table, following Figure 14.19.
   c. What conclusions do you draw from these comparisons?

References

Aldrich, J., and Nelson, F. "Linear Probability, Logit, and Probit Models," Sage University Paper 45, Sage, Newbury Park, N.J., 1984.

Goldberger, A. S. *Econometric Theory.* New York: Wiley, 1964.

Madalla G. S. *Limited-Dependent and Qualitative Variables in Econometrics.* New York: Cambridge University Press, 1983.

The State of the World's Children 2001, UNICEF, New York, Dec. 2000.
   [http://www.unicef.org/sowc01/tables/#].

GLOSSARY

#DIV/0! An Excel error message caused by trying to divide by 0.

#NAME? An Excel error message generally denoting the misspelling of an Excel function name.

#NUM! An Excel error message generally caused by trying to perform an undefined mathematical procedure, such as taking the square root of a negative number, or by requesting a result that exceeds Excel's limits, such as =FACT(171).

#VALUE! An Excel error message generally caused by including a nonnumerical value in a mathematical operation.

=AND() Excel function that returns the result of two comparisons, TRUE if both comparisons are true and FALSE if either comparison is false.

=AVERAGE() Excel function that returns the mean of a series of data.

=BINOMDIST() Excel function that returns the probability for the appearance of any value from a binomial distribution, given the number of trials and the outcome probability for a single trial.

=CHIDIST() Excel function that returns the probability of a chi-square value, given degrees of freedom.

=CHIINV() Excel function that returns the chi-square value, given the probability of the chi-square value and degrees of freedom.

=CHITEST() Excel function that returns the probability of a chi-square value, given the observed and expected values.

=COUNT() Excel function that returns the number of values in a series of numerical data.

=COUNTIF() Excel function that returns the number of times a given value appears in a series of data.

=EXP() Excel function that returns the value of e (approximately 2.718282) raised to the power of the number in the parentheses.

=FACT() Excel function that returns the factorial of the number in parentheses. Limited to numbers less than 171.

=FDIST() Excel function that returns the probability of an F value, given degrees of freedom.

=FINV() Excel function that returns the F value, given the probability of the F value and degrees of freedom.

=FREQUENCY() Excel function that returns a frequency distribution for a series of data in terms of series of categories.

=IF() Excel function that returns the result of an if-then decision.

=MAX() Excel function that returns the maximum value in a series of data.

=MDETERM() Excel function that returns the determinant for a square matrix.

=MEDIAN() Excel function that returns the median value for a series of data.

=MIN() Excel function that returns the minimum value in a series of data.

=MINVERSE() Excel function that returns the inverse of a matrix (array).

=MMULT() Excel function that returns the product of two matrices (arrays).

=MODE() Excel function that returns the modal value for a series of data. If the data have more than one mode, will return the value of the numerically smallest mode.

=NORMDIST() Excel function that returns probability for any value from a normal distribution, given the mean and standard deviation of the distribution.

=OR() Excel function that returns TRUE if either or both of two comparisons is true, and FALSE if both comparisons are false.

=POISSON() Excel function that returns the probability of a appearance of any value from a Poisson distribution, given the mean of the distribution.

=RAND() Excel function that returns a uniform random number between 0 and 1.

=RANDBETWEEN() Excel function that returns a uniform random number between two selected numbers.

=ROUND() Excel function that returns the selected number rounded to the number of decimal places specified.

=SQRT() Excel function that returns the square root of a number.

=STDEV() Excel function that returns the standard deviation of a series of data assumed to represent a sample.

=STDEVP() Excel function that returns the standard deviation of a series of data assumed to represent a population.

=SUM() Excel function that returns the sum of a series of data.

=SUMPRODUCT() Excel function that returns the sum of the product of the values of two series of data.

=SUMSQ() Excel function that returns the sum of the squares of a series of data.

=TDIST() Excel function that returns the probability of a t value, given degrees of freedom and a one- or two-tailed test.

=TINV() Excel function that returns the t value, given the probability of the t value and degrees of freedom.

=TRANSPOSE() Excel function that returns the transpose of a matrix (array).

=TRUNC() Excel function that returns the integer portion of a number.

=TTEST() Excel function that returns the probability of a t value, given a data set with a numerical dependent variable and a two-level categorical independent variable.

=VAR() Excel function that returns the variance of a series of data assumed to represent a sample.

=VARP() Excel function that returns the variance of a series of data assumed to represent a population.

=YEARFRAC Excel function that returns the number of years between two calendar dates.

Alpha The level of Type I error, usually set by the researcher at .05 or .01. (See Type I error.)

Analysis of variance (ANOVA) A test used to determine whether a numerical variable is independent of one or more categorical variables that may take on more than two values.

Analysis tool pak Package of statistical procedures that can be added in to Excel to perform such things as t tests, ANOVA, random sampling, and regression.

A priori probability Likelihood of the occurrence of and event that can be determined from the nature of the process that generates the event.

Array A set of data in contiguous rows and columns. An Excel designation of a matrix. In Excel, it often refers to a set of cells that are linked so that no one can be changed independently of the others.

Bartlett test A test for homogeneity of within-group variance between more than two groups.

Bell-shaped curve The shape of a normal distribution.

Bernoulli distribution A probability distribution that contains only values of 1 or 0, the number of which depend on the probability of 1.

Best-fitting line A line determined by an independent variable that passes closest to the values of a dependent variable in a two-dimensional graph. Usually defined as the line that minimizes the sum of squared differences between the line and the values of the dependent variable for all values of the independent variable.

Beta The level of Type II error, usually not known unless a specific value is stated for an alternative hypothesis. (See Type II error.)

Between-group variance Variance that exists among the means of some value for two or more groups.

Binomial distribution A probability distribution that represents the accumulation of a Bernoulli distribution for any number of trials and any value of the probability of 1.

Bins Excel designation for the categories into which the =FREQUENCY() function accumulates a data series.

Categorical variable A variable whose values are logically classified by names (that is, male, female), as opposed to numbers. May be coded as numbers, however.

Causal variable A variable whose values are assumed to influence the values of other variables in a given analysis but assumed not to be affected by these others.

Causality The concept that the value of one variable may be a cause of the value of another variable.

Central tendency A way of referring to the central or midpoint around which a data series clusters. Measured by the mean, median, or mode.

Chart Wizard Set of windows invoked by the chart icon on the Formatting menu bar that provides step-by-step direction in creating Excel graphs.

Chi-square statistic A statistical test that assesses whether a categorical variable is independent of one or more other categorical variables.

Cluster sample A sample drawn by first dividing the total population into several mutually exclusive and all-inclusive groups and then selecting some of the groups from which to take all members of the group or a sample of the group.

Conditional probability The probability of some outcome, given knowledge of some other event. For example, the likelihood that a person will arrive at an emergency room with a true emergency, given that the person arrives during the night.

Confidence interval Interval on the number scale within which a population value is expected to lie with some predetermined probability, such as 95 percent.

Constant A number or characteristic that is assigned to members of a sample and that is identical for every member of the sample.

Contingency table Simultaneous distribution of two usually categorical variables. (See cross-tabulation.)

Continuous numerical variable A numerical variable that can, theoretically, be infinitely divided, such as blood pressure.

Control group Those persons in an experiment who do not receive the actual experimental intervention. They generally receive some placebo intervention that mimics the actual experimental intervention but is expected to have no effect.

Correlation A value derived from a statistic that describes the relationship between two variables. May range from –1 for a perfect negative relationship to 1 for a perfect positive relationship. Zero indicates no relationship.

Critical value The value of a test statistic (chi-square, t value, F), above which the hypothesis of interest is rejected.

Cross-tabulation (or Cross-tab) Simultaneous distribution of two usually categorical variables. (See the contingency table.)

Cumulative frequency Frequency distribution that shows the accumulation of values from the lowest category to the highest.

Data range A set of generally contiguous cells that represent data to be included in some Excel operation.

Degrees of freedom A value that designates the number of options that can be exercised before no others are available.

Delimited Refers to one of two ways that data may be stored in a .txt file. Each data element is followed by a common character that designates or delimits the end of that data element. (See fixed-length.)

Dependent variable A variable whose values are assumed to be affected or modified by the value of other variables in a given analysis.

Determinant A single number that can be used to describe a square matrix. For a two-by-two matrix, equal to the product of the main diagonal elements minus the product of the off-diagonal elements.

Diagnostic-related group (DRG) A categorization of medical conditions used for determining payment by Medicare and Medicaid.

Discrete distribution An Excel option that allows the user to define the probability of the selection of any value from a predetermined set of values.

Discrete numerical variable A numerical variable that cannot be divided into units smaller than integers, such as the number of persons in a waiting room.

Dispersion A way of referring to the variability in a set of data. Measured by the variance or standard deviation.

Double-blind random clinical trial An experimental design in which neither the subjects under study, the persons administering the intervention of the study, nor the persons assessing the results of the study know which group or groups received which intervention.

Dummy variable A categorical variable that takes on two values and is coded 1 and 0. For example, the two colors blue and red could be coded 1 for blue and 0 for red. They would then represent a dummy variable.

Dust Bowl empiricism Term applied to the use of statistics to sift through data to find the best relationships, independent of theory.

Empirical probability The likelihood of the occurrence of an event that can be determined only on the basis of historical data about similar events that have occurred in the past.

Event The occurrence in a stochastic process to which a probability can be assigned.

Excel function A built-in Excel option that will produce the result of a formula or algorithm. Accessible on the Formatting menu bar.

Exponential model A regression model that is based on converting the dependent variable to its logarithmic value, either natural or base 10.

Factorial design Analysis that includes more than one independent variable. Usually used in reference to analysis of variance.

Finite population correction (fpc) A multiplier for reducing the standard error of a measure taken from a finite population when the sample is large relative to the size of the population.

Fisher's exact test An alternative to chi-square for two-by-two tables with extremely small expected values (less than 5) in any cell.

Fixed-length Refers to one of two ways that data may be stored in a .txt file. Each data element is the same length. (See delimited.)

Formula bar See formula line.

Formula line The line at the top of the Excel spreadsheet that shows the content of the currently selected cell.

HDI (Human Development Index) A composite number ranging from 0 to 100, developed by UNDP for each country of the world, from per capita income, literacy, and life expectancy.

Header row The row at the top of a column that contains the name of data in the column.

Histogram A graph that shows data values as vertical columns.

Homogeneity of variance Equal within-group variation across two or more groups.

Hypothesis A statement of belief about a population to be assessed, using data from a sample.

ICD-9 (International Classification of Diseases, ninth revision) A coding scheme maintained by the World Health Organization that provides a code to classify mortality data from death certificates.

Identity matrix A square matrix with 1 in the main diagonal cells and 0 in all other cells.

Independence Formally, the understanding that conditional probabilities equal marginal probabilities. The recognition that two variables or two events are not dependent on one another.

Independent variable A variable whose values are assumed to be unaffected by other variables in a given analysis. (See, also, causal variable, predictor variable.)

Information matrix A matrix derived from Logit analysis that provides an intermediary step in the calculation of standard errors of coefficients derived using Logit.

Interaction effect The joint effect of two or more independent variables on a dependent variable. (See main effect.)

Interval scale A numerical variable scale that has no real zero point, such as IQ or temperature measured in centigrade or Fahrenheit.

Inverse The value by which a number must be multiplied for the product to be 1 or a matrix must be multiplied for the product to be an identity matrix. For a scalar (single number), the inverse of x is $1/x$.

Joint probability The likelihood of two simultaneously occurring events. For example, the likelihood that a person will come to an emergency room during the day and will come for a true emergency.

Likert scale An ordinal scale that is usually constructed with categories such as "Strongly agree," "Agree," "Undecided," "Disagree," and "Strongly disagree."

Linear probability model A regression model derived by using ordinary least squares to estimate regression coefficients for a dichotomous dependent variable.

Linear regression A statistical technique for relating a dependent numerical variable to an independent numerical or two-level categorical variable that generally assumes a straight-line relationship.

Logarithmic model Regression analysis in which the x axis variable is converted to a logarithm, either natural or base 10.

Logit An analysis method that allows for the assessment of whether a two-level categorical variable is independent of one or more numerical or two-level categorical predictor variables. Based on maximum likelihood.

Main effect The direct effect of a single independent variable on an independent variable. (See interaction effect.)

Marginal probability The probability of some outcome without regard to any other event. For example, the likelihood that a person who arrives at an emergency room will come for a true emergency versus a nonemergent condition is a marginal probability.

Matrix A set of data in contiguous rows and columns (see array).

Maximum likelihood The estimation of regression coefficients based on the maximization of a likelihood function (rather than the minimization of the sum of squared errors).

Mean The overall average of all values for a single variable. Calculated by summing all values and dividing by the total number of values.

Median The midpoint of the values of a single variable. Calculated by finding the value for which half the observations are larger and half the observations are smaller.

Medicare A program administered by the federal government that pays specified medical expenses, primarily for persons over sixty-five.

Mode The most commonly occurring number in a series of data.

Monte Carlo technique A method of simulating the results of an analysis or process, using randomly assigned values.

Moving average model A regression-like model that is generated, based on the average of two or more previous time periods.

Multicolinearity A term descriptive of the relationship between two—usually independent or predictor-variables that vary together or are highly correlated with one another.

Multiple regression A technique for determining whether a single numerical variable is independent of two or more other numerical or two-level categorical variables.

Mutually exclusive Two or more outcomes of a stochastic process that cannot simultaneously occur.

Nested functions Two or more Excel functions in the same cell. Generally used for multiple decisions.

Nominal variable A categorical variable that is not ordered.

Nonlinear relationship A relationship between two variables that does not show evidence of a straight-line relationship.

Normal distribution A probability distribution in which values near the mean are more likely than values farther from the mean. Often referred to as a bell-shaped curve.

Numerical variable A variable that is measured on a number scale. May be continuous or discrete.

Ordinal variable A categorical variable that is ordered by magnitude or intensity (that is, good, better, best).

Ordinary least squares (OLS) The least complex multiple regression technique.

Outcome The results of the events in a stochastic process.

Parameter Measure of a characteristic of a population.

Pareto Chart A graph that shows actual frequencies as a histogram and cumulative frequencies as a line graph. Always ordered from the largest data category on the left of the graph to the smallest on the right.

Patterned distribution An Excel option that allows the user to generate a series of values in any pattern selected. Not a probability distribution.

Pivot Table Wizard Set of windows invoked by selecting Data/Pivot Table. Allows the creation of frequency distribution or cross-tabulations for categorical data.

Pivot table An Excel designation for a frequency distribution or cross-tabulation created by using the Excel Pivot Table Wizard.

Poisson distribution A probability distribution that represents the likelihood of a rare event.

Polynomial model A regression analysis in which a single independent variable is converted to its square, cube, fourth power, and so on to describe a dependent variable.

Population The group of persons or organizations about which there is an interest.

Power model Regression model in which both the independent and the dependent variables are converted to a logarithmic value, either natural or base 10.

Predictor variable A causal variable. A variable whose values are predictive of the values of other variables in a given analysis.

Probability The term used to describe the likelihood of an outcome of an event.

Probit An analysis method that allows for the assessment of whether a two-level categorical is independent of one or more numerical or two-level categorical predictor variables. Based on maximum likelihood.

Pseudo-random number A random number generated by a computer. Called pseudo-random because any computer generation scheme inevitably incorporates some selection pattern.

R square (R^2) Proportion of variance in a dependent variable that can be accounted for or explained by knowledge of variation in an independent variable or variables.

Random number table A table of numbers arranged in rows and columns. Each number is randomly ordered with respect to all other numbers in the table. Used to select random samples before the advent of computers.

Random sample A subset of a larger population selected in such a way that every member of the larger population has a known and nonzero likelihood of being included.

Ratio variable A numerical variable that has a real zero point. May be continuous, such as weight, or discrete, such as the number of persons in a physician's waiting room.

Regression analysis A statistical analysis that seeks to determine whether a given numerical variable is independent of some set of other numerical variables or two-level categorical variables.

Regression coefficient A value by which an independent variable can be multiplied to predict the values of a dependent variable.

Repeated measures More than one measure of a variable on the same group of subject (persons, organizations).

Sample space All possible outcomes of a stochastic process.

Sample A subset of a population about which there is an interest. Selected to determine the values of interest for the population.

Sampled population The population that is actually sampled. May or may not be the same as the target population.

Scalar A way of referring to a single number when discussed in the context of matrices or arrays.

Scatter graph, (scatter plot) A graph that shows the simultaneous distribution of the data points for two variables. Also called an XY graph.

Simple random sample A sample drawn in such a way that every possible sample of a given size has an equal probability of being selected.

Skewed left A designation for a data distribution that has a median value greater than its mean and a "tail" of data to the left side of the distribution.

Skewed right A designation for a data distribution that has a median value less than its

mean and a "tail" of data to the right side of the distribution.

Solver An Excel add-in that solves a wide variety of optimization problems.

Spreadsheet A computer-generated sheet of rows and columns. The area in Excel where work is done. (A set of 65536 numbered rows and 256 columns designated A through IV.)

Standard deviation A measure of overall variation in a set of data, the square root of the variance (see variance).

Standard error A measure of the overall variation in the means from samples of a given size taken from a population. Equals the standard deviation divided by the square root of the sample size.

Statistic Measure of a characteristic of a sample. Estimates a parameter.

Statistical significance Refers to a statistical test result that leads to the rejection of the implicit or explicit hypothesis of independence between two or more variables.

Stepwise regression A technique for using regression analysis to find a model that accounts for the largest possible share of the variance in the independent variable while eliminating variables that do not contribute to the prediction. Can be forward inclusion or backward elimination.

Stochastic process A series of events, the outcome of any one being determined by some probability.

Stratified sample A sample drawn by first dividing the total population into two or more mutually exclusive and all-inclusive groups and then drawing samples from each of these groups.

Sums of squares The addition of the difference between all values for a particular data set and the mean value for the data. May be calculated.

Systematic sample A sample drawn by dividing the population into several ordered groups, and then randomly selecting a first member of the sample from the first group and selecting each comparable member from all other groups.

T distribution A probability distribution similar to the normal distribution but having fewer values near the mean and more in the tails, depending on degrees of freedom.

t test A test that compares an estimated value from a sample to the standard error for that value. Used to determine whether a numerical variable is independent of a two-level categorical variable.

Target population The population of interest, the population from which a sample is desired.

Text import wizard A set of windows invoked by the attempt to load a non-Excel file into an Excel spreadsheet that provides step-by-step direction in turning the non-Excel file into an Excel file.

Transpose Operation by which the columns of an array (matrix) become rows and the rows become columns.

Trend line The single line through an XY scatter plot that provides the best linear or nonlinear fit to the data.

Type I error The likelihood of rejecting a hypothesis when it is true. Always set by the level of confidence selected.

Type II error The likelihood of not rejecting a hypothesis when it is false. Known only if a specific value of an alternative hypothesis is given.

Uniform distribution A probability distribution in which any number in a given range is equally likely. Often called a flat distribution.

Variable A measure of some attribute for a set of entities, persons, or organizations that takes on more than one value.

Variance A measure of overall variation in a set of data that represents the average squared difference between each value in the data set and the mean of all values.

Vector A matrix (array) made up of a single row or a single column.

Weighted least squares (WLS) A regression technique that takes account of possible unequal variation in the dependent variable at different levels of the predictor variables.

Within-group variance Variance that exists among the values for a specified group.

Workbook An Excel computer file consisting of one or more spreadsheets.

X axis A horizontal axis in a graph or chart. Usually considered to be the independent variable.

X variable A variable generally considered to be the independent or causal variable.

Y axis A vertical axis in a graph or chart. Usually considered to be the dependent variable.

Y variable Variable generally considered to be the caused or dependent variable.

Yates's correction A modification of the chi-square formula for two-by-two tables with expected values less than 10.

ADDITIONAL RESOURCES

Berk, K. N., and Carey, P. *Data Analysis with Microsoft Excel.* Pacific Grove, Calif.: Duxbury, 2000.

Brightman, H. J. *Data Analysis in Plain English with Microsoft Excel.* Pacific Grove, Calif.: Duxbury Press, 1999.

Cochran, W. G. *Sampling Techniques.* (2nd ed.) New York: Wiley, 1963.

Gujarati, D. N. *Basic Econometrics.* New York: McGraw-Hill, 1987.

Human Development Index (HDI), United Nations Development Program (UNDP). 1999. [http://www.undp.org/hdro/statistics/downloadtables.html].

Kaluzny, A. D., and Veney, J. E. *Health Service Organizations: A Guide to Research and Assessment.* Berkeley, Calif.: McCutchan Publishing, 1980.

Levine, D. M., Stephan, D., Krehbiel, T. C., and Berenson, M. L. *Statistics for Managers Using Microsoft Excel.* (3rd ed.) Englewood Cliffs, N.J.: Prentice Hall, 2002.

Middleton, M. R. *Data Analysis Using Microsoft Excel.* Boston: PWS-Kent, 1997.

Orvis, W. J. *Excel for Scientists and Engineers.* (2nd ed.) San Francisco: Sybex, 1996.

"Sudan: Results from the Demographic and Health Survey." *Studies in Family Planning,* 1992, *23*(1), 66–70.

Wonnacott, R. J., and Wonnacott, T. H. *Econometrics.* (2nd ed.) New York: Wiley, 1979.

INDEX